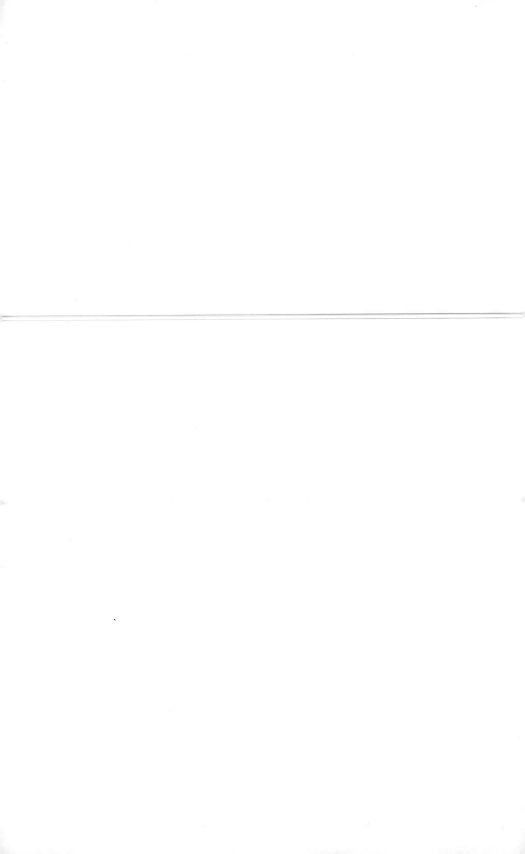

Brief Therapy for Couples

TREATMENT MANUALS FOR PRACTITIONERS
David H. Barlow, *Editor*

Recent Volumes

Brief Therapy for Couples
Helping Partners Help Themselves

W. KIM HALFORD

Series Editor's Note by David H. Barlow

Foreword by Howard J. Markman

THE GUILFORD PRESS
New York   London

© 2001 The Guilford Press
A Division of Guilford Publications, Inc.
72 Spring Street, New York, NY 10012
www.guilford.com

Printed in the United States of America

This book is printed on acid-free paper.

Last digit is print number: 9 8 7 6 5 4 3 2 1

Library of Congress Cataloging-in-Publication Data

Halford, W. Kim
  Brief therapy for couples : helping partners help themselves /
W. Kim Halford ; foreword by Howard J. Markham.
      p. cm. — (Treatment manuals for practitioners)
  Includes bibliographical references and index.
  ISBN 1-57230-179-1
      1. Brief psychotherapy—Handbooks, manuals, etc. 2. Marital
psychotherapy—Handbooks, manuals, etc. I. Title. II. Series
RC480.55 .H34 2001
618.89′156—dc21   2001018803

The practice of couple therapy blends the deeply personal with professional practice. I dedicate this book to my mother, Bev; to the memory of my father, John; and to a great couple therapist, researcher, and friend, Bob Weiss. My mother and father shared their lives, created the loving family in which I was raised, and loved and supported me across life's journey. Bob has given freely of his wisdom, wit, and friendship over many, many years. He helped me to develop faith in my professional knowledge and skills. Thank you to three special human beings.

About the Author

W. Kim Halford, PhD, is Professor of Clinical Psychology in the School of Applied Psychology at Griffith University, in Brisbane, Australia. Professor Halford earned his doctorate in clinical psychology from Latrobe University in Melbourne, Australia, in 1978. He has worked in a series of positions in academia and in clinical practice over the ensuing 20 years, including Head of Psychology at Griffith University for the last 6 years, and prior to that, in the Department of Psychiatry at the University of Queensland and Chief Psychologist at the Royal Brisbane Hospital. Over the last 15 years, his practice and clinical research have focused predominantly on work with couples. He coedited, with Professor Howard Markman, the *Clinical Handbook of Marriage and Couples Interventions*, published by John Wiley and Sons, and wrote the report *Australian Couples in Millennium Three*, which provided a review of research and development on marriage and relationship education for the Australian Department of Family and Community Services. He maintains an active practice in work with couples, and has presented clinical workshops on his approach to couple therapy in Australia, New Zealand, the United Kingdom, the United States, Canada, and Mexico.

Series Editor's Note

It is a well-worked but fundamentally true cliché, that the hardest thing we do in our lives is attempt to fulfill the goal of making a relationship permanent. The difficulties one encounters in achieving this goal do not make the pages of DSM-IV or ICD-10 and have been overlooked by many professionals because of this fact. And yet, the emotional and behavioral ravages of a relationship gone bad are every bit as severe as some of the most incapacitating psychological disorders. For this reason, any fresh insights on alleviating suffering in this area are welcome.

Now we have an important new contribution to brief couple therapy representing 15 years of clinical and research experience on the part of W. Kim Halford, an internationally known expert in this area, and his associates. The approaches presented in this book have strong empirical support but also the flexibility necessary for integration into any skilled couple therapist's repertoire. The stepped-care approach presented in some detail in this volume will ensure that therapists get maximum results as quickly and efficiently as possible. This protocol is a welcome addition to the Treatment Manuals for Practitioners series.

DAVID H. BARLOW

Acknowledgments

In the last 15 years, I have been fortunate to develop friendships with a number of excellent couple therapists, and they have taught me much. First and foremost, I am grateful to my longtime friend and collaborator, Matthew Sanders, who encouraged me to enter the world of clinical research, and with whom I first began to develop the notions of brief and self-regulatory couple therapy. I have been extremely fortunate to work closely with Bob Weiss, Howard Markman, Don Baucom, and Kurt Hahlweg over many years. Each of them taught me many valuable lessons on how to work with couples (and how to enjoy conferences), and each of these people is a great friend and professional colleague. In the last few years, I have begun a collaboration with Keithia Wilson. Her wisdom about adult learning processes has informed my thinking and her influences are reflected in my approach in this book. My work also has been greatly influenced by a circle of professional colleagues whose willingness to share their ideas and dedication to understanding the dilemmas of distressed relationships have enriched my thinking. A special thank you to Tom Bradbury, Steve Beach, Andy Christensen, Mark Dadds, Frank Fincham, Rick Heyman, Amy Holtzworth-Munroe, Hy Hops, the late Neil Jacobson, Jan Nicholson, Pat Noller, Dan O'Leary, Tammy Sher, Doug Snyder, and Dina Vivian. I am grateful for the exciting discussions and debates each of these people shared with me at various times, and in various exotic locations, over the last 15 years.

I have worked with many very gifted and dedicated students, and the ideas developed in the pages of this book owe much to their creativity. I particularly want to acknowledge the contributions of Brett Behrens, Ruth Bouma,

Adrian Kelly, Liz Moore, Sue Osgarby, Jenn Scott, Suzie Sweeper, and Kathy Skuja. Each of these people taught me valued lessons.

Hundreds of couples have entrusted me with the challenge of helping them to enhance their relationships. Some couples came as volunteers in research projects; others simply sought me out for help. Their openness to consider the possibilities of change instilled in me a fundamental optimism about improving distressed relationships that sustains me through the challenges of therapy.

The genesis of this book came during a sabbatical leave at the University of Oregon with Bob Weiss. I wrote most of the book while on sabbatical leave at the University of North Carolina at Chapel Hill. I am most grateful to both psychology departments for hosting me, and particularly thankful to my friends and hosts Bob Weiss and Don Baucom. I also thank my longtime secretary, Rhoda Richardson, and the wonderful research support staff of Charles Farrugia, Kathy Eadie, Carmel Dyer, and Jill Smythe, who gave lots of diligent assistance with manuscript preparation, and yet again all went beyond the call of duty to get it done.

I received enormous and valued help from Barbara Watkins and the team at The Guilford Press. Barbara's patience and guidance helped me shape ideas formed over 15 years into a book. Her help was invaluable.

Finally, and most important, I want to thank my wife, Barbara, and sons, James and Chris, who gave me space and time to do this. I look forward to some extra time to spend with them now that it is done.

Foreword

This book is a gift. It is a ticket for a journey that all professionals who work with couples will want to take. Dr. W. Kim Halford is our tour guide as he presents to us a thoughtful, easy-to-use, and effective approach to helping couples based on his years of experience as one of the world's leading couple researchers and therapists. It is a rare treat when one of the leading researchers in the family field shares with us the results of his research and clinical experience in such a thoughtful and accessible manner.

Our trip starts with an overview of a new and exciting approach to helping couples change, which Dr. Halford calls self-regulatory couple therapy (SRCT). Three key themes set this book apart from others in the field. First is its focus on the couple's interaction as the source of knowledge about relationship problems and success, and one of the sources from which change springs. Second is its active, short-term approach to understanding and facilitating change. The third key principle is that the therapist is helping the partners create the type of great relationship that most people want, need, and deserve. Like Dorothy in *The Wizard of Oz*, Dr. Halford shows how couples have the power to attain happiness at home.

The book is special not only because of the insight, understanding, and effective tools it presents, but for the marvelous way Dr. Halford marries basic couple research with clinical practice. He has a knack for translating decades of outstanding research (much of which is his own) into a step-by-step handbook that therapists can follow to help troubled couples restore love, friendship, and happiness to their relationship as well as to help happy couples protect and preserve their love, commitment, and high levels of marital satisfaction.

While this book is essentially written for therapists, its warmth, humanity, clarity, and wisdom also speak to partners themselves who can follow the ideas of self-change to work on their own to improve their relationship. Thus, this book has the potential to be not only the best guidebook for therapists on how to conduct short-term, active, and empirically based couple therapy, but an extraordinary guidebook for couples to use as self-help in restoring love and happiness to their relationships.

So, fellow readers, fasten your seatbelts, relax, and get ready to enjoy the friendly skies of the world of relationships with the best possible guidebook in your hands. Enjoy your journey.

HOWARD J. MARKMAN, PHD
Professor of Psychology, University of Denver

Preface

Couple therapy is a challenging process, and I do not pretend to have all the answers to making couple therapy effective. However, over 15 years of research and clinical practice, I have developed an approach called self-regulatory couple therapy (SRCT). In this book I explain this approach, an approach intended to make therapy very brief when possible. I hope SRCT is useful to therapists who work with couples. I also hope that my writing captures the blend of applied science and humane practice that I think characterizes good therapy.

This book has nine chapters. The initial chapter is a description of the significance of and key influences on relationship problems. I provide a model to integrate the findings on the determinants of relationship problems. This model provides a framework within which to conduct SRCT. Chapter 2 is a review of empirically supported approaches to couple therapy. I begin by describing how the effects of couple therapy are assessed. I then review cognitive and behavioral, emotion-focused, insight-oriented, and brief self-regulatory couple therapies.

In Chapter 3, I describe SRCT in detail. One key characteristic of SRCT is that it is intended to be as brief an approach to therapy as possible. In Chapter 3, I describe a hierarchy of three approaches that constitute SRCT: brief self-change therapy (2 to 6 sessions), relationship psychoeducation plus self-change (usually 7 to 10 sessions), and therapist-guided change (usually 11 sessions or more).

Chapters 4 to 6 detail the process of couple therapy from the initial presentation to negotiating and defining the goals of therapy. Chapters 4 and 5 address assessment of couples, and Chapter 6 focuses on the feedback of assessment results and negotiating relationship goals. Once the needed changes are defined, some couples can implement self-change processes that achieve the desired relationship outcomes. Chapter 6 includes a description of how to assess whether brief self-change will suffice to meet the couple's needs. Chapter 7 addresses the details of how to assist the couple to implement self-change.

Chapter 8 provides a description of relationship psychoeducation, which involves active learning by partners about relationship themes and influences. When assessment and goal setting are insufficient to help the couple define self-change goals, this additional intervention can be enough to allow partners to define self-change goals, which they can then achieve through self-regulated efforts. Brief couple therapy incorporates procedures described in Chapters 4 through 8.

Chapter 9 describes therapist-guided change for partners who are unable, despite having clear self-change goals, to implement relationship change themselves. The chapter explains how therapist-guided change can help couples develop the relationship skills that allow them to change.

How to Use This Book

A great chef who prepares a sumptuous feast is more than someone with a good recipe book. A good recipe can identify key ingredients, suggest a good sequence for combining elements, and help the chef to have all the required materials at hand. However, great chefs have certain skills that bring all the components together, skills such as monitoring how a particular dish is coming together and making fine adjustments, a sense of timing in conducting crucial steps, and creativity in presentation. In an analogous way, no book can provide a rigid prescription of how to do couple therapy, and the therapist must have a range of skills to make any set of therapy guidelines work. Every couple is different, and each course of therapy needs to be attuned to the couple's needs. However, there are common dilemmas that couples and therapists face at various points in couple therapy. This book is my attempt to describe the most common of these dilemmas and a process by which couples can be helped to respond to these challenges.

One central element throughout this book is how to assess couple interaction in a manner that informs therapeutic change. Developing a working model of how a couple interacts is central to therapy. The development of a working model of the couple should be guided by theory and research about common problems encountered by couples, but for each couple the model has unique characteristics that are identified in the assessment process. A second central element is an emphasis on client self-regulation of the relationship. By this I mean that the couple therapy approach described in this book is focused on empowering partners to be proactive in defining and building the sort of relationship they want. I hope this book will stimulate your approach to therapy, but caution against using this as a recipe book or rigidly following a set of steps. Effective couple therapy requires the creative application of general principles to unique situations.

Contents

1

The Nature and Significance of Relationship Problems

Marriage is one of the most nearly universal of human institutions. No other touches so intimately the lives of practically every member of the earth's population.
—TERMAN (1939, p. 1)

I think a man and a woman should choose each other for life, for the simple reason that a long life with all its accidents is barely enough for a man and a woman to understand each other; and in this case to understand is to love.
—JOHN BUTLER YEATS

This book provides a detailed guide on how to conduct couple therapy using a self-regulation approach.[1] This self-regulated approach emphasizes helping each partner to focus on those aspects of the relationship that can be changed most readily—namely, his or her own behavior, thoughts, and feelings. To that end, self-regulatory couple therapy provides only as much therapy as is neces-

---

[1]Many couples, both heterosexual and homosexual, live together in committed relationships without being legally married. I believe that most of what is described in this book is applicable to enriching the relationships of couples in any form of committed relationship. However, a lot of the research has been on heterosexual, married couples. When the comments I am making are specific to married couples, I refer to married couples. When the intent is to refer to any couple, I use the term "couple" or "relationship."

sary to help partners to self-regulate change in their relationship. Couple therapy is conceived of as a hierarchy of three major options. The first option is self-change, which is brief therapy of approximately two to five sessions. In self-change the therapist assists the partners to define the self-change goals they wish to make in their relationship, and the partners then implement those changes largely independently from the therapist. The second option is relationship psychoeducation, which is a brief therapy of typically five to nine sessions. In relationship psychoeducation the therapist uses an interactive educational process to help the partners operationalize and implement their self-change goals. The third option is therapist-guided change, which is a therapy of more traditional duration, consisting of from 10 to 25 sessions. In therapist-guided change the therapist works intensively with the partners to assist them to develop relationship skills and then to implement self-change in their relationship.

The Significance of Relationship Problems

An overwhelming percentage of people become involved in intimate couple relationships at some point in their lives. In Western countries more than 90% of the population marries by the age of 50 (DeGuilbert-Lanotine & Monnier, 1992; McDonald, 1995). Even among those who choose not to marry, the vast majority engage in "marriage-like" relationships by living together in committed, couple relationships (McDonald, 1995). Regardless of whether or not couples are formally married, expectations of couple relationships are high. In Western cultures the vast majority of adults perceive their marital relationship as their primary source of support and affection (Levinger & Huston, 1990). Most young unmarried adults expect to marry at some point in their lives; they expect that marriage to be lifelong, and they expect that their partners will show sexual monogamy, honesty, expressions of affection, intimacy, and support (Australian Institute of Family Studies, 1997; Millward, 1990).

Given the high expectations that people attach to marriage, perhaps it is not surprising that many people find their relationships do not match these expectations. Almost all couples that marry report high levels of relationship satisfaction early in their relationship (Markman & Hahlweg, 1993). Unfortunately, for many couples their relationship satisfaction erodes over time (Bradbury, 1998). The most statistically reliable index of marital distress is divorce rates, and divorce has reached epidemic proportions in most Western societies. About 55% of U.S., 42% of English, and 37% of German marriages end in divorce (De Guilbert-Lantoine & Monnier, 1992). As painful as the experience of divorce is for many people, the majority of individuals who divorce subsequently remarry (Glick, 1989). The divorce rates of second marriages (in which at least one partner has been married previously) is even higher than for first marriages (Glick, 1989).

Divorce rates represent only a portion of the total population of couples experiencing significant relationship problems. Other couples have significant relationship distress but opt to stay together for various reasons, (e.g., the financial implications of divorce, and personal and cultural expectations about divorce). Surveys of representative samples of adults in the United States suggest that at any given time approximately 10 to 15% of married people report significant relationship problems (Beach, Arias, & O'Leary, 1986; Eddy, Heyman, & Weiss, 1991; Gallup, 1990; Stanley & Markman, 1996).

There is some evidence that many of the 85 to 90% of currently married adults who report they are satisfied with their current relationship are making unrealistically positive comments and predictions about their relationship functioning (Fowers, Lyons, & Montel, 1996). For example, the majority of satisfied partners believe there is zero probability that they will ever divorce, despite the well-publicized evidence of how common divorce is (Fowers et al., 1996). Furthermore, of the married people who report high relationship satisfaction, 40% also report having seriously considered leaving their current partners at some point (Gallup, 1989). Thus it seems that, even within those couples that define themselves as satisfied in their relationship, problems occur. All these figures converge on the point that relationship distress is a common problem in most Western societies.

Defining Relationship Problems

Most problems with which mental health professionals assist people are defined primarily by the phenomenology of the experience of the person. This is also the case with relationship problems. However, unlike many other clinical problems, there are few observable behaviors that indicate degree of relationship distress (Weiss & Heyman, 1997). Relationship distress can be operationalized as the report of significant, ongoing dissatisfaction with the relationship by at least one partner. The term "significant" means that the level of dissatisfaction is such that the functioning of that partner is compromised. The use of the term "ongoing" is meant to connote more than transient upset experienced from a disagreement, and to focus on a persistent state of dissatisfaction.

The foregoing definition of relationship distress requires only one partner to feel dissatisfied. Dissatisfaction is strongly correlated between partners, and asynchrony in satisfaction is unusual. However, in some instances there can be marked differences between partners in their relationship satisfaction. For example, O'Farrell and Birchler (1987) found that wives of men drinking heavily were much less satisfied with the relationship than were the men. Even if one partner is not dissatisfied currently, if he or she is in a relationship with someone who is dissatisfied with the relationship, then negative effects from the partner's dissatisfaction are likely to occur. For example, marriage in most Western cultures is subject to veto by one partner. In other words, if one partner wishes to terminate the relationship then the relationship is over, regardless of how the other partner feels about that decision. The implication for therapy is that if one partner is distressed, both partners have a relationship problem.

Attempts to define and measure relationship problems have taken relationship (marital) satisfaction, as assessed by self-report inventories, as the ultimate criterion (Weiss & Heyman, 1997). The most widely used self-report inventories are the Locke–Wallace Marital Adjustment Test (Locke & Wallace, 1959) and an expanded revision known as the Dyadic Adjustment Scale (Spanier, 1976). These two scales, and many similar scales, have been subjected to repeated criticism (e.g., Heyman, Sayers, & Bellack, 1994) for confounding relationship satisfaction—measured by items such as "Overall how would you rate your marital happiness?"—with adjustment processes alleged to influence satisfaction—measured by items such as "How often do you and your partner disagree about finances?" Although the collapsing of the constructs of relationship satisfaction and adjustment seems conceptually unsound, factor analyses of measures of marital adjustment and dissatisfaction consistently show that partners make unidimensional, global evaluations of their relationship problems (Eddy et al., 1991; Heyman et al., 1994). In essence, partners who are dissatisfied with their relationships tend to report that just about anything that could be negative about their relationship *is* negative.

The finding that relationship distress reflects an overriding negative, global evaluation of the relationship does not mean that relationship quality is unidimensional. Recent work shows that couples distinguish between dissatisfaction about negative aspects of the relationship (e.g., the level of distress associated with conflict) and satisfaction with positive aspects of the relationship (e.g., the sense of satisfaction with expressions of love) (Fincham, Beach, & Kemp-Fincham, 1997). Some couples present with severe relationship distress and little positive feeling about their partner or the relationship. Other couples are distressed by the negative aspects of the relationship associated with dissatisfaction but still retain some positive feelings about the partner. The latter group of couples seems to benefit more from couple therapy (Hahlweg, Schindler, Revenstorf, & Brengelmann, 1984). In either group of couples their initial focus often is on reducing negative behaviors associated with dissatisfaction, but successful therapy also needs to prompt couples to attend to developing positive aspects of the relationship.

Occasionally outsiders define a couple's relationship as dysfunctional, even if the partners do not report distress. For example, Hafner (1986) described a number of cases in which he believed marital dysfunction had a deleterious effect on the wife, though many of the women initially did not report relationship distress. As a second example, there is a small but nontrivial proportion of couples in which severe violence occurs between the partners, but neither partner reports relationship dissatisfaction (Weiss, 1989). Sometimes the safety or well-being of a partner or dependent children may be perceived as at risk from such aggression, and police or welfare agencies may intervene in such cases.

Reports of relationship problems overlap with, but are not synonymous with, separation and divorce. Some partners consider separation or divorce without clear signs of relationship problems. In a survey of people presenting with relationship problems at a community relationship counseling agency, about 15% of people scored in the nondistressed range of the Dyadic Adjustment Scale, a global measure of relationship satisfaction (Halford & Osgarby, 1993). Many of these so-called nondistressed partners were contemplating separation or had actually separated.

Relationship dissolution with little or no relationship distress occurs but is the exception rather than the rule. Most couples who separate or divorce go through a sustained period of significant relationship distress, then contemplate separation, then proceed to actual separation, and finally divorce (Gottman, 1993a). However, some couples remain together despite severe, ongoing relationship distress. A complex range of factors determine the rate at which a couple proceeds through the steps toward divorce, and whether they proceed at all. These factors include the beliefs each partner holds about divorce; the financial position of each partner in the marriage, and the likely financial position of each partner after divorce; the presence of children, and the partners' beliefs about the effects of divorce on children; and the perceptions held about the alternatives to marriage available to each partner.

In summary, relationship distress is defined by the subjective evaluations of the relationship by the participants. Relationship dysfunction is a judgment made by someone outside the relationship that the relationship has deleterious effects. Ongoing relationship distress often is associated with steps taken toward separation and divorce. However, some couples separate with mild relationship problems, while other couples stay together despite severe relationship problems. Couple therapy usually, though not always, is a response to relationship distress.

Consequences of Relationship Problems

Most people experience relationship problems as extremely stressful. In fact, after a death in the immediate family, marital distress and divorce are the most severe commonly occurring stresses adults experience (Bloom, Asher, & White, 1978). Relationship problems are the most common presenting problem in adults seeking psychological services (Overall, Henry, & Woodward, 1974). Relationship distress is associated with increased risk for development of a range of individual psychological disorders including depression, particularly in women (Bebbington, 1987a, 1987b; Coyne, Kahn, & Gotlib, 1987; Hooley, Orleay, & Teasdale, 1986); alcohol abuse, particularly in men (O'Farrell, 1989); higher rates of sexual dysfunction in both sexes (Zimmer, 1983); and increased behavioral problems in the couples' children, particularly conduct disorders in boys (Emery, 1982; Emery, Joyce, & Fincham, 1987; Grych & Fincham, 1990).

The causal connection between relationship distress and psychological disorder is not just one way. Long-standing and severe psychological disorder reduces the chance of someone developing a satisfactory relationship. For example, patients diagnosed with schizophrenia or severe personality disorders are much less likely than the rest of the population to get married and are much more likely to get divorced if they do marry (Lange, Schaap, & van Widenfelt, 1993). People who abuse alcohol before meeting their partner are equally likely to get married as the rest of the population but are much more likely to get divorced (Reich & Thompson, 1985).

In cases of coexisting relationship problems and depression, the relationship problems often antedate the onset of depression (Birchnall & Kennard, 1983). Even when treatment produces an improvement in depressed mood there is limited effect on relationship distress (Dobson, 1987; Klerman & Weissman, 1982; O'Leary & Beach, 1990), and the ongoing relationship problems are associated with poor prognosis for the depression (Rounsaville, Weissman, Prusoff, & Herceg-Baron, 1979). Similarly, relationship problems stimulate excessive drinking (Davis, Berenson, Steinglass, & Davis, 1974), precipitate relapse by abstinent alcoholics (Maisto, O'Farrell, Connors, McKay, & Pelcovits, 1988), and are predictive of poor prognosis in alcohol treatment programs (Billings & Moos, 1983; Vannicelli, Gingerich, & Ryback, 1983). Thus, a simple unidirectional model of causality is inadequate; relationship problems and psychological disorder reciprocally influence each other (Halford, Bouma, Kelly, & Young, 1999).

In addition to psychological maladjustment, relationship problems also are correlated with poorer physical health. Individuals in satisfying and supportive relationships are less likely to have major illnesses, and they recover better when they do become ill, than are individuals in distressed relationships (Burman & Margolin, 1992; Schmaling & Sher, 1997). The mechanisms linking poor physical health to relationship distress are complex and only partially understood. Relationship distress has some indirect effects mediated through health-related behaviors, such as low adherence to medical treatment regimens by those in distressed relationships (Schmaling & Sher, 1997). There also are well-documented correlations between pain and coping behaviors in chronic illness and inadvertent reinforcement of illness behavior in distressed relationships (Schmaling & Sher, 1997). Furthermore, there are some direct effects of marital distress on physiological processes. For example, relationship conflict is associated with immunosuppression (Kiecolt-Glaser et al.,

1988), elevated blood pressure in people with essential hypertension (Ewart, Taylor, Kraemer, & Agras, 1991), and possibly arteriosclerosis (Gottman, 1990; Medalie & Goldbourt, 1976). Each of these physiological effects is likely to increase risk for serious health problems.

Violence is another means by which relationship problems have a major effect on health. About 25% of all marriages have at least one episode of interspousal physical aggression at some point (O'Leary et al., 1989; Straus, Gelles, & Steinmetz, 1980), and this violence almost always is associated with relationship distress. Nearly three-quarters of distressed couples presenting for therapy report having experienced violence by one partner toward the other in the previous year (O'Leary & Vivian, 1990). Men and women are equally likely to engage in physical aggression such as hitting, pushing, or slapping (O'Leary et al., 1989; Straus & Gelles, 1986). However, men are much more likely to engage in severe violence, and women are at particular risk for being injured or even killed by their partner (Stets & Straus, 1990). In Australia, about 25% of all homicides and 20% of all reported offenses against persons result from violence between partners (National Committee on Violence, 1990). In the United States, female homicide victims are murdered more often by their partners than by any other class of assailant (Browne & Williams, 1993). In the United States, up to 40% of women presenting to accident and emergency services have been the victims of domestic violence, with as many as 10% of these presentations linked to an assault by the partner (Stark & Flitcraft, 1988).

Even when physical injuries are less severe, violence has negative consequences for the victim and other members of the family. Women repeatedly assaulted by their partners have a high risk of depression, alcohol abuse, and psychosomatic disorders and are high users of the health care system (Cascardi, Langhinrichsen, & Vivian, 1992; Jaffe, Wolfe, Wilson, & Zak, 1986; Stets & Straus, 1990). Interpartner aggression also is linked to child abuse (Grych & Fincham, 1990), development of antisocial behavior in male offspring (Grych & Fincham, 1990), and increased risk of children entering a violent relationship as an adult (Widom, 1989).

Satisfying relationships convey a variety of advantages to the partners and their offspring. These advantages include enhanced mental and physical health of partners and their offspring as well as increased resilience to life stress. Relationship problems are a major risk factor for mental and physical health problems.

The Development of Relationship Problems

There are more than 100 published studies assessing the longitudinal course of couple relationship satisfaction and stability (Karney & Bradbury, 1995).

Bradbury (1995) offered a heuristic model by which this comprehensive literature usefully can be summarized. He suggested that there are three broad classes of variables that affect the etiology of relationship problems: adaptive processes within the couple system, stressful events impinging upon the couple, and enduring individual vulnerabilities of the partners. I believe this model is useful, but two modifications make it even more useful. "Individual vulnerabilities" as a concept refers to individual differences that make relationship problems more likely. However, I prefer the term "individual characteristics" as some individual characteristics have positive effects on relationships (e.g., gender role flexibility). A second modification to Bradbury's model is that I add a fourth class of factors that influence relationship outcomes: contextual variables.

Adaptive Couple Processes

BEHAVIOR EXCHANGE

Adaptive processes refer to the cognitive, behavioral, and affective processes that occur during couple interaction. Certain deficits in these adaptive processes seem to predispose couples to relationship problems. Specifically, positive day-to-day interactions predict sustained relationship satisfaction (Weiss & Heyman, 1997). In contrast, high rates of negative behaviors, and reciprocity of negativity (Karney & Bradbury, 1995; Weiss & Heyman, 1997) predict distress. Sharing positive, mutually enjoyable activities also is important to the experience of relationship closeness (Hill, 1988; Reissman, Aron, & Bergen, 1993). In particular, sharing new mutually enjoyable activities enhances couples' sense of intimacy (Baumeister & Bratlavsky, 1999).

AFFECTION

Active expression of affection and other positive emotions is associated with sustained relationship satisfaction (Weiss & Heyman, 1997). In contrast, certain patterns of emotional expression are predictive of relationship problems. Showing contempt, disgust, fear, or emotional withdrawal toward partners during interaction is predictive of relationship deterioration and taking steps toward separation (Gottman, 1994).

COMMUNICATION, CONFLICT MANAGEMENT, AND AGGRESSION

Deficits in communication and conflict management observed in engaged couples prospectively predict divorce and relationship dissatisfaction over the first 10 years of marriage (Markman & Hahlweg, 1993). Dysfunctional communication in engaged couples also predicts the development of relationship verbal and physical aggression in the first few years of marriage (Murphy & O'Leary, 1989; O'Leary et al., 1989), at least for mild to moderate severity aggression. Relationship aggression often is established early in the relationship, usually continues and escalates once established (Murphy & O'Leary, 1989; O'Leary et al., 1989), and is associated with declining relationship satisfaction and increased risk of relationship breakdown (Rogge & Bradbury, 1999).

It is noteworthy that the communication deficits observed in some engaged couples do not correlate with their reported relationship satisfaction at the time (Markman & Hahlweg, 1993; Sanders, Halford, & Behrens, 1999). It seems that these communication difficulties do not stop couples from forming committed relationships, but the difficulties may predispose couples to develop relationship problems later (Pasch & Bradbury, 1998). In couples who have been married for some time, these same communication difficulties predict deterioration in relationship satisfaction, and decreased relationship stability (Gottman, 1993b, 1994).

ROLE FUNCTIONING

Role functioning refers to the completion of core tasks essential to sustaining a couple's life together and includes such tasks as household chores, parenting, food purchase and preparation, garden and house maintenance, and money management. Role responsibilities that place substantially greater burden on one partner increase the risk of relationship problems (Belsky & Rovine, 1990; Goodnow & Bowes, 1994; Margolin, Fernandez, Talovic, & Onorato, 1983). A common pattern predictive of relationship distress, particularly in women, is for the woman to do the majority of household chores when both partners are in paid employment (Goodnow & Bowes, 1994; Julien, Arellano, & Turgeon, 1997). Women often report feeling conflict in trying to sustain both their relationship and work responsibilities, and such work–relationship conflict is associated with deteriorating relationship satisfaction and stability (Thompson, 1997).

MUTUAL SUPPORT

Providing support for each other is crucial in sustaining relationship satisfaction. Support can be both at the practical level (e.g., assisting with completion of role responsibilities) and emotional support (e.g., listening sympathetically to a partner's concerns). The level of emotional and practical support partners communicate to each other prospectively predicts their relationship satisfaction across the early years of marriage (Pasch & Bradbury, 1998).

SEX

As might be expected, there is a strong relationship between relationship satisfaction and sexual activity and satisfaction (Schenk, Pfrang, & Raushe, 1983; Spence, 1997). This strong association probably reflects that similar factors influence both sexual and overall relationship functioning. For example, communication between the partners predicts both relationship satisfaction and sexual satisfaction (McCabe, 1994). However, early satisfaction with the sexual relationship is a strong predictor of later relationship satisfaction and stability (Fowers & Olson, 1989; Olson & Fowers, 1986; Olson & Larson, 1989). This suggests that sustaining a satisfying sexual relationship is important in sustaining a generally satisfying relationship.

BELIEFS AND EXPECTATIONS

The beliefs and expectations individuals have when entering into relationships predict the risk of relationship distress and divorce in the first few years of marriage (Olson & Fowers, 1986; Olson & Larsen, 1989). Couples characterized by unrealistic expectations and beliefs in areas such as importance of communication, appropriate methods of conflict resolution, importance of family and friends, and gender roles have higher rates of erosion in relationship satisfaction than couples not so characterized. Moreover, these same expectations predict changes in relationship satisfaction of couples married for some time (Fowers & Olson, 1989). Negative attributions in which partners ascribe blame for relationship problems to stable, negative characteristics of their partner also prospectively predict deterioration in relationship satisfaction (Bradbury & Fincham, 1990).

Life Events

Life events refer to the developmental transitions and changing circumstances that impinge upon the couple or individual partners. Relationship problems are more likely to develop during periods of high rates of change and stressful life events (Karney & Bradbury, 1995). For example, the transition to parenthood sometimes is associated with a decline in couple relationship satisfaction (Cowen & Cowen, 1992), as is an increase in work demands (Thompson, 1997). Retirement is another major transition for couples which can be associated with relationship distress (Dickson, 1997). One partner developing a major health problem also puts couples at increased risk for relationship and sexual problems (Schmaling & Sher, 1997).

A common stressful transition worthy of special mention is entering a second marriage. Second marriages in which there are dependent children from an earlier relationship break down at very high rates (Booth & Edwards, 1992; Martin & Bumpass, 1989). Negotiating parenting roles in stepfamilies is a common source of interpartner conflict, and unresolved differences in this area are the most common stated reason for relationship breakdown in stepfamilies (Lawton & Sanders, 1994).

Couples with less robust adaptive processes are believed to be particularly vulnerable to the negative effects of a range of stressful events (Markman, Halford, & Cordova, 1997). In particular, couples that lack communication skills or have inflexible or unrealistic expectations of relationships find it hard to negotiate the changes required in adapting to major life transitions. For example, I, along with colleagues, have been studying couples in which the woman was recently diagnosed with breast or gynecological cancer. In couples with good communication and effective mutual support the adversity of cancer diagnosis and treatment seems to bring the couples closer together and reinforce the relationship bonds. In contrast, couples with poor adaptive processes show deterioration in their relationships and poor individual coping with the cancer (Halford, Scott, & Smythe, 2000).

Individual Characteristics

Individual characteristics refer to the stable historical, personal, and experiential factors that each partner brings to a relationship (Bradbury, 1995). Family-of-origin experience has been widely studied as an historical factor that correlates with risk of relationship problems. For example, the adult offspring of divorce are more likely than the rest of the population to divorce (Glenn & Kramer, 1987), and interparental aggression is associated with increased risk for being in an aggressive relationship as an adult (Widom, 1989). The mechanism by which exposure to parental divorce or aggression may have an impact subsequent adult relationships is becoming clearer. Exposure to parental divorce is associated with more negative expectations of marriage (Black & Sprenkle, 1991; Gabardi & Rosen, 1991) and with observable deficits in communication and conflict management in couples prior to marriage (Sanders et al., 1999). Adult offspring of parents who were aggressive also show deficits in communication and conflict management skills in dating and marital relationships (Halford, Sanders, & Behrens, 2000; Skuja & Halford, 2000). Negative expectations and communication deficits may well be learned from the parents' relationship, and subsequently this learned behavior has a negative impact on the adult relationships of the offspring. The argument that communication difficulties may be acquired through observation and interaction with parents is supported by the finding that couple communication style assessed at the beginning of adult relationships predicts subsequent communication style when the partners become parents and are interacting with their children (Howes & Markman, 1989).

The association between personality variables and relationship problems has been widely studied. Most normal personality variations do not seem to contribute much variance to relationship satisfaction (Gottman, 1994; Karney

& Bradbury, 1995). Two exceptions are that low ability to regulate negative affect (high neuroticism) consistently has been found to predict higher risk for relationship problems and divorce (Karney & Bradbury, 1995), and insecure attachment style has been associated with relationship problems (Feeney & Noller, 1996). How neuroticism affects relationship problems is not yet understood, but there is significant research on attachment style.

ATTACHMENT STYLE

Bowlby (1969) originally proposed the concept of attachment. He argued that early childhood experience of intimate relationships leads people to form schemas, also referred to as cognitive working models, of intimate relationships. Bowlby argued that close emotional bonds with parental figures lead to secure attachment, meaning that the child develops an attachment style in which intimate relationships are experienced as a source of positive closeness. On the other hand, negative, emotionally distant, or punitive early relationships lead the person to develop an insecure attachment style. People with insecure attachment are asserted to experience close relationships as uncomfortable and often associate closeness with an anxiety over being abandoned.

The assessment of attachment in adults is a matter of some controversy (Feeney & Noller, 1996), though there seems to be some agreement about the value of at least two broad dimensions of adult attachment: the degree of comfort with closeness and the extent of anxiety over abandonment. Individuals with low levels of comfort with closeness are asserted to avoid high levels of intimacy because their relationship schema lead them to interpret high levels of closeness as distressing. High anxiety over abandonment also leads people to interpret relationship events in terms of the possibility of being abandoned.

In the earliest formulations of attachment theory, attachment style was seen as relatively unchangeable after childhood. More recently it has been recognized that a range of relationship experiences, such as very positive or very negative committed relationships, can modify attachment style (Furman & Flanagan, 1997). However, attachment style is still argued to be hard to change because responses to subsequent relationships are influenced significantly by attachment style. For example, the person with very high anxiety over abandonment may avoid intimate relationships in order to reduce the risk of abandonment. This avoidance prevents experience of positive, intimate relationships in which abandonment does not occur. Thus, the schema sets up a pattern of behavior that prevents experience altering the schemas.

PSYCHOLOGICAL DISORDER

A major risk indicator for relationship distress and divorce is past or present history of psychological disorder. Higher rates of relationship problems and divorce consistently have been reported in populations with severe psychiatric disorder (Halford, 1995), and in people with depression, alcohol abuse and some anxiety disorders (Emmelkamp, De Haan, & Hoogduin, 1990; Halford et al., 1999; Halford & Osgarby, 1993; O'Farrell & Birchler, 1987; Reich & Thompson, 1985; Ruscher & Gotlib, 1988; Weissman, 1987). As described earlier in this chapter, relationship problems and individual problems both can exacerbate each other (Halford et al., 1999). In addition, certain personal vulnerabilities may dispose people to both psychological disorders and relationship problems. For example, deficits in interpersonal communication and negative affect regulation are risk factors that predict the onset of both alcohol abuse (Block, Block, & Keyes, 1988) and relationship problems (Markman & Hahlweg, 1993). This common risk factor might be part of the explanation for the common co-occurrence of relationship and alcohol problems.

GENDER

There are important differences between how men and women function within relationships. For example, relative to men, women are more likely to report dissatisfaction with a lack of emotional closeness in their marriages (Clements & Markman, 1996; Julien et al., 1997), to be more emotionally expressive when discussing relationship issues (Weiss & Heyman, 1997), to report greater conflict between their work and family roles (Thompson, 1997), and to initiate divorce (Wolcott & Glazer, 1989). There also is evidence that men and women experience intimacy somewhat differently. Women are more likely to experience self-disclosure of feelings as high in intimacy, whereas men are more likely to experience shared activity as intimacy (Markman & Kraft, 1989). Couple therapy needs to provide the couple with means of managing conflict and enhancing intimacy that accommodate men's and women's needs.

Context

Couple interaction occurs within broader contexts that can serve to promote relationship satisfaction or undermine relationship functioning. Many approaches to couple therapy do not include specific attention to these contextual variables, but these factors often are crucial to helping couples.

THE SOCIOCULTURAL CONTEXT

As noted earlier, marriage and similar relationships occur within a cultural context that defines how marriage should be. While there are certain general assumptions shared across Western cultures, there also are important variations between those cultures. For example, German couples without relationship problems engage in levels of verbal negativity similar to that of Australian distressed couples (Halford, Halweg, & Dunne, 1990), suggesting that greater levels of negativity are more acceptable and less dysfunctional in the German than Australian cultural context. Even within one country there is great diversity in acceptable relationship behavior. Winkler and Doherty (1983) found that verbal conflict was reported as more common in New York couples who were born in Israel than in Anglo couples living in New York. However, verbal conflict was less often associated with physical aggression or relationship distress in the Israeli-born couples than in the Anglo couples. Thus, the cultural appropriateness and functional impact of behavior varies considerably even within Western cultures.

It can be important to assess the cultural context within which relationship standards develop and may be reinforced. Partners who differ in their ethnic, racial, or cultural background often differ in their expectations and beliefs about relationships (Jones & Chao, 1997). This diversity in partner assumptions and beliefs can be a source of great strength for a relationship when the partners are able to draw on the wisdom and strengths of different cultural traditions. At the same time, substantial differences in expectations can be a significant source of conflict between the partners (Jones & Chao, 1997).

OTHER RELATIONSHIPS AND ROLES

While the partner role is central to most adults in couple relationships, this is not the only relationship or role that the partners have. Other relationships and roles of each partner are part of the context in which couple interaction occurs, and these other relationships and roles can have a positive or negative impact on the couple relationship. For example, work often provides extra stimulation and ideas to enrich the relationship, but work demands also can compete for time with the partner (Thompson, 1997). Friends may provide support and shared activities that complement the relationship and reduce the chance of excessive dependence on the partner. However, friendships also can take away time from the partner. Parenting, sports, hobbies, and community service activities all have the capacity to enrich or erode relationship quality. Couple therapy targeted on relationship interaction often involves secondary change in other relationships and roles because they have an impact on the couple relationship.

SETTING VARIABLES

Most couple therapy is conducted within the therapist's office. Typically the layout and routine within a therapist's office is structured to reduce distractions and to provide privacy. The context in which couple interaction normally occurs is quite different. Couples may be sharing their home with children, other members of the extended family, or other people. At home telephones ring, people come and go, and tasks must be done. In the therapist's office all these factors are removed. To the extent that we assume what we see in our offices is representative of the couple's usual behavior, we are ignoring the impact of context on interaction. Implicitly we are assuming that the partner is the only important stimulus that elicits relationship interaction and that the whole spectrum of settings within which interaction occurs are relatively homogeneous. This assumption is wrong. Instead, couple interaction is strongly influenced by settings (Halford, Gravestock, Lowe, & Scheldt, 1992).

Relationship conflict occurs more often in particular settings. High-risk settings for distressed interaction include being in particular physical locations, when either partner is busy or distracted, when there are time pressures, or if either partner is stressed by events outside the relationship (Halford et al., 1992). Furthermore, the topics about which couples have conflict often are directly related to the settings in which those interactions occur (Halford et al., 1992). For example, disagreements about parenting often arise when one or both partners are engaged in child care, and conflict about household chores often occurs when performing those tasks.

In addition to the impact of settings on conflict, settings also have an impact on a couple's chance to develop intimacy within their relationship. For example, couples with young children often report difficulty in getting private couple time. Lack of privacy in the parental bedroom can inhibit the couple's sex life. Lack of a quiet, private time at home can inhibit the couple's communication. The difficulties and expense of going out as a couple when child care is hard to arrange can inhibit the couple's opportunities to share positive experiences.

Couples in distressed relationships often minimize or ignore the impact of settings on their relationships. As noted earlier, relative to satisfied couples distressed couples more often attribute problems in their relationship to their partner and perceive their partner as choosing to behave in ways that are displeasing to them (Bradury & Fincham, 1990). In contrast, happy couples are more likely to attribute negative behaviors to transient setting variables (Bradbury & Fincham, 1990).

Processes That Maintain Relationship Problems

The factors that influence the development of a relationship problem are not necessarily the factors that maintain that relationship problem. Once distress emerges there are often couple adaptive processes that sustain or exacerbate that distress. As an example of this distinction, consider a typical pattern of onset and maintenance of relationship distress. Many couples report that after the birth of their first child there is a decrease in the time they have for shared couple activities. Couples that lack communication skills find it hard to negotiate the lifestyle changes needed to adapt to the new demands of parenthood. If one partner has an individual vulnerability (e.g., the man copes with negative affect by excessive drinking), this may further exacerbate the problems. The context within which the couple is interacting also will influence the relationship. For example, suppose one partner comes from an ethnic background in which the extended family are seen as central to the couple's life together, whereas the other partner values privacy and believes any relationship problems should be kept strictly between the partners. In this context the presence of extended family may constitute a setting within which destructive conflict is likely to occur. A stressful life event (the transition to parenthood) interacts with poor adaptive processes (lack of communication skills), individual characteristics (the alcohol abuse), and the context (ethnic differences about the involvement of extended family). This is the etiology of a relationship problem.

Now consider the same couple 1 or 2 years later when they present for couple therapy. Their unsuccessful attempts to negotiate change may establish highly negative affective responses to each other. Over time their experience of the relationship has shifted. Initially their experience may have been of fun, mutual support, and positive affect, which was associated with active attempts to enhance this state (planning ahead to schedule in shared activities, doing small things to express positive feelings, etc.). Later the experience of the relationship shifts to a mutual negative struggle to avoid pain. There may be conflict over sharing parenting responsibilities and over the man's drinking, and feelings of hurt and pain accumulate after destructive conflict. Avoidance of discussion of difficult issues becomes habitual, which reduces immediate distress but prevents resolution of the dilemmas confronting the relationship. In turn, these ongoing problems result in more negative and less positive interactions. Efforts to support each other and to plan positive shared activities decrease. Their sex life deteriorates. By the time the couple present with relationship distress their whole focus may be on the pain, hurt and conflict, and the need to reduce these problems.

It can be useful to think of all couples as needing to negotiate a series of lifespan developmental transitions. Although not all couples experience exactly the same transitions in the same sequence, all couples must adapt to a number of transitions. For example, early in most relationships couples make the transition from casual dating to commitment. Usually, though not always, this transition is associated with exclusivity in dating. Increasing commitment to the relationship usually is associated with commencing sexual relations, living together, and getting married. The order in which these various transitions occur varies somewhat from culture to culture and from couple to couple. The transition to parenthood often occurs in the first 5 to 10 years of a committed relationship. It is possible to then trace the relationship through commonly occurring changes such as the transition of any children into adolescence, which often is associated with increased independence from the parents, children leaving home, middle age for the couple, and aging and retirement. Each of these phases of the couple's relationship brings changes in work, family, and recreational patterns, which in turn have an impact on the couple's relationship.

Effective couple therapy needs to change those factors that maintain relationship problems. Once this is achieved, the original etiological factors that put the couple at risk of relationship problems may need to be addressed in order to prevent relapse of relationship problems. This section takes a closer look at the specific couple adaptive processes most closely associated with relationship distress. These are the behavioral, cognitive and affective factors that usually are the targets of couple therapy.

Negative Behavior

A common complaint of couples seeking relationship therapy is the negativity of their day-to-day interactions (Halford, Kelly, & Markman, 1997; Weiss & Heyman, 1997). Using behavioral checklists in which people monitor their partners' behavior, there is a well-replicated finding that monitored daily behaviors correlate with relationship satisfaction (Birchler, Weiss, & Vincent, 1975; Halford & Sanders, 1988a; Jacobson, Follette, & McDonald, 1982; Johnson & O'Leary, 1996). Specifically, relative to satisfied couples, distressed couples report higher rates of negative and lower rates of positive behaviors by their partner (Birchler et al., 1975; Halford & Sanders, 1988a; Jacobson et al., 1982; Johnson & O'Leary, 1996). Moreover, distressed couples tend to reciprocate on a "quid pro quo" basis the negative behaviors of their partner. In other words, in a distressed relationship if one partner behaves negatively, the other responds negatively (Birchler et al., 1975; Jacobson et al., 1982). In contrast, satisfied couples' behaviors are less contingent on the preceding behaviors of their partner; satisfied couples are more positive irrespective of their partner's prior actions.

Weiss (1984) suggested that the exchange of behaviors within a relationship is analogous to a bank account. Positive behaviors add credit to the account, while negative behaviors draw on that credit. In satisfied couples the history of positive behavior results in the relationship account being positive, and partners tend to overlook or not respond to negativity. In contrast, in distressed couples a history of negative behavior results in the relationship account being in deficit. Under these circumstances partners tend to reciprocate negativity, and this high rate of reciprocated negativity becomes self-sustaining. A challenge in therapy is then to have partners be positive toward each at higher rates to build up the positive relationship credit associated with satisfying relationships.

Lack of Shared Positive Activities

As noted earlier, a low rate of shared positive activities, and in particular a failure to develop new shared activities, predicts relationship deterioration. Positive shared activities generate positive affect, and trying new positive activities enhances intimacy. In contrast, low rates of positive activity lead to dysphoric mood and depression in vulnerable individuals. This in turn can lead to loss of effort in planning future activities, and alienation and lack of fun come to pervade the relationship. Helping couples bolster their creativity to generate new, pleasurable activities is therefore crucial in couple therapy.

Lack of Intimacy

Another marker of relationship distress is lack of intimacy. Intimacy refers to the occurrence of interaction between the partners that leads them to feel close, loving, and cared for. There are a diversity of ways in which intimacy is developed. For some people intimacy is felt most intensely when self-disclosing intimate feelings, for others when sharing positive experiences, and for others when having sex. A common element to most relationship distress is that the couple is not meeting each other's needs for intimacy, and there is a need to revitalize the manner in which intimacy is promoted within the relationship.

Behaviorally a lack of intimacy is evident in distressed couples in a number of ways. Distressed couples do not talk about positive aspects of their relationship together or self-disclose about their feelings as much as other couples do (Osgarby & Halford, 2000a). Distressed couples show low rates of expressions of caring and intimacy toward each other on a day-to-day basis (Halford & Sanders, 1988a; Weiss & Heyman, 1997). Bolstering intimate talk and the expression of affection is central to couple therapy.

Poor Communication and Conflict Management

Problems in communication are the most frequently cited specific complaint by couples seeking therapy, with up to 90% of distressed couples citing these difficulties as a major issue in the relationship (Bornstein & Bornstein, 1986). Both independent observers and partners report that communication deficiencies are associated with relationship distress (Weiss & Heyman, 1997). When discussing problem issues distressed partners often are hostile and criticize and demand change of each other (Christensen & Shenk, 1991; Gottman, 1993b, 1994; Gottman & Krokoff, 1989; Halford et al., 1990; Heavey, Christensen, & Malmuth, 1995). Distressed couples also do not actively listen to their partner when discussing problems (Halford et al., 1990; Jacobson, McDonald, Follette, & Berley, 1985; Weiss & Heyman, 1990), and tend to withdraw from problem discussions (Christensen & Shenk, 1991; Gottman, 1994; Gottman & Krokoff, 1989; Halford et al., 1992; Heavey et al., 1995). Contentious relationship issues are less likely to be resolved by discussion in distressed couples than in nondistressed couples (Halford et al., 1992).

In observational studies of communication the conditional probabilities of distressed partners responding with hostility to their partner's hostility is much higher than the conditional probabilities for nondistressed partners (e.g., Halford et al., 1990). In addition to this negative reciprocity, relationship distress also is associated with high levels of psychophysiological arousal during interaction (e.g., Gottman & Levenson, 1988). This arousal is aversive, which may explain the higher rates of withdrawal during problem-focused discussions by distressed partners (Christensen & Shenk, 1991; Gottman & Krokoff, 1989). In any case, both the extent of arousal and the frequency of withdrawal prospectively predict deterioration in relationship satisfaction (Gottman, 1993b; Gottman & Krokoff, 1989; Heavey, Layne, & Christensen, 1993; Heavey et al., 1995).

While conflict is often the most obvious element of the initial presentation of relationship problems, relationship distress and severe conflict are not interchangeable concepts. Some distressed couples report and demonstrate little overt conflict (Gottman, 1994). Gottman (1993b) showed that there is considerable variety in how both distressed and nondistressed couples manage conflict. Some distressed couples avoid discussion of conflict topics, at least as far as practicable. Such couples may report few arguments but major dissatisfaction with the relationship. However, the common problem to almost all distressed relationships is ineffective conflict management.

Ineffective communication and conflict management have several effects that sustain relationship problems. Poor communication reduces partners' understanding of each other. This makes it difficult for the partners to support each other and to recognize and attempt to meet each others' needs, or to understand the other person's perspective about conflict issues. Ineffective conflict management means that important relationship issues remain unresolved, and hence the issues often become the source of repeated conflict. Many distressed couples report that they have the same, or similar, arguments around a given topic without resolving the problem.

Inequitable Role Functioning and Lack of Mutual Support

Inequitable role functioning is one of women's most common relationship complaints and is a frequent source of couple conflict (Julien et al., 1997). Excessive role loads on partners, particularly on women, is associated with stress and depression (Thompson, 1997). In turn, stress and depression exacerbate and maintain relationship problems (Halford et al., 1999).

Lack of support from the partner is a common component of unsatisfactory couple relationships (Baxter, 1986), and higher perceived level of support by one's partner is correlated with higher relationship satisfaction (Acitelli & Antonucci, 1994). Direct observation of couples discussing issues that are stressful for one of the partners shows that positive emotional and instrumental support behaviors are associated with high perceived supportiveness in that discussion (Cutrona & Suhr, 1992; Pasch, Bradbury, & Davila, 1997). Greater frequency of these positive support behaviors during couple interaction is correlated with higher current relationship satisfaction (Cutrona & Suhr, 1992) and with longitudinal stability of high relationship satisfaction in couples (Pasch & Bradbury, 1998).

Evolutionary psychologists argue that couple relationships are pervasive to all human cultures because these pairings confer adaptive advantage to the partners (Baumeister & Leary, 1995; Buss, 1994). In other words, partners help each other in crucial processes in surviving and raising offspring. Inequitable role functioning and lack of social support in the relationship violate these fundamental processes and make life more generally stressful for the partners. To the extent that couple therapy can promote equitable and sustainable roles for each partner and help them to support each other, it is likely to enhance relationship satisfaction and stability.

Poor Sex

Sex is an important means for couples to experience intimacy. Good sex is associated with sustained relationship satisfaction while infrequent or unsatisfactory sex is a common source of hurt and conflict in distressed couples (Spence, 1997). Gender differences may exist regarding the role of sex in maintenance of relationship problems. In my experience it is common for partners to agree that they both lack closeness and have a poor sex life. However, the best way to manage these problems often is a source of disagreement. Typically, though not universally, the male recommends that the couple work on improving their sex life, and he asserts that an improvement in sex would have a positive effect on the relationship. Equally as frequently the woman will assert that the sense of closeness must be built first, and then sex will improve after that. The challenge in couple therapy is to find a means acceptable to both partners to enhance both sexuality and other aspects of the relationship.

Perceptual Biases

In some of the earliest empirical research on the interactions of distressed couples the researchers hoped they would be able to identify which behaviors were associated with relationship distress and then teach couples to do those behaviors in order to enhance relationship satisfaction (Weiss, Hops, & Patterson, 1973). However, as research accumulated it was found that observed behavior accounted for only a modest percentage of the variance in relationship satisfaction (Weiss & Heyman, 1997). This leads to the question of what else is influencing relationship distress.

As Weiss (1984) has pointed out on numerous occasions, it is important to distinguish between the insider's (participant's) and outsider's (e.g., observer or therapist's) perspectives on couple interaction. Research has identified a number of influences on the insider's perspective of relationships that make it diverge from outsiders' perspectives. We know that distressed couples have systematic biases in how they perceive events in their relationships. Relative to outsider observers, distressed couples selectively attend to the negative behaviors of their partners and have negative biases in their perception of those behaviors (Eidelson & Epstein, 1982; Floyd & Markman, 1983; Jacobson & Moore, 1981; Notarius, Benson, Sloane, Vanzetti, & Hornyak, 1989). In contrast, satisfied people tend to overlook negative behaviors by their partner (Gottman, Markman, & Notarius, 1977; Notarius et al., 1989) and to have an unrealistically positive view of their partner and their relationship (Fowers, Applegate, Olson, & Pomerantz, 1994). Furthermore, distressed couples selectively remember negative relationship events, while satisfied couples tend to selectively remember positive relationship events (Osgarby & Halford, 2000a, 2000b).

Once a negative perceptual bias develops in someone's perception of his or her partner or relationship, it can become difficult to enhance satisfaction by behavior change alone. For example, many couple therapists report that increases in positive behavior during therapy are ignored or discounted by distressed partners (e.g., Baucom & Epstein, 1990). A challenge in couple therapy is to change the manner in which partners appraise their partner and relationship so that positive behaviors are attended to and valued.

Negative Emotion

The lack of objectivity in perceiving one's own relationship is due to many factors. Two important influences are the impact of intense negative emotions and cognitions. At the positive end of the emotional spectrum love, respect, support, and passion often are expressed with greatest intensity toward our partner. Such strong positive feelings are associated with overlooking the human failings of our partner, particularly early in relationships (Notarius & Markman, 1993). At the negative end of the emotional spectrum anger, fear, contempt, jealousy, depression, and rage are all common emotions displayed during relationship interaction (Gottman, 1994). Arousal of these emotions leads people to focus on negative aspects of their partner and their relationship, and often to revert to automated, almost reflexive negative responses to their partner (Bradbury & Fincham, 1987).

Johnson and Greenberg (1994) describe the psychological functions of emotion as directing behavioral tendencies. By this they mean that arousal of given emotions tends to potentiate broad classes of response. For example, when feeling afraid, people selectively attend to threat cues, may misperceive neutral stimuli as evidence of threat, and are likely to respond with attack or withdrawal in response to perceived threat cues. In Johnson and Greenberg's (1994) view, the essence of relationship distress is the negative emotion elicited in interaction with the partner and the effect that this negative emotion has in maintaining attention to negativity in the relationship.

Weiss (1984) coined the term "sentiment override" to describe essentially the same phenomenon as that described by Johnson and Greenberg (1994). Sentiment override is the notion that partners develop a global sentiment (general emotional state) about their relationship which is either positive or negative. He argues that people perceive their partners and their relationships in terms of that global sentiment. In other words, if you have a negative sentiment, you will perceive most of the behavior of your partner as being negative. On the other hand, if you had a positive sentiment you would tend to see exactly the same behaviors as positive.

Negative Cognition

In addition to these emotional characteristics, distressed couples also have a number of characteristic cognitions. Distressed couples hold unrealistic beliefs about relationships and partners. Specifically, relative to happy couples, distressed couples are more likely to believe that any form of disagreement is destructive, that change by partners is not possible, and that rigid adherence to traditional gender roles is desirable (Eidelson & Epstein, 1982). Distressed couples also report that their relationships often violate standards about how they think their relationship should be (Baucom, Epstein, Daiuto, et al., 1996). For example, distressed women report that their partners do not share power within the relationship in the manner the women believe they should, and men believe their partners should invest more time and energy in the relationship than they do (Baucom, Epstein, Daiuto, et al., 1996).

Another cognitive characteristic of distressed couples is attribution of the causes of negative behavior by partners to stable, internal, negative characteristics of the partners (Bradbury & Fincham, 1990; Fincham & Bradbury, 1992). These negative attributions are associated with more blaming of the partner for relationship problems by distressed than by satisfied couples (Bradbury & Fincham, 1990). For example, a partner arriving home late from work may be perceived as "a generally selfish person who doesn't care about the family" by a distressed partner. The same behavior may be attributed by a satisfied person as the partner "struggling to keep up with a heavy load at work, being subject to lots of pressure from the boss." The process of attributing much or all of the relationship problems to their partner leaves most people with relationship distress feeling powerless to improve their relationship (Vanzetti, Notarius, & NeeSmith, 1992). A key element of couple therapy is to enhance each partner's sense of relational efficacy or capacity to improve the relationship through his or her own actions (Halford, Sanders, & Behrens, 1994)

Other cognitive characteristics of distressed couples are that they expect negative outcomes from interaction with their partners and have negative biases in their memory of relationship interactions. Distressed couples report that prior to a discussion, they expect not to be able to resolve problems in their relationship (Vanzetti et al., 1992). In anticipation of a problem-solving discussion, distressed partners show high physiological arousal (Gottman, 1994) and negative affect and become primed to access negative evaluative judgments about their partner and the relationship (Fincham, Garnier, Gano-Phillips, & Osborne, 1995). When asked to describe past interactions they remember the interactions as being more negative then their perceptions immediately after the interactions (Osgarby & Halford, 2000b).

The cognitive characteristics of distressed couples mediate their subsequent behavior toward their partners. For example, the occurrence of negative attributions is associated with subsequent behavioral negativity (Bradbury & Fincham, 1992). In unhappy couples, negative thoughts about the partner predict future negative behaviors better than do predictions from previous behavior (Halford & Sanders, 1990), suggesting that these cognitions are more than just the consequences of negative marital behavior. In other words, distressed partners seem to respond to their subjective perceptions and memories of relationship interactions, and these perceptions and memories are negatively biased.

A Model of Couple Relationships

Figure 1.1 is a schematic representation of the factors influencing couple relationships. It portrays the interactions between partners, the life events that have an impact on the partners, the individual characteristics the partners bring to their relationship, and the broader context within which couple interaction occurs. The model of relationships I propose has interaction between the partners (i.e., couple adaptive processes) as the central element. This is depicted schematically in Figure 1.1 by placing interaction at the center of the diagram. However, interaction that we can observe as outsiders is only part of the process. The internal state of each partner during interaction also is important to understanding the interaction. Both the cognitive appraisal each partner

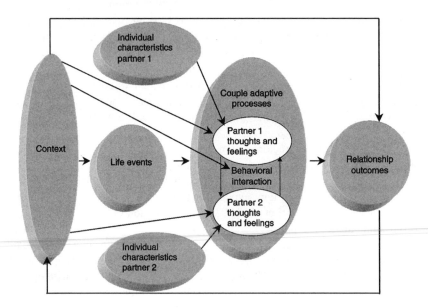

FIGURE 1.1. Schematic diagram of the influences on couple relationships.

makes of the interaction and his or her emotional responses determine what happens in the interaction.

Relationship outcomes refer to the satisfaction with the relationship experienced by both partners and the stability of the relationship. Couple therapy primarily is focused on changing couple adaptive processes, which includes observable interaction (the outsider's perspective) and the emotional and cognitive processes of the couple (the insiders' perspectives), to promote more positive relationship outcomes. Couple therapy begins with the assessment of distressed couple adaptive processes and with the gathering of data on individual characteristics, life events, and context affecting couple adaptive processes. Couple therapy proceeds if change in couple adaptive processes seems likely to be achieved by working directly on the couple interaction. In some instances changes in individual characteristics, stressful events, or context might be achieved outside couple therapy, and these changes can produce desired changes in distressed interaction. For example, working with one person to reduce an individual partner's heavy drinking might enhance relationship interaction and promote relationship satisfaction.

The couple therapy approach described in this book is focused on helping partners to self-regulate change in the adaptive processes within their relationship. Each partner is assisted to produce self-change in his or her adaptive processes. The promotion of self-regulation is achieved through the development of a series of relationship metacompetencies that promote self-change. Chapter 3 details these metacompetencies, which include appraising the relationship context, the life events affecting the relationship, and one's own adaptive processes within the relationship; setting self-change goals for adaptive processes that will promote relationship satisfaction and stability; implementing self-change strategies; and evaluating the effects of these self-change efforts.

2

Approaches to Couple Therapy and Their Effectiveness

Couple therapy is defined by the use of conjoint therapy sessions to alter the relationship between the partners. Many forms of individual psychotherapy have been adapted to couple therapy format, and some new psychotherapy approaches have been developed that are specific to couple therapy. Given the diversity of couple therapy approaches for relationship problems, how does the therapist determine which approach to take? For me, an important influence on therapeutic approach is the empirical evidence about what works. However, only a small number of couple therapy approaches have been subjected to empirical evaluation (Baucom, Shoham, Mueser, Daiuto, & Stickle, 1998).

In the last 10 years or so there has been a concentrated effort to define criteria for judging whether psychological treatments have reasonable empirical evidence that they are efficacious (American Psychological Association, 1993; Chambless & Hollon, 1998). A widely used definition is that a treatment is empirically supported if two methodologically sound, independently conducted, controlled trials show that treatment is superior to no treatment or placebo treatment (Chambless & Hollon, 1998). A treatment is regarded as possibly empirically supported if just one methodologically sound trial has been conducted (Chambless & Hollon, 1998). There are more than 40 published, well-controlled trials of couple therapy (Baucom et al., 1998; LeBow & Gurman, 1995), and several meta-analyses have been published summarizing this body of literature (e.g., Hahlweg & Markman, 1988; Shadish et al.,

1993). By far the most thoroughly researched couple therapy is behavioral couple therapy (BCT), with nearly two-thirds of all published studies evaluating couple therapy examining BCT (Baucom et al., 1998). Moreover, there are many studies of BCT examining the variability and clinical significance of therapeutic change, and the mechanisms of therapeutic change. This chapter is a review of those approaches for which there is at least one controlled trial evaluating efficacy. They are behavioral couple therapy, cognitive couple therapy, emotion-focused therapy and insight-oriented therapy, and self-regulatory couple therapy.

Defining Success in Couple Therapy

Defining and evaluating the effects of couple therapy is difficult. Consider the case of Chris and Norma, who presented to me with relationship distress. At presentation both partners reported severe ongoing conflict and ambivalence about whether they wished to remain in the relationship. Chris reported that he drank alcohol quite heavily over the last 12 months, averaging approximately six standard drinks a day. Norma reported that she was depressed over the last year. She completed the Beck Depression Inventory and had a score of 22, indicating moderate depression. Furthermore, both Chris and Norma reported that their 7-year-old son John had witnessed a number of marital conflicts between them recently, and that John was showing evidence of severe distress in response to these conflicts. John's teacher recently had reported deteriorating performance in John's school work.

I saw Chris and Norma for 12 sessions of couple therapy. At initial presentation both partners completed the Dyadic Adjustment Scale (Spanier, 1976), with scores for Chris and Norma of 79 and 75, respectively. These scores are indicative of moderate to severe relationship distress. At the end of treatment they completed the Dyadic Adjustment Scale again, and each obtained scores of 94. A score of 100 is often used as the cut-off to indicate normal relationship satisfaction, so each of the partners was still distressed at the end of treatment though improved relative to their pretreatment scores. Furthermore, both Chris and Norma reported substantial improvement in their individual adjustment. Chris reported moderating his drinking so that he was now having one to two standard drinks a day. Norma's report of substantial improvement in her depression was supported by a score on the Beck Depression Inventory of 8 at the end of therapy, which is within the normal range. Finally, both partners reported reduced marital conflict particularly in front of their son.

Three months later Norma and Chris re-presented to me. They said that their conflict was still low but that each of them still felt significantly dissatisfied with their relationship. After reassessment of their relationship over two sessions, they reached a mutual decision to separate. Therapy then focused on negotiation of shared parenting and financial arrangements after separation. Three therapy sessions produced a mutually acceptable agreement about separation. While each found the negotiation process harrowing at the time, they reported being pleased to have negotiated a low-conflict separation. A subsequent follow-up 12 months later affirmed that they had separated but remained on amicable terms. Each of them was doing well individually, Norma was not depressed and Chris was drinking at moderate levels. Each felt pleased with the coparenting arrangements that they had negotiated, and with their individual coping with the separation.

Should the case of Chris and Norma be regarded as a therapeutic failure? In most couple therapy research, success is defined in terms of whether the couple remains together, and if they do, whether their relationship satisfaction is significantly improved. Thus, the foregoing case would be classified as a failure. However, given the substantial improvements in individual functioning of each of the partners, and the decreased impact of their relationship distress on their son, there are a number of reasons why this intervention might be regarded as at least partially successful.

Measuring Success in Couple Therapy

In the research on couple therapy, relationship satisfaction usually is measured on a global self-report inventory (Heyman et al., 1994). For example, the Dyadic Adjustment Scale (Spanier, 1976) is a widely used global assessment of relationship satisfaction. Relationship stability is another possible outcome index for couple therapy. Stability can be operationalized in terms of separation or divorce, though even in distressed couples the rates of actual separation and divorce within a limited period after therapy usually are low, and therefore this may not be a sensitive index of therapy outcome. To circumvent this limitation, Weiss and Cerreto (1980) developed the Marital Status Inventory. The Marital Status Inventory is a 14-item Guttman-type rating scale in which people respond true or false to statements that they have made a series of steps toward relationship dissolution. Total scores are indicative of separation or divorce potential.

Therapy also has been evaluated in terms of relationship processes. For example, in numerous studies communication and conflict management have been assessed before and after therapy (e.g., Halford, Sanders, & Behrens, 1993; Snyder & Wills, 1989). Even in those couples that decide to separate, assessment of relationship adaptive processes is relevant. The negotiation of low-conflict separations may be a positive outcome because ongoing conflict is associated with poorer adjustment both for the separating ex-partners (Walsh, Jacob, & Simons, 1995) and for dependent children from the relationship (Baris & Garrity, 1997).

Even if no changes in interaction between the partners were to occur as a result of couple therapy, other positive changes may occur as the result of therapy. As in the example of Chris and Norma, sometimes there can be significant improvements in individual functioning even when a relationship does not improve dramatically. If a couple seeks therapy, improvement in individual adjustment may well constitute a meaningful therapeutic gain. Unfortunately, little attention has been paid in the couple therapy outcome research to the impact on individual adjustment or negotiating low-conflict separations. With that caveat, I now review what we do know about the effects of couple therapy.

Empirically Supported Approaches to Couple Therapy

Behavioral, Cognitive, and Cognitive-Behavioral Couple Therapy

BCT is the most widely researched approach to couple therapy (Baucom et al., 1998). BCT is conducted in a conjoint format with the goal of altering the interaction between partners (Baucom & Epstein, 1990; Jacobson & Margolin, 1979). In BCT the maladaptive interaction is viewed as the relationship problem. BCT emphasizes the use of behavior exchange and training in communication and problem solving to promote change in dyadic interactions (Baucom & Epstein, 1990; Halford et al., 1993; Jacobson & Margolin, 1979).

The emphasis in BCT is to assess the patterns of key interactions between the partners. A demand–withdraw communication pattern is one example that is common in distressed couples (Christensen & Shenk, 1991). This pattern consists of one partner approaching and making requests for change of the other, while the spouse responds by withdrawing. This repetitive pattern is often self-sustaining and has been shown to lead to deterioration in couple relationships. From a BCT perspective the goal of therapy is to overcome this pattern by training couples in new forms of communication which circumvent this maladaptive style, and which promote effective conflict resolution. This could involve some combination of communication and problem-solving skills training.

Cognitive couple therapy involves the application of the general cognitive model of distress developed by Beck (1976) to couple relationship problems. In this approach it is assumed that the cognitions of partners mediate their emotional and behavioral responses to one another. Irrational relationship beliefs such as "any form of disagreement with my partner is destructive to the relationship" or "people cannot change the way they are in relationships" are believed to underlie negative emotions in relationships. Similarly unhelpful, partner blaming attributions such as "he/she does these negative things just to annoy me" also are believed to mediate negative emotions in relationships. When relationship negativity is excessive, emphasis is placed on identifying and changing these sorts of maladaptive cognitions (Baucom & Epstein, 1990).

Cognitive-behavioral couple therapy (CBCT) combines the behavioral and cognitive therapy approaches. In CBCT the therapist combines behavior change strategies such as behavioral contracting and communications skills training with cognitive restructuring. The aim is to modify both the couple's behavioral interactions and their individual cognitive appraisal of that interaction.

There are now more than 25 controlled trials of BCT in which BCT consistently has been shown to be superior to no treatment or to therapist contact control in reducing relationship distress (Hahlweg & Markman, 1988; Shadish et al., 1993). Specifically, BCT improves couples' communication skills, reduces destructive conflict, enhances the positivity of day-to-day interactions, increases the positivity of couples' cognitions about their partners and their relationships, and enhances relationship satisfaction (Hahlweg & Markman, 1988; Halford et al., 1993; Shadish et al., 1993). BCT is a powerful intervention. In two meta-analyses of outcome studies conducted, the magnitude of the effect size for BCT is in the order of 0.9 to 1.0 standard deviations on key outcome measures such as relationship satisfaction (Hahlweg & Markman, 1988; Shadish et al., 1993). This constitutes a large effect size and is comparable to the effect sizes obtained for the most effective psychological interventions.

Despite the replication and magnitude of the observed effects of BCT, there are significant limitations to its effects. Approximately 25 to 30% of couples show no measurable improvement with BCT, and as many as a further 30% improve somewhat from therapy but still report significant relationship distress after treatment (Halford et al., 1993; Jacobson, 1989; Jacobson et al., 1984). Even among those couples that initially respond well to BCT, there is substantial relapse toward relationship distress over the next few years (Jacobson, Schmaling, & Holtzworth-Munroe, 1987; Snyder, Mangrum, & Wills, 1993; Snyder, Wills, & Grady-Fletcher, 1991a). There is a consistent finding that the longer couples have been distressed and the more severe their relationship dissatisfaction, the poorer their response to BCT (Jacobson & Addis, 1993; Snyder et al., 1993; Whisman & Snyder, 1997).

Recognition of the limitations of BCT led to efforts to enhance its efficacy. Cognitive interventions alone modify maladaptive relationship cognitions and improve relationship satisfaction (e.g., Emmelkamp, van Linden, van den Heuvell, Ruphan, et al., 1988). Cognitive interventions were added to traditional BCT (consisting of behavior exchange and communication and problem-solving skills training) but did not significantly increase relationship satisfaction gains from BCT (Baucom & Lester, 1986; Baucom, Sayers, & Sher, 1990; Halford et al., 1993). However, demonstrating greater efficacy of one active intervention over another is notoriously difficult, as large sample sizes are required to provide adequate statistical power to detect the differential effect (Kazdin & Bass, 1989). Given that BCT is efficacious for many couples, the failure to demonstrate additive effects of cognitive interventions to BCT may be due to a lack of statistical power in the designs of studies. Moreover, even if cognitive interventions do not add to the average efficacy of BCT across distressed couples, cognitive interventions may be useful to a particular subset of distressed couples. Notwithstanding this possibility, it has to be conceded that despite the enormous research effort into cognitions within BCT since the early to mid-1980s, there is no evidence that we have improved on the efficacy obtained 20 years ago in BCT.

The focus of CBCT on behavior exchange, communication and problem-solving skills training, and cognitive interventions includes an implicit assumption that changes in some or all of these aspects of couple adaptive processes mediate improvements in relationship satisfaction resulting from therapy. However, there is inconsistency in the findings on the association between changes in couple adaptive processes and relationship satisfaction. In two studies little association was found between changes in communication skills and relationship satisfaction (Halford et al., 1993; Iverson & Baucom, 1990), and in one study a modest association was found between these two variables across the course of therapy (Sayers, Baucom, Sher, Weiss, & Heyman, 1991). Changes in cognitions consistently have *not* been found to covary with changes in relationship satisfaction across the course of CBCT (Emmelkamp, van Linden van den Heuvell, Sanderman, & Scholing, 1988; Halford et al., 1993). In summary, there is little evidence that BCT produces therapeutic improvement by the means assumed in the traditional models of BCT.

Typically, BCT as reported in the literature involves anything from 12 to 20 sessions of conjoint therapy. If changes in behavior exchange, communication and problem solving, or cognitive restructuring are the crucial mechanisms of change, and if this number of sessions is required to achieve such changes, it would be expected that change in these variables would be gradual across the course of therapy. Yet, in several intrasubject evaluations of BCT, striking changes were observed in behavior, cognitions, and self-monitored relationship satisfaction in the first few sessions of therapy, with modest or no gains evident in the later phases of therapy (e.g., Behrens, Sanders, & Halford, 1990; Kelly & Halford, 1995). If the hypothesized mechanisms of therapeutic gain during BCT require substantial therapist input across large numbers of therapy sessions, then these observed rapid improvements are hard to explain.

Emotion-Focused and Insight-Oriented Couple Therapy

Another extensively researched approach to couple therapy is emotion-focused therapy (EFT). EFT was developed by Johnson and Greenberg (1995) and is targeted at the couple's interaction as the locus of therapeutic change. The EFT approach originally was described as drawing largely from existential and humanistic psychotherapies (Greenberg & Johnson, 1988), but in more recent writings greater emphasis has been placed on the psychodynamic concept of attachment (Johnson & Greenberg, 1995). EFT asserts that there is reciprocal influence between couple interaction and internal emotional experience. Specifically, distressed relationships are seen as the result of insecure attachment bonds. The goal of EFT is to access and reprocess the emotional responses underlying negative couple interactions, which is believed to lead to the development of more secure attachment styles and different patterns of couple interaction. The conjoint format allows development of empathy by each partner for the other's experiences, and allows the development of new patterns of couple interaction.

In insight-oriented couple therapy (IOCT), the traditional psychodynamic transference issue has been reframed so that the major therapeutic focus is on how the individual spouses project their own unresolved conflicts onto each other rather than onto the therapist (Snyder & Wills, 1989). It is assumed that earlier relationships lead the partners to respond emotionally in unhelpful ways toward each other. This being the case, IOCT pays a good deal of attention to the growth of each individual spouse, and to the impact of developmental processes on the interactions between the partners. The assumption is that emotional reprocessing and insight gained through such exploration alters the partners' affective and behavioral responses to each other. This allows the couples to overcome destructive conflict.

An element common to both IOCT and EFT is the emphasis on high negative emotion within the relationship being attributable to individual vulnerabilities in the partners. As a consequence, couple therapy within these frameworks is focused on changing internal affective responses to the partner. In both approaches developmental processes in previous relationships are believed often to drive current negative responses to the partner.

EFT has been evaluated in at least five controlled trials (Baucom et al., 1998), and has been found to significantly improve relationship satisfaction relative to no treatment or placebo controls (Greenberg & Johnson, 1988; Johnson & Greenberg, 1985). Consequently, EFT meets the criteria for an empirically supported therapy. There also is one well-designed study which found that IOCT significantly improved couple communication and enhanced relationship satisfaction (Snyder & Wills, 1989; Snyder et al., 1991a). IOCT meets the criteria for a probably empirically supported treatment, but replication of the one controlled trial is needed.

EFT and IOCT share the BCT focus on conjoint therapy to change couples' adaptive processes but do not place the same emphasis as BCT on behavioral skills training or rational approaches to cognitive change. Both EFT and IOCT emphasize changing partners' subjective emotional experience of relationship interactions through corrective emotional experiences, or through insights gained into the individual significance of particular relationship events (Greenberg & Johnson, 1988; Snyder, Wills, & Grady-Fletcher, 1991b). Blind expert ratings of couple therapy sessions show that IOCT is different in therapeutic process and content from BCT (Wills, Faitler, & Snyder, 1987). However, there is no research on whether IOCT and EFT sessions are distinctive.

There has been research examining the mechanisms of change within EFT. The EFT approach hypothesizes that as partners access and reprocess their emotional experiences of the relationship, there should be changes in their emotional expressions within sessions. Specifically, EFT argues that therapy should facilitate the expression of positive affiliative emotions, greater expressions of vulnerability, and reduced expression of hostility and rejection (Greenberg & Johnson, 1988). However, the evidence to support these theoretical expositions is inconsistent. In one study the extent of change within sessions on these variables predicted modest variance in changes in relationship satisfaction after therapy (Johnson & Greenberg, 1988), but in a more recent study no significant association between these variables was evident (Johnson & Talitman, 1997). Thus, like BCT there is little evidence that EFT produces change via the mechanisms proposed by the developers of the therapy.

Self-Regulatory Couple Therapy

Self-regulatory couple therapy (SRCT) is the application of behavioral self-control theory (Kanfer, 1970; Kanfer & Karoly, 1972; Karoly, 1993) to relationship problems. The emphasis in SRCT is on helping each partner in a distressed relationship to learn metacompetencies to change problematic patterns of behavior, cognition, and affect and thereby to enhance their relationship. Specifically, being able to self-regulate relationships depends on individuals possessing a number of separate but interconnected metaskills including relationship appraisal, goal setting, self-change implementation, and evaluation of self-change attempts. My colleagues and I (Halford et al., 1994) used the idea of self-regulated change as an integrating framework within which to understand the efficacy of existing approaches to couple therapy.

The central concept of SRCT is that partners, not therapists, produce long-term change in couple relationships. Couple therapy is successful to the extent that it engages partners in self-regulated change processes. Self-regulation begins by helping both partners to appraise their relationship and, based on this appraisal, to self-select personal goals for change. This process involves the use of structured assessment and discussion of assessment results to help each partner define personal change goals intended to enhance the relationship. For some couples, once the partners are able to define specific personal change goals, they are able to successfully implement these self-regulation goals (Halford, Osgarby, & Kelly, 1996). In other words, one implication of the self-regulated approach to couple therapy is that brief couple therapy, usually consisting of assessment and goal setting, can be sufficient to achieve relationship improvement for some couples.

Some couples need more extensive therapy than goal setting to achieve their relationship goals. Extended SRCT makes use of behavioral, cognitive, emotion-focused and insight-oriented procedures to enable the couple to achieve relationship change. In the SRCT application of procedures derived from other approaches, emphasis remains on promoting a focus on self-change. For example, suppose the assessment process has identified the demand–withdraw pattern as characteristic of a couple's negative interactions. In the self-regulated change process, each partner is encouraged to self-select goals for change that might overcome this problem and to attempt to implement these goals. If the couple were able to produce the desired relationship changes with this and other self-selected personal change goals, then brief therapy would have been successful.

If the partners were unable to select communication self-change goals successfully, or unable to implement those goals successfully, then therapy would move to more extended therapy. This more extended couple therapy might include communication skills training. In traditional BCT the therapist would train the couple in a range of skills and encourage the couple to apply these skills in their communication. In self-regulated couple therapy each partner would be assisted to self-evaluate his or her use of various communication skills and to self-select new ways of interacting that both wished to implement. The idea is that couples not only learn helpful communication but also learn to self-change unhelpful communication when it arises. In Chapter 3, I explain the nature of SRCT in greater detail.

There have been at least two published evaluations of brief SRCT. The first was not specifically labeled by the authors as SRCT, but Worthington et al. (1995) did evaluate the effects of assessment and goal setting on enhancement of relationship functioning of couples. As described in detail in Chapter 3, assessment and goal setting are central elements to brief SRCT. In a randomized controlled trial Worthington et al. (1995) found that assessment, feedback, and goal setting produced significantly greater increases in relationship satisfaction than assessment alone. Couples in the study were only mildly distressed relative to couples in many other couple therapy treatment studies, but the study showed that couples can self-direct changes in their relationship and enhance their satisfaction.

In a second study, a quasi-experimental evaluation of brief SRCT was tested with severely distressed couples. In the brief therapy condition couples went through a systematic assessment of their relationship across three sessions, which culminated in feedback and goal setting. In the feedback, partners were encouraged to identify specific actions each could take to enhance the relationship. Some couples also were given brief self-regulated skills training in the last part of the third session, if that was indicated. All couples received a copy of the book *Living and Loving Together* (Montgomery & Evans, 1989). This is a popular book published in Australia that describes the key elements of a cognitive-behavioral approach to understanding and changing relationships. The partners were encouraged to read the book, and specific chapters were identified as being particularly relevant for the couple, based on the self-defined change goals.

Couples who received the brief SRCT were reassessed on their relationship satisfaction 3 months after the assessment and goal-setting sessions. There was a significant increase in relationship satisfaction relative to pretreatment measures. The increase was of a comparable magnitude to the change in relationship satisfaction reported by couples that had been through a full course of 15 sessions of traditional BCT (Halford et al., 1996). This study had some significant limitations, notably that the assignment of couples to conditions was not random. However, it was striking that only three sessions of assessment, feedback, and goal setting achieved substantial increases in relationship satisfaction in severely distressed couples.

The two foregoing studies show that brief SRCT, involving structured assessment and goal setting, meets the criteria for a probably empirically supported couple therapy. The other empirical findings suggest that assessment, goal setting, and self-directed change are important elements of observed therapeutic effects of all empirically supported couple therapies. Assessment, feedback to the partners, and goal setting are common to each of the empirically supported couple therapies of BCT and emotion-focused and insight-oriented therapies. In studies of the mechanisms of change in BCT and emotion-focused couple therapy, skill acquisition and changes in emotional expression account for either none or very modest proportions of the variance in relationship satisfaction outcomes. Moreover, in studies of the process of change in BCT, changes occur primarily in the first few sessions of therapy. All this evidence converges on the point that the process of promoting self-regulated change through assessment, feedback, and goal setting can improve relationship satisfaction for at least some couples. Moreover, these processes probably account for at least some of the efficacy of all empirically supported couple therapies.

Relative Efficacy of Different Approaches to Couple Therapy

There is limited research on the relative efficacy of the various empirically supported, or probably empirically supported, approaches to couple therapy, though the effect sizes obtained from the various approaches across all published studies seem similar (LeBow & Gurman, 1995; Shadish et al., 1993). In one study EFT was compared with a form of BCT including only communication skills and problem-solving training (CPST) (Johnson & Greenberg, 1985). The EFT produced a large treatment effect size of 2.19, which was significantly larger than the BCT effect size of 1.12. However, in this study the behavior exchange component from the BCT was excluded and worked with only mildly distressed couples. In an uncontrolled evaluation of EFT with more distressed couples, the effect size was still substantial at 1.26 (Johnson & Talitman, 1997), but the magnitude of this effect size is similar to the effect sizes reported for BCT. Further research is needed to determine the relative efficacy of EFT and BCT.

Snyder et al. (1991a) compared BCT, including behavior exchange and CPST, with IOCT, and the latter was found to have greater long-term efficacy than BCT. The interpretation of the study as supporting greater efficacy of IOCT was challenged on the grounds that the treatment in the BCT condition allegedly was not state-of-the-art BCT, and that the insight-oriented therapy included much of what should be included in BCT (Jacobson, 1991). Snyder et al. (1991b) rebutted these criticisms and showed that their versions of insight-oriented and BCT treatments were distinctive and included the elements they intended (Wills et al., 1987).

In the quasi-experimental comparison of three sessions of brief self-regulated change and 15 sessions of traditional BCT, no significant differences were found between the approaches (Halford et al., 1996). The number of couples per treatment condition was modest, so there was low power to detect moderate magnitude differences in efficacy. Assessment of the variability and clinical significance of the self-regulated change treatment showed that its effects were comparable with those reported for BCT. Given that there is only one study comparing BCT with EFT, one comparing BCT with IOCT, and one comparing BCT with brief SRCT, it is premature to conclude that any particular empirically supported couple therapy truly is more effective than any other. However, SRCT is not intended as an alternative to replace the other couple therapy approaches. Rather, I see SRCT as offering a broad framework to understand couple therapy. This framework can be used to apply procedures drawn from other approaches that have been empirically supported. SRCT also provides some new interventions for assisting distressed relationships.

Predictors of Response to Couple Therapy

Couple therapy works better for some couples than for others. The majority of studies of predictors of response to couple therapy have assessed predictors of response to BCT. Socioeconomic status generally has not been found to predict response to BCT (Baucom & Hoffman, 1986), though most subjects in the research were of middle to upper socioeconomic status and the limited variability may obscure some modest effect of low socioeconomic status.

In general, the more severe the relationship problems at presentation the poorer the response to couple therapy. Low levels of presenting relationship satisfaction (Jacobson, Follette, & Pagel, 1986; Johnson & Talitman, 1997; Whisman & Jacobson, 1990) are associated with poorer response to BCT, EFT, and IOCT. Negative patterns of couple interaction typically become entrenched over time and resistant to change (Markman, Floyd, Stanley, & Storaasli, 1988; Raush, Barry, Hertel, & Swain, 1974). More severe problems in managing conflict (Snyder et al., 1993) are associated with poorer response to BCT and IOCT. Erosion of positive feelings between the partners and relationship disengagement often follow from prolonged distress. Low levels of emotional affection, such as little tenderness or low frequency of sex, predict poor response to BCT and IOCT (Hahlweg et al., 1984; Jacobson & Addis, 1993; Snyder et al., 1993). Active consideration of separation also is predictive of poorer response to couple therapy (Weiss & Heyman, 1997).

Among couples that present for therapy, long-term negative effects of relationship distress often are evident in deteriorating individual functioning (Bloom, 1985). For example, alcohol abuse and depression are common in partners seeking couple therapy, as are behavior problems in the couple's children (Halford & Markman, 1997). These individual problems predict poor response to couple therapy (Jacobson & Addis, 1993; Snyder et al., 1993).

High initial valuing of intimacy in relationships, particularly by the male partners, is predictive of a stronger response to couple therapy. Male partners who report high needs for affiliation and closeness, and who exhibit more feminine gender role behaviors of valuing relationships, show the greatest gains from BCT, EFT, and IOCT (Baucom & Aiken, 1984; Johnson & Talitman, 1997; Snyder et al., 1993). Women having high affiliation and relationship needs show a modest association with therapy outcome for BCT and IOCT (Baucom & Aiken, 1984; Snyder et al., 1993) but no association with outcome in EFT (Johnson & Talitman, 1997). In couples in which the female is high on affiliation and the male is high on autonomy, the couple tends to respond more poorly to BCT (Jacobson et al., 1986). In other words, if the couple hold traditional gender roles in which the woman seeks high affiliation and the male does not, couple therapy seems to be less effective.

A strong therapeutic relationship predicts better response to couple therapy. Specifically, when the therapist and partner rate the relationship as positive, and the therapist is perceived as warm and expert, there are stronger effects of BCT and EFT (Holtzworth-Munroe, Jacobson, DeKlyn, & Whisman, 1989; Johnson & Talitman, 1997).

In summary, existing approaches to couple therapy are most efficacious for couples that have less severe distress and that retain positive affect between the partners. This suggests that early intervention in distress is desirable so that the negative impact of prolonged distress does not erode relationship positivity. Second, the impact of therapy has more efficacy with partners who value relationships characterized by emotional closeness and flexibility in gender roles. Addressing these issues more directly than is typical of current couple therapy approaches might enhance efficacy of couple therapy. Finally, a warm therapeutic relationship with the partners predicts better outcome.

Effectiveness of Couple Therapy

Psychotherapy research draws an important distinction between efficacy and effectiveness. *Efficacy* refers to the empirical status of psychological treatments as they are evaluated in research, most commonly within controlled trials. *Effectiveness* refers to the impact of psychological treatments on clients who present to routine treatment services. Although there is a lot known about the efficacy of couple therapy, much less is known about its effectiveness (Halford, 1997). There are a number of reasons to suspect that the efficacy research reviewed previously does not provide a clear picture of the effectiveness of couple therapy in routine service delivery.

Almost all couple therapy efficacy research is conducted within universities. Usually therapists are highly trained in the specific treatments being evaluated and deliver the therapy in those research settings. Couple therapy delivery in research settings usually is delivered following written treatment manuals, with predefined content being covered in sessions, and with a set number of therapy sessions of treatment. In addition, the delivery of therapy often is individually supervised and carefully monitored. For example, in many efficacy studies couple therapy sessions are videotaped and subsequently coded for their adherence to treatment protocols. Moreover, the clients in research settings must agree to the conditions of research. For example, clients usually must agree to be randomly assigned to therapy conditions, to attend sessions (both partners) from the beginning of therapy, and for sessions to be recorded. In efficacy research, the assessment of clients is extensive, and clients have to agree to this assessment before entering the study. Finally, often the clients of the therapy conducted within research settings are restricted to those with particular defined characteristics, such as only one presenting disorder of relationship distress and no comorbid conditions. Each of these characteristics of efficacy studies is intended to maximize the internal validity of the research, allowing demonstration that the couple therapy produces observed clinical change. At the same time, these characteristics may limit the generalizability of research efficacy findings to effectiveness in routine service delivery.

In most service settings the training of the couple therapists delivering psychological treatments rarely is standardized in the manner typical of research settings. The content and duration of couple therapy often are highly variable, and frequently are determined by negotiation between therapist and client. Routine checks of the content or process of therapy delivery are rare.

Moreover, the means by which clients present to treatment agencies, the presenting problems of clients, and the existence of comorbid problems probably make the clients in service delivery settings substantially different from the clients in research settings.

Couple therapists in routine service delivery seem only marginally influenced by published research in the approach they take to therapy (Halford, 1997). While BCT, EFT, IOCT, and SRCT are the approaches with some empirical evidence supporting their efficacy, most practicing couple therapists do not espouse these approaches as their preferred mode of couple therapy (Boughner, Hayes, Bubenzer, & West, 1994; Hahlweg & Klan, 1997; Wolcott & Glazer, 1989). Moreover, while all couple therapies with empirical support involve use of a wide range of systematic assessments including interview, self-report inventories, self-monitoring, and behavioral observation, most couple therapists in routine service delivery rely exclusively on unstructured clinical interviews to assess couple relationships (Boughner et al., 1994). Given the evidence of the impact of assessment, feedback, and goal setting on relationship satisfaction, the absence of wide-ranging, systematic assessment is likely to undermine the effectiveness of couple therapy.

Hahlweg and Klan (1997) evaluated the effectiveness of couple therapy in routine clinical service in Germany and Austria. Only 50% of couples agreeing to participate in the study provided posttherapy assessment data. For those who did provide data, there was a small to moderate mean effect size on relationship distress of 0.37. Moreover, only 20% of clients who provided data were in the nondistressed range on relationship satisfaction after therapy. Given that people declining to provide data in outcome studies are generally believed to have an overrepresentation of people with poor outcomes, these data probably overstate the effectiveness of couple therapy. The estimated effect size of 0.37 reported by Hahlweg and Klan (1997) is substantially smaller than the effect sizes reported in meta-analyses of couple therapy efficacy studies (e.g., Hahlweg & Markman, 1988—effect size = 0.90; Shadish et al., 1993—effect size = 0.60).

An important index of the value of couple therapy is the satisfaction of clients with the service they receive in that therapy. *Consumer Reports* has its readers complete a survey every year. In one of its surveys the magazine asked about satisfaction with psychotherapy, including couple therapy (Seligman, 1995). As it is a voluntary survey, the representativeness of the respondents is questionable. However, the study does provide the largest sample size survey of consumer perspectives on couple therapy. The results were positive in terms of the effects of psychotherapy from the consumers' point of view. However, consumers expressed less satisfaction with couple therapy than with any other form of therapy. When one thinks about the goals of couple therapy, it makes sense that there is less satisfaction from the consumers' point of view. Often partners use couple therapy as a way of exiting the relationship. In a survey conducted in Colorado (Stanley, Lobitz, & Markman, 1989), couple therapists reported that about one-third of the relationships they saw in practice ended in separation or divorce. Interestingly, the therapists rated 80% of the therapy in which the relationships ended in divorce as successful, presumably on the grounds that people achieved goals such as reaching a considered decision to end the relationship, negotiating a low-conflict separation, or improvement in individual partner outcomes. Consumer satisfaction with couple therapy may be low because people expect therapy to lead to relationship reconciliation and improvement and do not see other positive outcomes as valuable.

Aside from which therapy is delivered and how it is delivered, effectiveness also is influenced by the proportion of individuals with psychological problems who will seek and remain in the treatment offered. In the United States, about 14% of the adult population have ever sought any form of relationship counseling (Gallup, 1996). It is unclear what proportion of people have ever had relationship problems, but given that 40% of currently married individuals report that they have considered separation from their current spouse at some time (Gallup, 1996), it is clear that the majority of people who have relationship problems do not seek professional assistance. In Australia, less than 10% of couples who divorce ever seek couple therapy or counseling (Wolcott & Glazer, 1989). Thus, if we are to increase the effectiveness of couple therapy it must be more accessible to people with relationship problems.

Conclusions

There is strong evidence that BCT has efficacy within controlled trials, and that it is a powerful treatment, at least in the short term. EFT also is a well-replicated efficacious treatment. SRCT and IOCT have empirical evidence supporting their efficacy. However, there is insufficient evidence to draw conclusions about the relative efficacy of these different couple therapy approaches. The mechanisms of change in couple therapy are not well elucidated but probably are not the mechanisms proposed by the proponents of CBT, EFT, or IOCT. The processes of assessment, feedback, and goal setting are common to all empirically supported couple therapies and probably contribute significantly to the efficacy of these approaches. In routine service delivery when assessment and goal setting often are absent, the observed effect sizes of couple therapy are small.

Brief forms of couple therapy rarely have been seriously considered in the couple therapy literature. Most written descriptions of couple therapy include large numbers of conjoint sessions, typically anywhere from 12 to 30 sessions of therapy. Implicit in these descriptions seems to be an assumption that any form of change of significant relationship problems will take a protracted period of time, and sizable input from an expert therapist. However, as noted previously, there is considerable evidence that relationship functioning changes after assessment and goal setting with little or no additional therapist input, at least at times. Two independent studies found positive effects of three sessions of brief couple therapy on relationship satisfaction (Halford et al., 1996; Worthington et al., 1995). In two national surveys of couple therapy in routine practice in Australia and Germany the mean number of sessions attended was low relative to the number of session reported in efficacy studies (Hahlweg & Klan, 1997; Wolcott & Glazer, 1989). The number of sessions attended was unrelated to the satisfaction with the service or the magnitude of change in relationship satisfaction (Hahlweg & Klan, 1997; Wolcott & Glazer, 1989).

All this evidence has led me to believe that traditional couple therapies are a good beginning to helping couples, but that a new model of couple therapy is needed. Moreover, much of the evidence converges on the point that brief couple therapy does work for some couples. I am not asserting that brief therapy can be effective for all distressed couples, only that brief therapy is effective for some distressed couples. A cost-effective approach to couple therapy provides brief therapy to couples who can benefit from this approach and offers more extended courses of therapy only to those couples who will not benefit from brief therapy. In Chapter 3, I spell out a self-regulatory couple therapy model that elaborates on a framework for providing couple therapy that is only as extended as is really required.

3

Self-Regulatory Couple Therapy

Self-regulatory couple therapy (SRCT) is both an extension of cognitive-behavioral couple therapy (CBCT) and an attempt to provide an integrating framework for applying other empirically supported couple therapies. Like CBCT, the procedures used in SRCT are developed from the substantial data on the determinants of relationship problems. That is, SRCT is aimed at changing patterns of behavior, cognition, and affect (couple adaptive processes) that are well established as associated with relationship distress. However, the emphasis in SRCT is on promoting metacompetencies for self-change. Once these metacompetencies are acquired, partners have the skills to change their adaptive processes within the relationship.

SRCT is intended to be brief couple therapy. Partners receive as few sessions of therapy as allows them to achieve their self-selected relationship goals. If partners struggle, then procedures developed within cognitive-behavioral, emotion-focused, and insight-oriented therapies are adapted to assist partners to produce self-directed change.

Self-Regulation and Couple Therapy

Concept of Self-Regulation

The terms "self-regulation," "self-control," "self-management," and "self-guidance" have been used extensively, and sometimes interchangeably, in the psychological literature to describe a process of self-directed change. Kanfer and colleagues (Kanfer, 1970; Kanfer & Karoly, 1972; Karoly, 1993) first

42

used a behavioral analysis to explain how individuals exercise control over their own behavior and then introduced these concepts into behavior therapy. In a comprehensive review of the research on self-regulation, Karoly (1993) highlights how self-regulatory concepts have pervaded many diverse areas of contemporary psychological inquiry, including personality theory, motivation and emotion, social, developmental, and health psychology, to name a few. Although there are clearly several alternative conceptual frameworks used to interpret and understand self-regulatory phenomena, much of the research into the component processes has been dominated by cognitive social learning theories (Bandura, 1977, 1986), operant theory, and control (cybernetics) frameworks (Karoly, 1993). For the purpose of the present discussion, the definition of self-regulation provided by Karoly is useful.

> Self-regulation refers to those processes, internal and or transactional, that enable an individual to guide his/her goal directed activities over time and across changing circumstances (contexts). Regulation implies modulation of thought, affect, behavior, or attention via deliberate or automated use of specific mechanisms and supportive metaskills. The processes of self-regulation are initiated when routinized activity is impeded or when goal directedness is otherwise made salient (e.g., the appearance of a challenge, the failure of habitual patterns; etc.). . . . (p. 25)

This definition emphasizes that self-regulatory processes are embedded in a social context that not only provides opportunities and limitations for individual self-direction but implies a dynamic reciprocal interchange between the internal and external determinants of human motivation. From a therapeutic perspective, self-regulation is a process whereby individuals are taught skills to modify their own behavior. There have been several comprehensive formulations of self-control phenomena and the role of self-generated events in the regulation of human behavior (Bandura, 1977, 1986; Catania, 1975; Karoly, 1993; Mahoney & Thoreson, 1974; Skinner, 1953). Although several self-control theorists acknowledge the interdependent nature of self-generated and externally imposed influences on behavior, the assumption that individuals can regulate their own behavior remains central to the overall conceptualization of self-regulatory processes.

A key characteristic of SRCT is an emphasis on a process that empowers individuals to change their relationship. Let me explain how this emphasis is similar to, but also substantially different from, the traditional CBCT approach to process. Descriptions of traditional CBCT emphasize that assessment serves multiple purposes (e.g., Baucom & Epstein, 1990; Beach, Sandeen, & O'Leary, 1990). For example, assessment goals include identifying and measuring the problem behaviors, establishing the environmental controlling variables, selecting intervention strategies, developing a therapeutic relationship with the client, and developing a conceptualization of the problem that is acceptable to the client and that promotes therapeutic change. A particular challenge in couple therapy, relative to individual therapy, is that the assessment process needs to achieve these assessment goals with both partners.

Within traditional behavioral couple therapy (BCT) assessment, typically there is an attempt to refocus each partner from reporting on dissatisfactions with his or her partner toward a more dyadic collaborative conceptualization of his or her problems. For example, if one person wants an increase in the amount of time that the couple spend together while the other partner requests a decrease, this issue could be phrased as follows: "The two of you have not yet achieved a mutually acceptable agreement about how much time you spend together." This formulation prompts both partners to attend to mutually acceptable goals and helps the therapist select therapeutic interventions relevant to the couple. The therapy goal in this case might be to develop the communication and problem-solving skills believed necessary to formulate a mutually acceptable agreement. Although this dyadic conceptualization may encourage the partners to think of their relationship problem in a more collaborative and less blaming manner, it fails to help either individual identify what to do to produce change. Implicitly the clients must wait on the therapist to conjointly teach them new ways to interact.

In the self-regulation approach, a dyadic problem formulation may still be used, but it would be followed by each partner self-selecting behavior change goals for him- or herself. For example, if the agreed problem was difficulty in communication about time spent together, a partner may decide that his current methods of communicating about concerns needed to be changed. A second possibility is that the manner in which the concerns of the partner are listened to needs changing. An important characteristic of the self-regulation approach is that the development of the skills to self-appraise one's relationship behaviors and to select and implement self-change is the explicit goal of therapy. Construing relationship problems in a dyadic manner can be an intermediate step in achieving this goal, but goals for personal change are the ultimate objective. These personal goals may include altering how one attempts to influence one's partner. Thus the partner's behavior is not ignored, but the emphasis remains on what the individual can do about aspects of the relationship that are distressing.

In emphasizing partner self-regulation, I am not advocating that the therapist passively accept whatever goals the client may generate. If a client stated that he or she would avoid any discussion of a difficult topic as a self-selected goal, this strategy might be self-evaluated as successful if it reduced immediate conflict. However, I highlight that the long-term consequences of avoiding conflict topics are likely to be continuing dissatisfaction and a deteriorating relationship and encourage a self-selected goal which achieved better long-term outcome. In other words, self-regulatory processes such as self-selection of goals and realistic self-evaluation of the effects of behavior are skills the therapist helps the client develop across the course of therapy.

SRCT is focused on self-regulation for two reasons. First, most distressed partners inaccurately attribute most or all of their relationship problems to their partner's negative behavior (Bradbury & Fincham, 1990; Fincham & Bradbury, 1992). As they have no direct control over their partner's behavior, this often leads partners to feel powerless to produce any change in a distressed relationship (Vanzetti et al., 1992). The focus of SRCT on self-change empowers the partners to do something constructive about their relationship. Second, the focus on self-regulation promotes metacompetencies that not only allow the partners to change the interactions that are current relationship problems but also help them to produce self-change, which enhances the relationship in the future.

The Metacompetencies for Self-Regulation of Relationships

Self-regulation within the context of relationships refers to partners engaging in self-change processes to enhance their relationship satisfaction and stability. Self-regulation can be thought of as a set of metacompetencies that allow effective self-change. Table 3.1 summarizes the metacompetencies needed for relationship self-regulation (Halford et al., 1994). They are self-appraisal, self-directed goal setting, self-implementation of change, and evaluation of change efforts.

SELF-APPRAISAL

Self-appraisal of relationship functioning involves being able to articulate current relationship functioning, and the major influences on that functioning, in a manner that facilitates relationship enhancement. In practice, that means being able to analyze the relationship adaptive processes in terms of both the helpful cognitions, affect, and behavior one is doing and what is unhelpful. It also means being able to identify stressful events, personal vulnerabilities, and contextual variables that influence relationship adaptive processes. Examples of poor relationship self-appraisal are the common pattern of distressed partners focusing on partner-blaming attributions for relationship problems and ignoring the impact of contextual factors and life events on couple adaptive processes. The assessment process in SRCT is designed to facilitate self-appraisal in the couple.

The following is a concrete example of effective and ineffective relationship self-appraisal. Grace and Mick undertook *in vitro* fertilization in an attempt to overcome long-standing problems in fertility. The recurrent visits to the medical system, the need for Mick to provide sperm samples for fertiliza-

TABLE 3.1. Self-Regulation Metacompetencies

Metacompetency	Definition	Example
Self-appraisal	To accurately define key strengths and weaknesses of own behavior, and of interactions with spouse, in specific instances. To describe contextual factors, key stressful events and individual vulnerabilities which may lead to the development of current patterns of own and partner's behavior without blame or hostility.	After an argument with the spouse the partners identify the pattern of interaction that occurred and identify behaviors, thoughts, and actions of their own which were helpful and unhelpful in the interaction.
Self-directed goal setting	Individual defines specific actions he or she can take which can enhance relationship functioning.	Individual identifies specific behaviors or thoughts which he or she will attempt to use in managing the conflict in the future (e.g., person might resolve to attempt better conflict management by restarting conversation but stating desire to hear partner's perspective, to listen more effectively by not interrupting, asking open questions, and to focus on thought "I need to hear my partner's perspective.")
Self-change	Individual describes and then carries out specific plan to enact self-selected goals.	Individual resolves to initiate discussion at appropriate time and then carries through with intention.
Self-evaluation of change efforts	Individual self-appraises the extent to which the desired changes were actually implemented, and appraises the functional impact of those changes that did occur.	Individual evaluates correctly that she or he did start discussion as planned, asked open questions, but then interrupted partner during discussion. Notes that discussion began well but deteriorated to anger again.

tion attempts on just a few hours' notice at the optimal ovulation time, and the repeated waits to see if Grace became pregnant were taking their toll on the couple. When they presented to me they were considering separation, they had not had sex together for months, and both were overwhelmed by the stress of the attempts to become pregnant. Both partners gave vague descriptions of the relationship problems in terms of "arguing lots, and just not getting on anymore" and attributed these relationship problems primarily to their partner.

The initial phase in therapy was helping them (1) to identify the current thoughts, feelings, and actions of each partner, and their patterns of interaction; (2) to analyze how these had changed in the last few years; and (3) to identify what was helpful and unhelpful. At the point of presentation the couple were so stressed they could not do this self-appraisal. After two sessions of assessment they were able to articulate the behaviors, thoughts, and feelings that were problems, and they began to view their problems as an outgrowth of a complex of factors. These factors included long-standing difficulties with conflict management, the stress of the *in vitro* fertilization process, Grace's inability to imagine life without being a mother, and Mick's inability to respond constructively to women who were highly distressed.

SELF-DIRECTED GOAL SETTING

Self-directed goal setting is the process of defining specific, actionable goals for change in oneself, based on the self-appraisal of relationship functioning. The revised appraisals of Mick and Grace allowed them to consider goals for self-directed change. For example, Grace defined a goal of changing her thoughts and feelings so that if having a child proved not to be possible for them, she could still have a positive relationship with Mick. Mick defined improving his ability to support Grace when she was upset as a key skill he needed to learn.

SELF-IMPLEMENTATION OF CHANGE

Self-implementation of change is the process of each partner taking active steps with the aim of changing future adaptive processes. For example, Grace resolved to read a book on the effects of cognitions on feelings and to attempt to apply these ideas to her current feelings about the possibility of not being able to have children. Mick resolved to have a series of conversations with Grace about the *in vitro* fertilization process and how upsetting she found the process. He also resolved to ask Grace for feedback on what he did that she found supportive.

SELF-EVALUATION

Self-evaluation is the process by which the individual appraises the extent to which the desired behavior change was achieved and then the extent to which that change produced the desired relationship changes. In Grace's case she did buy the book and read it. She said the ideas made sense to her, and she applied an idea in the book called rational self-analysis, which involved writing down her negative thoughts about not being a mother. Grace found identifying and reflecting on these negative thoughts upsetting, and then she became discouraged and did not complete the process of self-change. The therapist reviewed her attempts at self-change and noted how Grace had successfully identified negative thoughts but had not proceeded to identify or apply positive coping thoughts. Based on this discussion Grace's evaluation was that she had made significant progress but still needed to complete the rational self-analysis process to evaluate if it would help her. Thus, in each step the partners are prompted to develop self-regulatory skills to self-direct relationship change.

Structure of Self-Regulatory Couple Therapy

In the self-regulation approach to couple therapy a typical course of therapy can range from only 1 or 2 to as many as 20 conjoint sessions. SRCT is structured hierarchically so that partners receive the smallest number of sessions of therapy necessary to produce the desired relationship changes. Table 3.2 summarizes the typical content of SRCT at three different levels of intervention: brief self-guided change consisting of 1 to 6 sessions, relationship psychoeducation and self-guided change consisting of 7 to 10 sessions, and therapist-guided change consisting of 11 to 25 sessions.

Brief Self-Change

Minimizing the number of therapy sessions is achieved by focusing therapy initially on developing partners' self-regulation metacompetencies of relationship appraisal and goal setting. The processes of assessment and structured feedback are attempts to promote adaptive relationship appraisal and goal setting (Chapters 4 to 6 describe in detail how to do this). The assessment process is a structured, interactive examination of the key factors discussed in Chapter 1 that influence a couple's relationship. This form of assessment plus collaborative goal setting are key steps in promoting self-regulatory change. The process of assessment described in Chapters 4 and 5 is intended to prompt and reinforce each partner's attempts to appraise the context, life events, and adaptive processes in the relationship. Ultimately this is intended to promote a functional self-appraisal of the relationship. By functional I mean an appraisal that effectively guides self-directed change. After completion of assessment, the therapist uses a collaborative process of sharing assessment results to help each partner develop a functional self-appraisal of the relationship, define self-change goals, and develop self-change strategies. Chapters 5, 6, and 7 describe the process of feedback and negotiation.

I believe that commitment to self-change is necessary to achieve relationship improvements in distressed couples, and for many distressed couples this

TABLE 3.2. Structure of Self-Regulatory Couple Therapy

Structure of couple therapy	Stage	Tasks
Brief self-change (1–6 sessions)	Engagement (Chapter 4).	Building empathy with individual partners; identifying immediate threats to individual or relationship; building positive therapeutic expectations.
	Assessment (Chapters 4–5).	Building shared understanding of relationship problems to facilitate change; assessing individual vulnerabilities and problems; evaluating feasibility of couple therapy.
	Feedback and negotiation of goals (Chapter 6).	Providing structured feedback of assessment; negotiating working model of relationships; identifying shared couple goals.
	Evaluating possibility of brief self-change (Chapter 7).	Assessing self-change competencies.
	Supporting self-change (Chapter 8).	Evaluating self-change outcomes; promoting generalization and maintenance.
Relationship psychoeducation plus self-change (7–10 sessions)	As for brief self-change: engagement, assessment, feedback and negotiation of goals, evaluating possibility of brief self-change.	As for brief self-change.
	Relationship psychoeducation (Chapter 8).	Interactive relationship psychoeducation; assessing self-change competencies.
	Reevaluating possibility of self-change.	Testing self-directed change outcomes.
	Supporting self-change.	Evaluating self-change outcomes; promoting generalization and maintenance.
Therapist-guided change (11–25 sessions)	As for brief self-change: engagement, assessment, feedback and negotiation of goals, evaluating possibility of brief self-change.	As for brief self-change.

(continued)

TABLE 3.2. (*continued*)

Structure of couple therapy	Stage	Tasks
	Behavior exchange (Chapter 9).	Self-directed change of key relationship behaviors.
	Cognitive change (Chapter 9).	Rational self-analysis; cognitive restructuring.
	Intimacy (Chapter 9).	Intimate communication; shared positive activities.
	Support (Chapter 9).	Emotional support; practical support.
	Conflict management (Chapter 9).	Communication skills; patterns of conflict management.
	Supporting self-change.	Evaluating self-change outcomes; promoting generalization and maintenance.

commitment is necessary and sufficient to achieve relationship improvement. For those couples for whom commitment to self-change goals is necessary and sufficient for relationship improvement, brief couple therapy of three to four sessions can be effective. For other couples more extended courses of therapy sessions may be necessary. If couples produce the desired changes in their relationship at this point (Chapter 6 describes in detail how to assess this), this may be all the therapy required. This is brief self-guided change and most often takes three to six sessions.

Relationship Psychoeducation and Self-Change

Therapy includes relationship psychoeducation if couples are unable to self-appraise their relationship or to define self-change goals. Relationship psychoeducation assists couples in exploring themes in their key relationship adaptive processes and how individual characteristics, context, and life events might influence those processes. The goal is to facilitate more effective self-appraisal and goal setting.

In using the term "relationship psychoeducation" I am not suggesting that the therapist give the couple extensive didactic lectures about research on couple relationships. Rather, relationship psychoeducation uses such processes as guided discovery, cognitive-affect reconstruction, and guided reading with discussion. (Chapter 8 describes each of these processes). For example, I routinely explore with couples issues such as the work–family interface, the impact of interactions with extended family, and family-of-origin and cultural influences on the development of expectations and behavior in relationships as a means of helping couples appraise their relationship difficulties in a more helpful manner.

A key notion in relationship psychoeducation is that partners' inability to implement self-change reflects one of two problems. One problem is that strong negative thoughts and feelings interfere with self-change. For example, some couples agree that reducing conflict is a desired relationship goal but find that they repeatedly escalate into destructive arguments about key issues. In this instance relationship psychoeducation focuses specifically on exploration of these negative thoughts and feelings in an attempt to help the couple understand their negative responses to each other, move away from partner blaming, and then to move toward self-change. A second problem is that the partners lack knowledge of what constitutes really helpful self-change to address their relationship goals. For example, in stepfamilies many partners agree that developing a good stepparent–child relationship is important but are unsure what are reasonable expectations for such a relationship.

The aim of relationship psychoeducation is to help the partners develop the thoughts, feelings, and knowledge that enable them to operationalize how they will self-implement their desired relationship goals. Once this is achieved, often the couple are then able to self-change. (Chapter 8 describes in detail the nature and content of relationship psychoeducation.) Typically, relationship psychoeducation occurs after the feedback and negotiation session and consists of three or four sessions. The couple would then attempt self-change, as described in Chapter 7, or if self-change looked unlikely, the couple would be offered therapist-guided change. A typical course of relationship psychoeducation plus self-change would last from 7 to 10 sessions.

Therapist-Guided Change and Self-Change

If, after relationship psychoeducation, the partners still are unable to produce the desired relationship changes, then therapist-guided change is used. The assumption in therapist-guided change is that the partners have either never learned or have forgotten important skills of couple interaction. In therapist-guided change selections of procedures are used from empirically supported couple therapies, particularly BCT. As in BCT, the goal in therapist-guided SRCT is to help partners develop skills that enhance the relationship. But in SRCT, procedures are adapted to a self-regulatory framework. For example, in the self-regulatory adaptation of behavior exchange, partners self-identify goals for change that they believe will enhance the relationship. The focus on self-defined change goals has two effects. First, self-direction promotes a sense of self-efficacy in being able to produce change. Second, the process promotes individual responsibility for the enhancement of the relationship. (Chapter 9 describes the procedures most often used in extended SRCT.) They are procedures for increasing positive day-to-day interactions, better communication, conflict management, and changing negative thoughts and feelings. Chapter 9 includes a number of specific exercises and handouts for teaching these skills.

Once the couple has developed the necessary relationship skills using therapist-guided change, the process reverts to self-change. Typically a course of SRCT that involves relationship psychoeducation, therapist-guided self-change, and self-change consists of 11 to 20 sessions. The first three to four sessions are assessment, feedback, and negotiation of goals; the next three or four sessions are devoted to relationship psychoeducation; then comes a series of sessions of therapist-guided change, culminating in a final few sessions of self-change.

For clarity of exposition, the different levels of intervention within SRCT are presented as if they are quite different. In practice, these levels of intervention form a continuum of increasing numbers of sessions and increasing therapist guidance in helping couples define and achieve their relationship goals. The ultimate goal in SRCT is to help partners to self-regulate their relationships. Some couples can move straight to self-change after assessment. Other couples need relationship psychoeducation or therapist-guided change, but for them therapy eventually shifts to promotion of self-change, as illustrated in Figure 3.1. Once the couple is successfully implementing self-change, the final step in therapy is promoting the generalization and maintenance of that self-change process.

At each level of intervention in SRCT, sessions usually occur at least weekly at the beginning of therapy and often become less frequent toward the end of therapy. The initial session establishes contact with the couple and determines whether therapy is an appropriate response to the couple's problems. A further one or two sessions usually are occupied by assessment. Assessment most often consists of a combination of interview, completion, and review of self-report and self-monitoring instruments and completion of interaction tasks. Next the therapist provides feedback of the assessment results to the couple and negotiates their relationship goals. The therapist then negotiates the structure of therapy to be used: self-change, relationship psychoeducation or therapist-guided change. In essence the therapist helps the couple test their capacity to self-change at that point. Relationship psychoeducation and therapist-guided SRCT are used only if self-change is not sufficient to achieve relationship goals.

Throughout the course of therapy, beginning with the first assessment session, couples are asked to complete various tasks between sessions. The essence of therapy is to help partners to alter their adaptive processes outside the therapy sessions, in the settings in which they usually interact such as at home, at friends' places, and so forth. To that end what happens in the therapy session is relevant only to the extent that it facilitates such change. Therefore the

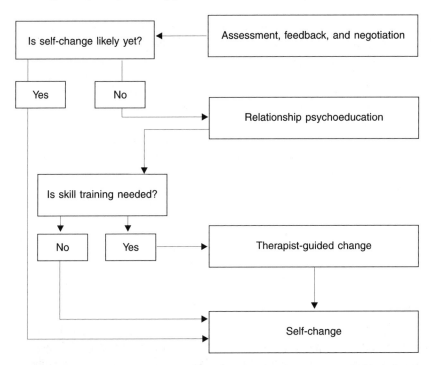

FIGURE 3.1. The decision-making process in negotiating the structure of self-regulatory couple therapy.

tasks undertaken between sessions are what are important in therapy. Therapeutic tasks in SRCT initially are related to assessment of problems (e.g., completion of questionnaires or self-monitoring forms). During therapy tasks are developed collaboratively by the therapist and clients as a means of the partners experimenting with new ways of responding to each other.

The Process of Self-Regulatory Couple Therapy: Making It Succeed

Couple therapy is effective to the extent that the partners are able to identify, implement, and sustain changes that enhance their relationship. But, there are a variety of potential barriers to achieving effective couple therapy. In this section I want to address how to structure therapeutic process to maximize the chance of making couple therapy effective. I use the concept of therapeutic momentum to describe how to establish and maintain change in couple therapy.

Therapeutic momentum is the rate and the strength of change processes occurring both within and between therapy sessions. High momentum is characterized by a high level of energy and involvement in therapeutic process and tasks by the partners and high levels of personal initiative being shown in generating positive change between sessions. Low therapeutic momentum is characterized by lack of engagement, anger, and hostility in therapy sessions; low levels of therapeutic effort; and failure to engage in tasks between sessions.

A number of the client behaviors I describe as low therapeutic momentum are similar to behaviors referred to as resistance or low adherence by other writers. I dislike the notions of resistance or adherence; to me these terms imply that the therapist drives the change process. Implicitly, the terms "resistance" and "nonadherence" attribute slow therapeutic progress to whether the client did as the therapist suggested. As I view couple therapy predominantly as driven by the self-change efforts of the partners, I think adherence and resistance are inappropriate constructs for considering the therapeutic process.

Establishing Therapeutic Momentum

Establishing therapeutic momentum is, in my opinion, important at the beginning of any therapy. It is particularly important in couple therapy. Many partners in distressed relationships present feeling discouraged about attempting to alter their relationship. Frequently, the long periods of relationship distress prior to presentation have left one or both partners ambivalent about whether to remain in the relationship and possibly skeptical about the possibility of relationship change. Early in couple therapy it is necessary to establish a sense of reasonable optimism about the possibility of positive change.

What might establish reasonable optimism at the beginning of couple therapy? First and foremost I believe each partner needs to feel understood in terms of the pain and suffering he or she is experiencing in the relationship. Typically in distressed relationships partners invalidate each other's experiences and partners rarely feel understood. In the initial interview structure described in Chapter 4, the therapist meets with each partner individually. This allows the therapist to join with each partner and then synthesize the two partners' individual experiences into a coherent whole.

In writings and workshops on couple therapy I have attended, I have heard therapists advocate the benefits of having only conjoint sessions. Those same couple therapists also describe a variety of strategies they use to help partners to relate their relationship pain in the presence of their spouse. A high degree of structure and effort seem necessary to avoid the expressions of individual hurt and anguish leading to destructive conflict in these initial conjoint sessions. Often the therapist is busy stopping partners' cross-talking or interrupting each other, or reframing and doing all sorts of verbal gymnastics to keep the couple on task. Conjoint sessions in which there is a high degree of therapist structuring can make it difficult to establish empathy and intimate personal contact between therapist and client. I find it easier to get to know someone intimately on a one-to-one basis. I find it much easier to empathize with complaints, hurt, and pain about the spouse if the spouse is not present at the time. Then I can focus on understanding the person's message to me, and I do not constantly have to play traffic cop to prevent the sessions from becoming acrimonious or unproductive.

SUMMARIZING CONCERNS IN A WAY ACCEPTABLE TO BOTH PARTNERS

Ultimately, one goal of couple therapy is to build a consensus about the nature of the relationship problems and their potential solutions. With the foundation of some understanding of each individual, I then bring the couple together and summarize the key things that each of them has told me. In Chapters 4, 5, and 6 I describe how these summaries reframe the individual concerns and complaints, complaints that usually are about the partner, in terms of relational processes. This reframing process makes the anguish of the partners accessible to each other.

To establish a personal, empathic relationship with each partner and to summarize the couple's major presenting concerns in a manner acceptable to each partner builds a major platform for therapeutic momentum. If the first therapy session allows the couple to express their concerns and pain without destructive conflict, this is a major achievement for many couples. For most distressed couples prior attempts to address their relationship problems only lead to pain, more hurt, and frustration. Avoidance often becomes a key means by which the couple deals with relationship pain. If the initial therapy session is full of anger, hurt, and pain, then the couple may seek to avoid any further such sessions, or at least to avoid raising the most difficult and painful relationship problems. If the initial therapy session gives them a sense that the issues can be raised without severe pain, their willingness to engage in therapy is likely to increase.

OFFER EVIDENCE FOR HOPE

Based on my established understanding of their feelings, often I can describe how one or both partners may feel discouraged and identify their sense of powerlessness to produce change. I then can offer research-based evidence for hope. Based on the research reviewed in Chapter 2, I state how many couples enter couple therapy feeling discouraged and ambivalent about the relationship, but that 80% or more of couples report significant improvement in their relationship across the course of couple therapy. Even those couples that do not report any relationship improvement often make an informed decision to leave the relationship, and many couples are able to negotiate low-conflict separations. In my experience, when these facts are presented by a therapist who relates this information to the couple in a personal manner, they become a powerful instigator of hope.

ENGAGE THE PARTNERS IN ACTION

I almost always give couples tasks to do between the first and the second therapy sessions. I do this for multiple reasons. One reason is to increase the efficiency of information gathering during the assessment phase. Another reason is that I wish to give the partners a sense that they can do something to shift the problems that until now they found intractable. I state the importance of the tasks, and I urge the partners to tell me if any task I suggest does not seem reasonable or useful. I check, by specifically asking each partner, whether he or she will complete the task(s) before the next session. In drawing out the partners' commitment to undertaking these tasks I am keen to develop their sense of excitement about the possibility of change.

In the second session I always follow up on the tasks that the partners agreed to do between sessions. Most people do the tasks, and I make a point of praising their commitment. To me the effort people expend, despite their often having a history of feeling powerless in their relationship, is an important sign of developing therapeutic momentum, and I point this out to the couple. Completing a few questionnaires between sessions rarely solves a 20-year relationship problem, but the couple's effort can be an important start to the change process.

The first two, or sometimes three, sessions are assessment sessions which build toward the feedback and goal-setting session. Across these sessions I typically spend an increasing proportion of the sessions with the couple conjointly. I adjust the proportion of time spent in individual versus conjoint sessions according to the extent to which the sessions allow exploration of difficult relationship issues in a constructive manner. I am keen to establish in each partner a view of therapy sessions as a safe environment in which risks can be taken in order to relate in a more intimate manner. As the partners experience, often for the first time for years, an ability to understand something about their relationship, an appreciation of the spouse's perspective, and a feeling of being understood, I find that positive expectations develop.

Maintaining Therapeutic Momentum

If assessment proceeds well and the couple have a shared understanding of the key relationship issues, then the possibility of brief self-change therapy needs to be considered. I probe the partners to establish the extent to which each can identify personal change goals relevant to achieving the desired therapy goals. (Chapter 6 describes details of this process.) If the partners do have clear self-change goals, and therapeutic momentum is high, I discuss the option of brief self-change therapy with the couple. Usually this means giving the couple a break of an agreed period between sessions to establish the extent to which partners can successfully implement their desired self-change goals.

If brief self-change is not appropriate, then brief therapy involving relationship psychoeducation may be appropriate, or therapist-guided couple therapy may be the treatment of choice. In SRCT, even if positive therapeutic momentum initially is established, maintaining that momentum across the course of couple therapy remains a challenge. Many couples experience setbacks across the course of therapy. Sustaining a positive self-change focus requires careful attention to process by the therapist. There are three important broad strategies of momentum maintenance: matching therapy process to partner affect, matching the sequence of therapy content to couple needs, and reviewing and highlighting therapeutic gains.

MATCHING PROCESS TO PARTNER AFFECT

Maximizing therapeutic momentum involves matching the therapeutic process in session to the affective states of the partners. For example, rational problem solving rarely works when one or both partners are really angry with each other. Rational problem solving requires a degree of acceptance of the perceptions of the problem by the partner and only moderate arousal of negative affect. Similarly, asking partners to expose their vulnerabilities to each other when one or both partners are feeling misunderstood by the therapist also is unlikely to work. Partners need to feel positive toward the therapist for this process to be effective. In both the foregoing examples, I would try to establish strong empathy with each partner before moving to rational problem solving or self-disclosure of vulnerabilities in the presence of the partner.

The therapist needs constantly to monitor the affective expression of the partners. In couple sessions this means constantly visually scanning the faces of both partners. It also means that if the therapist is speaking primarily with one partner, the therapist must monitor the reactions of the other partner. If the nonspeaking spouse is withdrawing or becoming hostile, the therapist needs to change strategies. Any time I see marked hostility or withdrawal by either partner, I am prompted to consider whether the therapy process needs adjustment at that time.

In my view good couple therapy often is emotionally intense, but the emotions should not be restricted to anger. A range of emotions should be evident in couple therapy: tenderness as the partners feel and express closeness for each other, humor as the partners see the absurdity of what we all do in our attempts to deal with problems, sadness for the losses and pain experienced, and joy as gains are made. If therapy is predominantly hot, negative emotions, then different approaches are needed. The therapist needs to enable the couple to experience the positive aspects of their relationship.

I find that establishing positive affect in the partners at the beginning and the end of sessions helps sustain therapeutic momentum. Positive affect at the beginning of the session sets the tone for partners' behavior during the session. A warm greeting by the therapist to each partner and asking the partners about the best aspects of their relationship over the last week often prompt attention to positive aspects of the partner. This can establish a positive frame for tackling negative aspects of the relationship. It is easy to allow sessions to begin with negativity and for this to establish the tone for the whole session. The negative bias of distressed partners means that if the therapist begins the session with an open question such as "How have things been in the last week?" often the partners focus on the most negative aspects of the relationship over that period. If the therapist draws the couple out on those problems, often this arouses the negative affect associated with the problems. Then couples find it difficult to access positive memories or feelings in the session.

MATCHING THE SEQUENCE OF CONTENT TO COUPLE NEEDS

Most couples present with complex relationship problems, and therapy typically involves addressing a number of goals. Therapy needs to sequence the order in which problems are addressed to enhance therapeutic momentum. Problems of high salience to partners that are resolved reinforce change efforts by the partners. Changes that increase positive experiences of the partner and interaction with the partner reinforce change efforts. In my work with couples I make these considerations explicit and negotiate with the couple the order in which we will tackle the goals they have established.

In common with many cognitive-behavioral approaches to therapy, I negotiate an agenda with the couple at the beginning of each session (e.g., Beck, 1995). I usually begin that process by summarizing where we are up to in therapy. That summary typically involves highlighting the number of sessions we have had so far, what we have done up to now, and what we have negotiated to do in future sessions. The goal of this process is to ensure that the content of the couple therapy is addressing those issues salient to the couple.

HIGHLIGHTING THERAPEUTIC GAINS

Every two to three sessions of couple therapy I review with the couple the progress in therapy to that point. In this summary I reinforce the positive efforts by the partners and underscore the successes in therapy to that point. I also ask questions intended to prompt partners' attention to the positive effects of their self-change efforts. For example, if the couple report a reduced level of conflict in their relationship, I often ask them what each has done to bring about this change, (e.g., "What have you done differently to bring about this reduction in arguing?"). I also draw out descriptions of the positive effects of changes on the relationship, (e.g., "What difference does it make when the arguments are not happening?"). This process is meant to support effort and sustain momentum.

Responding to Slowing Therapeutic Momentum

Extended couple therapy often proceeds in bursts, and rarely does the initial establishment of therapeutic momentum carry the couple through to a satisfied relationship without some periods of waning therapeutic momentum. The most obvious source of slowing momentum occurs when the spouses have a major argument. Often couples who were making reasonable progress and feeling good about the impact of therapy on their relationship feel very discouraged when a destructive argument occurs. In many instances I have had partners initially report they feel like giving up on therapy and the relationship after destructive arguments. Failure to complete agreed tasks is a second source and signal of slowing momentum. Both situations are described next.

RECOVERING FROM DESTRUCTIVE CONFLICT

The occurrence of a destructive argument can rekindle the negative feelings and hurts that brought the couple to therapy. The partners' focus can shift from self-directed attempts to promote positivity to self-protective strategies to reduce pain. The therapist's challenge is to reestablish therapeutic momentum again. If this occurs, the couple learns that their relationship can transcend the negativity which inevitably is a part of any long-term relationship.

I see three important steps in responding to destructive arguments that slow therapeutic momentum. First, the partners often need assistance to self-regulate their feelings about the argument. Second, the couple needs to appraise why one argument changed feelings about the relationship so dramatically. Third, each partner needs to select practical self-change goals that will help them better manage future arguments. For the first step, most often I use the guided cognitive-affect reconstruction procedure described in Chapter 9 to explore the strength of feelings that the argument elicited. The core underlying relationship themes need to be identified and resolved. The second step of reestablishing therapeutic momentum is to explore the partners' emotional response after the argument, to focus on why one argument changed the partners' feelings so dramatically. Guided-discovery cognitive procedures often can be useful here. Consider the following interaction that illustrates this process.

THERAPIST: Julie, we have talked about why you responded so strongly to Tony not coming down to see you Friday night. The argument and the feelings you had over the weekend make a lot of sense given that you were thinking that Tony did not want to spend time with you. The argument really got to you didn't it? You were still very upset about it when you came in here, and it's nearly a week later. Help me to understand why you are so upset. What is it about what happened that gets to you so much?

JULIE: It's, well, you know everything seemed to be on the mend. You know. Not perfect, but better. Tony was trying. I was trying. We were talking, starting to have fun together again. Then, well, he no-shows.

THERAPIST: And when he no-showed, what did that mean to you?

JULIE: It made me wonder if he was giving up on us. Just sort of feeling it was all too hard.

THERAPIST: So, after the no-show you thought that the marriage might just fall apart?

JULIE: Sort of. I thought Tony was throwing in the towel.

THERAPIST: Help me to understand this bit. How was the one argument showing that things would not work out?

JULIE: Well, I know that one argument does not mean the end of the world, but it was because we were supposed to be fixing things. So if he is not trying now, now we are in therapy, will he ever really try for us?

THERAPIST: So if anything goes wrong at this stage, that's really bad, really bad?

JULIE: Well, it feels bad. Look, I know things can't be perfect, no marriage is perfect.

THERAPIST: OK. So you seem to be saying that no relationship is perfect, that arguments are going to happen. No disagreement from me there. I never met a couple that did not argue sometime. So what made this one so bad?

JULIE: Timing, I guess. The changes we are trying to make, you wonder if things have really changed, if we can make it work. I thought we had, but then. . . .

THERAPIST: So an argument when you are feeling the relationship is brittle, when you are not confident. . . .

JULIE: Yeah, I am still scared we might blow it. And things seem to be fine, then wham we're back to the old arguments.

THERAPIST: Back to the old arguments. Has anything changed?

JULIE: Sorry?

THERAPIST: Do you think anything has changed in your relationship? Is it really exactly as it was 4 or 5 weeks ago?

JULIE: No. No. Tony and I are much better with each other. Politer you know. Even in the argument we did not tear strips off each other.

This transcript illustrates a common theme evident early in couple therapy: Many couples still feel unsure about the future of their relationship. An argument often prompts thoughts about the difficulty of change. Any positive gains from therapy may be overlooked when the couples are feeling negative. Here the therapist gently guides the partner to describe a more complete picture of therapy, recognizing the positive changes that have occurred, and the limitations of what has been achieved. Relationship psychoeducation can be useful at this point, highlighting how most couples struggle to reestablish a sense of certainty in the future of their partnership. It is important for partners to understand that some set backs are inevitable, and that such set backs do not necessarily reflect on the future of the relationship.

The final step in reestablishing therapeutic momentum is to have partners self-select goals for managing setbacks. Questions such as "What could you do to reduce the negative effect of arguments in the future?" are useful. Most couples understand that some arguments are inevitable in any relationship, and the help the therapist gives to partners to self-regulate their adaptive processes after conflict can be a crucial therapeutic achievement.

RECOVERING FROM FAILURE TO COMPLETE AGREED UPON TASKS

Another key index of slowing therapeutic momentum is the failure of partners to carry through on agreed tasks between sessions. I see this as a critical event in therapy. Self-directed change is the essence of effective therapy, and so the failure to attempt a given task is vital information concerning the therapeutic process. When supervising therapists I often have seen them minimize the importance of uncompleted tasks with such phrases as "Well, see if you can get around to it next week." However, this phrase implicitly carries the message that the task was not important. Most people have lots to do in their lives, and a therapist should only suggest tasks that are important and should convey a sense of the importance of self-directed effort. Many couple therapists dismiss or minimize uncompleted tasks because they are unsure of how to deal with the issue. Certainly the question "Why didn't you do as you said you would?" often leads to defensive explanations which do not advance therapy.

Shelton and Levy (1981) suggest responding to nonadherence to therapeutic tasks based on three possible reasons for noncompletion of tasks. Although I do not like the concept of adherence, I think their classifications of reasons for noncompletion is useful. Table 3.3 summarizes suggestions based on their classification system. The first reason people fail to carry out agreed-on tasks is that the task was unclear or the person lacked the skill to carry out the task. The therapist can ask the client to restate the task. This request provides a check on whether the client has a clear understanding of the task. If the task is one in which a skill deficit might explain the failure to complete the task, then the skill level can be assessed. For example, if the partner was supposed to initiate a problem-solving discussion with his or her spouse, the therapist can ask the partner to do this in the therapy session.

If it is established that the client did understand the task and had the skills to carry out the task, then negative cognitions may explain the failure to complete the task. The person simply may not see the value of the task or may believe negative consequences will result from completion of the task. Exploring the beliefs the person has about the task often helps clarify whether the task is indeed useful. Sometimes the task is useful but the therapist has not explained the rationale clearly to the client, or unhelpful thoughts by the client need to be restructured. Other times, the therapist may be persuaded by interaction with the client that the task is not appropriate, and it may be necessary to renegotiate that aspect of therapy.

Finally, if it is established that the partner can do the task, and wants to do the task, circumstances in the environment may prevent the task from being completed. For example, suppose one partner is asked to arrange a special outing for the couple but the spouse refuses to go, or work demands prevent time being set aside. This is important information for the therapist to understand; often it can initiate further problem solving.

A case example illustrates the process of how to respond to noncompletion of a client task. Gena (56) and Joseph (58) married 3 years ago. Joseph's first wife died 7 years ago, and Gena had been divorced 30 years earlier from her first husband. They were struggling in adjusting to being married to each other. Gena had a wide variety of community and social activities she was engaged in, while Joseph preferred to spend time at home. These preferences reflected how each had lived their lives before meeting each other. They often argued about how much to go out. Joseph did not like Gena going out without him; he wanted her to spend time with him at home. Gena was unhappy that Joseph rarely wanted to do things outside the home. Joseph had decided on the task of organizing a dinner out with friends as part of his attempt to be more outgoing and meet Gena's need for more stimulation in the relationship.

THERAPIST: In the couple of weeks since we last saw each other, Joseph, you were going to organize a dinner out with friends. What happened with that?

TABLE 3.3. Responding to Loss of Therapeutic Momentum through Failure to Complete Agreed-Upon Tasks between Sessions

Reasons for failure to complete	Recommendations for enhancement of therapeutic momentum
Type 1: The client lacks the necessary skills and knowledge to complete some or all of the tasks in the assignment.	The therapist should prompt the client to self-define goals that contain specific detail regarding response and stimulus elements relevant to the desired behavior. The therapist should give direct skills training when necessary. The therapist should prompt the client to begin with small homework tasks and gradually increase assignments. The therapist should encourage the client to use cognitive rehearsal strategies to improve success with assignments.
Type 2: The client has cognitions that interfere with completion of the assignment.	The therapist should have the client review the self-selected goals, and make a public commitment to complete the tasks if that is the goal. The therapist should help the client develop a private commitment to comply (e.g., prompting attention to the positive effects of previous behavior change). The therapist should try to anticipate and reduce the negative effects of task completion.
Type 3: The client's environment elicits failure to complete task.	Completions should be reinforced by the therapist and self-reinforcement encouraged. The therapist should introduce the client to appropriate self-control strategies such as cuing. The therapist should prompt the client to try to anticipate and reduce the negative effects of completion of the task. The therapist should explore with the client context changes that might enhance the completion of the task.

JOSEPH: Well, it was pretty hectic you know. So it didn't happen.

THERAPIST: I see. Look, when someone says, "I am going to do X, but then does not, I think that is important. Often I find there are important lessons to be learned here. Just to check that we all left with the same understanding, Joseph tell me what you intended to do.

JOSEPH: I was going to organize dinner for Gena, me, and some friends. Probably the Newtons.

THERAPIST: OK, and when were you going to do that?

JOSEPH: Oh, just in the next week or so.

THERAPIST: OK. Well that is what I remember as well. Now sometimes the ideas we come up with in therapy seem not very good later on. Sometimes people come up with lousy ideas to improve their relationships. Sometimes I make lousy suggestions. Other times I do not explain a good suggestion well enough. Let's check how we're thinking about this idea now. Joseph, do you think organizing a night out for you and Gena with friends is a good idea?

JOSEPH: Yeah. Yeah, I do. It's just that it was a busy week you know.

THERAPIST: Uh huh, sure. Sometimes things get in the way of something we really want to do. Was the dinner something you really wanted to do?

JOSEPH: Well, sort of, you know. I mean Gena wants to go out more, so I guess I should do this.

THERAPIST: It sounds like you are not sure this is for you. Is that true?

JOSEPH: Well, I never went in much for racing around. I am a kind of quiet home body, you know?

THERAPIST: So organizing this dinner is really something you are doing for Gena, it's not something you really want to do yourself, is that it?'

In this example, the therapist initially checks that Joseph had a clear understanding of the task and then explores the cognitions Joseph holds about the task. Initially Joseph restates that it was just a time thing, but the therapist pushed to check whether Joseph really wanted to do the task. At this point some of Joseph's underlying cognitions emerge. As the interaction proceeded, Joseph described his desire to make Gena happy. He saw becoming more outgoing as the only means to achieve that, yet he felt uncomfortable with that role. Ultimately he stated that he felt he could never be sociable enough to keep Gena satisfied, and that maybe she regretted marrying him.

This issue proved to be central to their relationship problems. When they were dating Joseph had gone out more, but he saw that as a transient phase of dating. Gena thought that their level of social activity during dating reflected how they would live their lives together. Joseph's failure to complete the task reflected his deep concern that he would not measure up to what he saw as Gena's need for an outgoing, sociable man. He described his fear that he could never measure up to Gena's expectations. The exploration of the failure to complete the task of organizing a dinner engagement allowed identification of this issue. (Postscript: As Gena came to see Joseph's reluctance to go out as his preference to spend time with her alone, her desire to get Joseph to go out more diminished. She came to place greater value on shared time together at home. Joseph came to see Gena's desire to go out as an individual difference based on prior experiences, such as her long period of time as a single woman, rather than a rejection of spending time with him at home. As his view changed he felt more comfortable with her level of independent activity and reduced his criticism of her activities. Joseph also did become somewhat more outgoing once he experienced decreased pressure to be more outgoing.)

The foregoing transcript above reflects a common experience of mine in couple therapy. The failure to complete agreed-on tasks often is important information. The three-step structure summarized in Table 3.3 is invaluable to responding well to a loss of therapeutic momentum.

Completion of Couple Therapy

Ideally self-regulatory couple therapy is completed when the couple has achieved their self-selected relationship goals and each of the partners has developed the metacompetencies to self-regulate change in their relationship in the future. In practice, therapy sometimes is terminated by a partner or partners before this point is reached. To optimize the timing of completion, the issue needs explicitly to be negotiated between the therapist and the partners.

To ensure that therapy meets a couple's needs and continues only for as long as is necessary, I usually raise the issue of completion of therapy in the first session of SRCT. I state that couple therapy is not appropriate for all couples, and the first session or two should help us to determine whether couple therapy is appropriate. (Chapters 4 and 5 describe in some detail the contraindications for couple therapy.) I also describe that many couples find they can work out what they need to change in their relationship in three or four sessions. I explain that once we have done an assessment together I will review with the couple the changes they want to achieve and their perceptions of their capacity to produce those changes. At that point they might want to attempt to make those changes themselves, and in that case I would support them, but this would take relatively few sessions. Alternatively, the couple might still feel unclear on their relationship goals, or how to achieve those goals. In that case we would negotiate a set number of sessions with a clear agenda for the goals of those sessions.

As described in the section on maintaining therapeutic momentum, every few sessions I review therapy progress with the couple. If the couple is getting close to having achieved their relationship goals, I discuss with them what else they feel they need to achieve before therapy is completed. I also would explore with them any concerns they have about the future of their relationship after the end of therapy. Chapter 7 provides details on promoting the generalization and maintenance of therapeutic change in couple therapy.

To this point I have provided a model and analysis of the nature of relationship problems, reviewed the empirically supported approaches to couple therapy, and presented an overview of self-regulatory couple therapy. That is enough of the preliminaries; a couple await us in the waiting room, and I do not like to keep my clients waiting. Thus, let us turn to assessing the needs of couples.

4

Assessment, Part I:
Overview and Initial Session

The process of assessment begins with the first contact the therapist has with a partner. When done well, assessment provides therapist and clients with an agreed-on working model of the relationship. The working model consists of three parts: (1) a list of the key strengths of the relationship, (2) a list of the key problem areas in the relationship, and (3) a list of the key influences on the development and maintenance of the relationship's key problem areas. Such a model is the basis for the participants to determine whether therapy is to proceed. Moreover the model provides the partners with a structure within which they can attempt self-regulated change of the relationship.

During assessment it needs to be established whether couple therapy is a suitable response to the distress of the presenting partner(s). The mere fact that a couple arrives together for therapy does not necessarily indicate that conjoint couple therapy is a good idea. Nor should initial presentation of just one partner lead the therapist to ignore the possibility of couple therapy being appropriate. Rather, the therapist and couple explore the presenting problems and together determine whether couple therapy is appropriate.

When couple therapy is appropriate, the separation of assessment and therapy is somewhat arbitrary. Assessment shapes partners' perceptions of their relationship and the relationship problems and their sources. This, in turn, shapes the partners selection of goals to improve the relationship. Much of this process can be seen as therapy that is building self-regulation meta-competencies. For example, often I ask couples to complete a structured task of discussing a problem in their relationship in the session. The task is introduced with the rationale of observing their communication. The process of assessing communication often prompts the couple to reflect on their current communication, which sometimes leads to self-appraisal, goal setting, and attempts at self-change with little additional therapeutic input. The whole process that is traditionally thought of as assessment can be defined as therapy because it helps partners develop self-appraisal and goal-setting skills. For some couples development of these metacompetencies are necessary and sufficient to resolve their relationship problems, and in such cases therapy can be quite brief.

Assessment usually takes two or three sessions but can take somewhat longer if there are crises to manage or complex individual problems are interacting with the relationship problems. This is the first of two chapters on assessment. This chapter begins with an overview of assessment: assessment structure, areas to assess, and assessment methods. It then focuses on the initial couple assessment session, its goals, and its structure. The chapter ends with strategies for management of couples in crisis, as crises often precipitate presentation, and the crisis usually becomes evident in the first or second assessment session. Chapter 5 is a description of the second and any subsequent assessment sessions.

Overview of Assessment

The two most common errors in the assessment of couples are doing too little or doing too much. Too little assessment and treatment commences with an inadequate understanding of the couple and often without the couple feeling understood. This often leads to inappropriate interventions and poor couple engagement in the processes of therapy. Too much assessment wastes everybody's time and makes therapy expensive. Excessive assessment makes couples feel that irrelevancies are being dragged into the process. Self-regulatory couple therapy (SRCT) has a core of assessment procedures that are used with almost all couples and a set of supplementary assessments that are used with some couples when these additional assessments are relevant to the couple.

Core assessment tasks include conjoint interviews, self-report inventories, self-monitoring tasks, and behavioral tasks. Any of these tasks can serve two key functions: the collection of information and the promotion of new ideas to the couple. New ideas can be promoted simply by completion of the task.

The goal of the assessment process is to develop a shared understanding among the partners and the therapist of the couple's relationship. This shared understanding needs to be consistent with each partner's experience of the relationship and to promote positive change. Throughout the assessment process the therapist is summarizing and reflecting the information gathered. This process serves two important functions: It builds empathy with the partners, and checks the accuracy of information gathered. The assessment process culminates in a feedback and goal-setting session. In this session the therapist presents an integrating summary of the results of the assessment to the couple using a guided participation process (described in detail in Chapter 6).

Structure of the Assessment Process

The initial session is usually about 90 minutes in duration. The session begins with a brief conjoint orientation for the couple that lasts approximately 10 minutes. A key goal of this initial orientation is to establish the structure of the session. This initial orientation is followed by individual consultations with each partner of approximately 25 minutes each. A primary goal of the individual consultations is to do a preliminary assessment of the areas of relationship concern for each partner. During these individual interviews the other partner completes some self-report inventories in another room. The self-report inventories are intended to provide an indication of the level of relationship distress, key areas of conflict, and the areas of change each partner desires in the relationship. The initial assessment session ends with a conjoint closing consultation of approximately 25 to 30 minutes. In this closing consultation the therapist summarizes key areas of concern to ensure that he or she understands the key problems and then describes the couple therapy approach. If couple therapy is deemed to be suitable, the therapist usually negotiates with the partners for them to complete some self-report or self-monitoring measures between the first and second sessions. Details of the objectives and procedure of this initial session follow later in this chapter.

The second and subsequent sessions usually are 60 minutes in duration. The therapist begins the second session by summarizing what was covered in the first session and negotiating an agenda. Usually the therapist needs to continue to gather further information about the partners and their relationship. As in the first session, this may involve individual interviews with each partner. The therapist also reviews the information gathered in individual interviews and from the completed self-report inventories and self-monitoring forms conjointly with the couple and uses the information to further explore the nature of the couple's relationship. The couple usually undertake specific structured tasks, such as problem solving or social support discussions, in the second or third session. Finally, the therapist closes the session with a summary and negotiation of any further assessment tasks to be completed between sessions. (Chapter 5 describes details of these procedures for the second and any subsequent sessions.)

Areas to Assess

At the end of Chapter 1 I presented a model of the influences on couple relationships. The center of that model was couple adaptive processes: the thoughts, feelings, and actions of the partners as they interact. SRCT focuses on helping distressed partners to change these adaptive processes to promote positive relationship outcomes, which usually is operationalized as a mutually satisfying relationship. Therefore, the assessment of couples substantially focuses on relationship outcomes and the couple's adaptive processes. At the same time, as noted in the model, context, stressful events, and individual partner characteristics influence couple adaptive processes. Consequently, the assessment of couples also needs to look at these factors to establish their impact on the couple's relationship. Table 4.1 sets out the variables that most often need to be assessed in couple therapy. It is not an exhaustive listing but does cover what needs to be assessed most often.

Methods of Assessment

In SRCT the core assessment methods are individual and conjoint interviews, self-report measures, and behavioral observation. In addition, self-monitoring

TABLE 4.1. What Needs to Be Assessed in Couple Therapy

Domain	Key variables
Relationship outcomes	Relationship satisfaction Dissolution potential
Couple adaptive processes	Behavior exchange Positive activities Intimacy and affection Couple communication Conflict management Aggression Role functioning Mutual support Sex Beliefs and expectations
Individual characteristics	Psychopathology
Life events	Parenting Work Recreation
Context	Culture, ethnicity Extended family Friendships

is sometimes used as a supplementary assessment method. Assessment sessions largely consist of both conjoint and individual interviews, with some behavioral observation of the couple in structured tasks. Partners are asked to complete self-report measures during sessions while the other partner is being interviewed individually. Additional self-report inventories and self-monitoring measures are completed between sessions. Information gathered from self-report inventories and self-monitoring tasks between sessions is reviewed and explored in subsequent assessment sessions (see Chapter 5).

Table 4.2 presents a range of assessment methods available to couple therapists. Each method has advantages and disadvantages. Some methods assess certain relationship domains better than others. For example, people usually can report reliably on the major issues that elicit conflict in their relationships (Haynes, Jensen, Wise, & Sherman, 1981), however it is less likely that they will be able to identify deficits in their intimate communication (Osgarby & Halford, 2000a). An assessment that uses multiple assessment methods allows better assessment of different areas of relationship problems and provides convergent evidence on the nature of relationship problems.

Most clients can complete paper-and-pencil inventories that assess a wide variety of relationship issues far more quickly than they could talk about those issues with a therapist. When couples complete inventories between ses-

TABLE 4.2. Some Methods for Assessment of Couple Relationships

Method	Advantages	Disadvantages
Conjoint interview	Allows therapist to demonstrate empathy, gather information, draw together perspectives of individual partners; allows therapist to facilitate partners hearing each other's perspective.	Distressed couples may argue, feel threatened, angry about partner's comments in conjoint interviews; reliability of information gained in conjoint interviews is low.
Individual interviews	Allows demonstration of empathy with individual, collection of information, gathering of sensitive data (e.g., aggression).	Possibility of one person disclosing "secrets"; need to build common understanding between partners is not addressed.
Self-report inventories	Increases efficiency of information gathering, can provide clients with new ideas for assessing their relationship; provides psychometrically sound assessments.	In isolation, filling in questionnaires does not inform each partner about the other's perspective or allow the therapist to show empathy.

sions, the efficiency of doing therapy increases. Hence, I advocate the use of a selection of self-report inventories early in the assessment process. These inventories allow the therapist to assess a wide range of areas for relevance in a particular case. When a domain of relationship functioning is identified as relevant to a particular couple, it can be explored further within the interview.

INTERVIEWS

Effective couple therapy depends on effective interviewing. In SRCT a mix of individual and conjoint interviews are used in assessment. Interviews with individual partners allow the therapist to assess issues not easily accessed in conjoint interviews (e.g., violence). Individual interviews also allow the therapist to assess and develop empathy with the complaints of each partner about the relationship and spouse, without those complaints leading to further hurt or pain to the spouse. Conjoint interviews are the major means by which the couple and the therapist can influence each other and negotiate a shared understanding of the relationship's strengths and weaknesses. However, unless the therapist carefully structures the process, conjoint interviews with distressed couples can deteriorate into hurtful interchanges between the partners. Later in this chapter I provide detailed suggestions for structuring conjoint interviews so that the process is constructive.

Exclusive reliance on interviews for assessment is unwise. Such reliance implicitly assumes that all that needs to be known about a couple's relationship can be reported by the partners within the therapy sessions. We know that biases in perception and memory of relationship interaction characterize relationship distress (Osgarby & Halford, 2000b); thus why would we assume that partners are able to present all the information a therapist might need? Other assessment methods are needed, such as self-report inventories, observation, and self-monitoring.

SELF-REPORT INVENTORIES

Completing self-report inventories can serve useful functions by having couples address issues they have not yet thought about and by educating them about relationships. Table 4.3 presents six core self-report inventories most often used in SRCT. Partners usually fill out the Dyadic Adjustment Scale (DAS) and Areas of Change Questionnaire (ACQ) when I am interviewing their spouse in session 1. I ask both partners to complete the Marital Status Inventory between sessions 1 and 2. I also might ask them to complete the Depression, Anxiety, Stress Scale (DASS) and/or the Communication Patterns Questionnaire (CPQ) before session 2. (If either partner has not completed the DAS and ACQ in session 1, I get them to complete those inventories as the

TABLE 4.3. Core Self-Report Inventories

Domain	Variable	Measure	Session number	Authors	Description
Relationship outcomes	Relationship satisfaction	Dyadic Adjustment Scale	1	Spanier (1976)	32-item self-report inventory of global relationship satisfaction
	Separation potential	Marital Status Inventory	1–2	Weiss & Cerreto (1980)	14-item true–false measure of steps taken toward divorce
Couple adaptive processes	Overall desired change in adaptive processes	Areas of Change Questionnaire	1	Weiss & Birchler (1975); Weiss & Halford (1996)	68 items rating desired changes from partner and self in specific behaviors
	Communication and conflict management	Communication Patterns Questionnaire	1–2, or 2–3	Christensen (1988)	23-item self-report measure of use of common patterns of conflict management
	Aggression and violence	Conflict Tactics Scale (Revised)	2	Straus, Hamby, Boney-McCoy, & Sugarman (1996)	39-item self-report measure of specific acts of aggression by partner or self in past 12 months
Individual characteristics	Individual psychopathology	Depression, Anxiety, and Stress Scale (DASS)	1-2, or 2-3	Lovibond & Lovibond (1995)	21-item self-report inventory yielding scores on depression, anxiety, and stress

first priority before session 2 and might have them complete the DASS and/or CPQ between sessions 2 and 3.) In session 2 I usually have the partners complete the Conflict Tactics Scale—Revised (CTS-R) while I interview their spouse.

OBSERVATION

Observation is another underutilized but important assessment method for couples. Particularly in the domain of communication, the therapist is able, through observation of interaction, to formulate hypotheses about the nature of a couple's problems. For example, I routinely ask couples to discuss an issue in their relationship in the clinic. I prefer to leave the room during this discussion, so my presence does not distract the partners. I watch the interaction via closed-circuit videotape. During the interaction I observe the process of communication, attending to such issues as who talks the most, who listens effectively, and what the evident patterns of interaction are. In my experience couples rarely can describe these interaction patterns for themselves.

SELF-MONITORING

Self-monitoring of relationship events is a supplementary assessment method. This involves partners undertaking an individual or joint task of monitoring relationship events over time. For example, the Marital Events Diary (Osgarby & Halford, 2000b) asks partners to report at the end of each day the number of half-hour blocks of time they spent together. Each half-hour block is described in terms of the predominant activity during that time (e.g., doing chores, talking, and watching television) and is rated for the pleasantness or unpleasantness of the time period. Any stressful or positive exchanges during the day are recorded separately. This assessment method allows the therapist and couple to build a picture of the couple's routines during the week and how they perceive those patterns.

Self-monitoring can be used to address the negative memory biases in distressed couples' recall of their relationship. Distressed partners tend to forget positive relationship events and to selectively recall negative relationship events (Osgarby & Halford, 2000b). Furthermore, they recall positive events less positively and recall negative events more negatively over time. When partners complete the Marital Events Diary, the therapist can ask each person to elaborate on positive events he or she recorded during the week. These events are often difficult for distressed couples to recall without written prompts.

The Initial Assessment Session

The most important goal in the first assessment session is to establish an appropriate therapeutic process in which the couple can explore the nature of their relationship without suffering further hurts and humiliation from each other. If the process generates acrimony, one or both partners may not come again. Details of content that are overlooked in the first session can be gathered in subsequent sessions or from a variety of self-report instruments. Therefore, gathering information is important but is a secondary goal. Table 4.4 summarizes the structure and goals of this initial session within SRCT. However, therapists must bear in mind that this is not a rigid prescription.

Process Objectives

There are three objectives that, when accomplished, help establish an appropriate therapeutic process. These objectives are to engage both partners, to separate the processes of assessment and goal setting, and to provide realistic levels of hope. The first process goal in working with couples is to engage both partners. Although the two partners usually have different views of the nature of their problems, they do have in common feelings of considerable pain from the relationship distress. It is my general assumption that few people attend couple therapy with the intent to deliberately destroy their relationship. Instead, they want to work on the relationship, but they feel unable to do

TABLE 4.4. Structure of Initial Couple Assessment Session

Content	Goals
Initial conjoint orientation (10 minutes)	Introductions Present structure of session Assess conjoint statement of problem
Individual interviews (25 minutes)	Assess areas of relationship difficulty Screen for violence, individual psychopathology
Completion of self-report inventories (done in separate room while partner is being interviewed)	Assess levels of distress, key areas of conflict, areas for change
Conjoint consultation (30 minutes)	Summarize individual concerns Describe couple therapy approach Review suitability of couple therapy Negotiate assessment tasks to be completed before next session

this. The challenge in the therapeutic process is to help each person to express pain, concerns, and unhappiness in a manner that gives the partners a chance to join with each other in working on the relationship.

Most couples enter therapy with each partner showing some willingness to acknowledge a degree of contribution to the relationship problems. When this acknowledgment is combined with an ability to listen to the other person's perspective, the initial interview might be conducted largely as a conjoint interview. More often the therapist needs to listen to each person separately in order to develop rapport and empathy with each partner and only then attempt to join these two stories into a cohesive whole. For this reason I typically structure the initial interview as a mix of conjoint and individual interviews.

A second process goal is a strategic separation of assessment and therapy. Many couples begin therapy with unrealistic expectations. For example, commonly, individual partners feel the need for instant answers ("Should I be in therapy?", "Can our relationship ever work?"). The therapist needs to attend to the importance of these questions while avoiding the trap of attempting answers on the basis of insufficient data. A second common unrealistic assumption is that the therapist will adjudicate on the correctness of partners' perceptions of the relationship ("Our real problem is that she expects too much, isn't it?", "I am sure you will agree that if he was just more expressive of his feelings, that would make a hell of a difference"). Again, the therapist needs to acknowledge the importance of the issue raised to the person but to avoid making pronouncements that are unjustified by available data or that will alienate either partner.

The strategic separation of assessment and therapy is an important means to promote the therapist's and the couple's attention to thinking collaboratively in developing a model of the relationship problems. With every couple I spell out the importance of initially assessing the relationship before attempting to define the goals of therapy. In the first few minutes of the first session I emphasize that the initial focus of therapy will be on assessment, with the objective of providing additional information for the couple to negotiate goals and to define a helpful intervention process to achieve those goals. I aim, through the process of working with the individuals and the couple together, to develop a shared commitment to being involved in the assessment process and to at least consider the possibilities of promoting change within the relationship.

A third important process objective in the first session is to provide realistic levels of hope for clients. In my view the couple therapist generally should be an advocate for the relationship. This does not mean that the couple therapist should always encourage clients to stay together. However, if people are considering separation they should be informed about other choices available to them, and the therapist should try to assist the couple to recognize the difficulties associated with separation.

Content Objectives

I have limited objectives in terms of information collection for the initial session. The most important objective is to assess domestic violence and ensure that no one is in immediate danger from violence. After that priority comes identification of the key presenting concerns of each partner. Specifically, I aim to find out each partner's most pressing relationship concerns. A related goal is to establish whether there is sufficient common ground in the individuals' concerns that conjoint therapy is feasible. Sufficient common ground for proceeding to couple therapy does not require total agreement on the nature of the couple's problems but, simply, an agreement by both partners that there is one or more identifiable relationship problems that both wish to work on.

In this initial session the therapist is a manager of change. In particular, the therapist is attempting to join with each partner and then to promote a relationship focus in the way in which the problems are viewed. All this is meant to anticipate and help develop a self-regulatory focus throughout therapy. By a self-regulatory focus I mean shifting the emphasis in the way in which each partner thinks about the relationship to focus on what that individual can do to improve the relationship. Probes such as "What do you need to do to make the relationship better?" are needed to assist the individual to develop a self-regulatory focus. The timing of the use of such probes is important. Used prematurely, the individual may feel blamed for the relationship problems and may become alienated from the therapist. It is important that the challenges to the individual to consider ways in which he or she can improve their relationship be based on a well-established empathy with the individual's current perspectives about the relationship. I now turn to the details of how to conduct this session. The discussion follows the four-point structure for the initial assessment session presented in Table 4.4.

Initial Conjoint Orientation

The initial session begins with a conjoint orientation. It starts with introductions, then a statement of the general structure and aims of the first session. In the first few moments of the consultation process I highlight the need to do assessment before goal setting can occur. I explain that this first session will be an attempt to develop some understanding of the key concerns and to decide whether a subsequent session is desirable. I explain that after this brief joint orientation I will meet separately with each partner while the other completes assessment forms in another room. Then we will meet jointly again at the end of the session.

I then ask an open question relating to the reasons for the couple seeking assistance, such as "What is it that brings you to therapy?" This question is intended to assess process rather than content. To make the question effective, the therapist should make eye contact with each partner while asking the question but then look at a point midway between the partners (i.e., as the inflection occurs at the end of the question). My interest at this point is the ability of the couple to collaborate in developing a coherent story to tell the therapist. If each partner shows respect toward the other and shared views are presented, then using a conjoint interview to assess at least some of the content of the relationship problems may be feasible. However, it is quite common for couples not to respond constructively to an initial probe about the nature of their relationship problems and to rapidly escalate to a disagreement about who has done what, who is to blame, and so forth. When this happens the therapist should intervene early to prevent therapy from becoming another site for destructive conflict.

If the therapist does need to stop the couple from arguing, I recommend that the therapist explain why he or she is interrupting at that point. I make explicit that I am trying to prevent therapy from becoming another situation in which the couple argues. If I feel comfortable using humor with the couple at this point, I might pose it in this way: "Have you two ever had an argument before?" This almost inevitably produces the response: "Of course we have." I can then follow up with "Do you feel the need to practice the arguments anymore, or are you quite good now at arguing together?" This often elicits a response of the general form "Yes, we do argue, and no there is not much more point in us arguing any further." With or without the use of humor it is important to point out the need for the couple to learn to talk to each other in more constructive ways. I underscore the importance of the couple agreeing to a basic therapy rule. When I, as the therapist, ask them to stop arguing, they must stop. I emphasize that this request is often difficult to fulfill but is an important part of learning self-control in managing destructive conflict. The ability to recognize that a discussion has deteriorated to destructive argument, then stopping to deal with the frustration of not immediately expressing one's point of view, is an important skill to learn. Ultimately, I want the couple to be able to do that without an outside person prompting their attention to the need to stop. As an interim step, I suggest to the couple that we agree that it is important to be able to do that in therapy.

Sometimes couples present important shared views about their relationship problems in a conjoint interview. For example, a couple recently reported that they lack the ability to control conflict from being destructive and they wanted help to improve this aspect of the relationship. In describing their difficulties with conflict management the couple was able to agree on the topic areas about which they argued most and the patterns of interaction evident when they argued destructively. In cases in which the couple is providing useful content information within a constructive process, the conjoint aspect of the interview might be extended to form more of the initial session. However, even if the couple is able to present their concerns in a constructive manner in the initial conjoint interview, I still routinely speak to each partner separately. There are some issues, such as violence, which are assessed more accurately only when one partner is present. During the initial conjoint phase I establish the role of confidentiality in couple therapy.

CONFIDENTIALITY OF INFORMATION

When conducting individual interviews with one partner in the context of couple therapy, the issue of secrets arises. That is, there can be information shared between the therapist and one partner that the other partner does not know about. I tell couples that I will assume that anything they tell me individually I may tell their spouse unless they ask me not to. In general, it is my preference for information to be shared among the therapist and both partners. Thus, if a partner raises something that he or she does not want the partner to know, I would explore the nature of his or her concerns about sharing the information with the spouse. Most of the time there is little real cost to sharing the information with the partner. However, there are two issues frequently raised by individuals that create challenges for the therapist: affairs and abuse. Suggestions for handling these issues are covered later in the chapter.

Completion of Self-Report Inventories In Session

As noted in Table 4.4, when interviewing one individual I ask the other to complete some self-report inventories in another room. Completion of these inventories is intended to gather information from the partners that provides an overview of their relationship and concerns. The process of completing the inventories also shapes the partners' descriptions of their relationship concerns to be more comprehensive and specific.

I usually ask the partners to complete the DAS (Spanier, 1976) and the ACQ (Weiss & Birchler, 1975; Weiss & Halford (1996). The DAS is 31-item inventory that is an updated and expanded version of the Marital Adjustment Test (Locke & Wallace, 1959). It is a global self-report measure of relationship satisfaction. The ACQ is a 68-item inventory on which people rate how much they want their partner to change on a list of 34 specific behaviors and then how much they believe they need to change those same behaviors. The ACQ provides a helpful overview of the areas of the relationship that partners believe need to change and the areas that are satisfactory. It also is a useful way to prompt people to consider improvement of the relationship as involving change by both partners.

Before completing the conjoint interview I usually give copies of both the DAS and ACQ to each partner. I explain my intent to ask them to complete these inventories as I talk with their partner. I then describe each instrument and check whether completing the forms makes sense to them. Then one partner leaves the room and I commence the individual interview. Some people do not complete both inventories in the time taken to conduct the individual interview with their partner. In that case I ask the person to take the form home and complete it before the next session. I collect the form(s) that are completed and review them before the next session. Chapter 5 describes the interpretation and use of these and other self-report inventories.

Individual Interviews

The individual interview is intended to establish key concerns and to develop an empathic relationship between the therapist and the client. Not all areas needing to be assessed for couple therapy presented in Table 4.1 are covered, as some areas are best assessed with other methods. Individual key concerns usually fall within the areas identified in Table 4.5. Not all these will be covered in the first interview, but the most immediately pressing concerns of each partner should be identified. I usually begin with an open question along the lines of "What would you see as the areas you most want to change?" Sometimes the person responds in great detail, covering most of the areas that are listed in Table 4.5; other times I need to probe to fill out the picture. The sequencing of areas in Table 4.5 is my preferred sequencing of probing, if probing is needed.

BEHAVIOR CHANGE FOR SELF AND PARTNER

I usually pose a question such as "In order for the relationship to be as you want it, what does your partner need to do differently?" This can be followed up with "What do you need to do differently?" Helping the person to be as specific as possible in his or her descriptions is helpful. Vague comments such as "be more affectionate" can be probed with how such affection might be expressed. The questions on self-change are the first attempts to assess the individual's ability for self-appraisal and goal setting, two key self-regulatory skills to be developed throughout the course of therapy.

COMMUNICATION AND CONFLICT MANAGEMENT

Communication is a central relationship concern for most distressed couples. A general question such as "Tell me about how you two communicate" can get things started. Many distressed partners focus their answers on conflict. Management of conflict is important, and I ask people to describe a typical conflict and go through what happened in some detail. In this exploration I want to establish the behaviors of each partner and the emotion(s) experienced

Table 4.5. Key Areas to Explore in Individual Interviews

Adaptive couple processes
   Behavior changes for partner and self
   Communication and conflict management
   Domestic violence
   Time use
   Social support
   Sex
   Relationship beliefs and expectations

Relationship outcomes
   Commitment and separation

Context and life stresses
   External stresses

Individual characteristics
   Individual problems

by the person I am interviewing. It also is important to establish to what extent the pattern described is representative of their arguments. A question such as "Do disagreements always follow this pattern?" can be useful. In addition to conflict management, it is helpful to know how the couple communicates more generally. If the person does not describe this specifically, I ask about how often the couple has an interesting conversation together and the extent to which they share feelings and experiences.

DOMESTIC VIOLENCE

Perhaps the most important area to assess in the initial individual interviews is the occurrence of violence within the family. Approximately 70 to 75% of couples presenting for couple therapy have had an incident of physical aggression within the relationship in the previous 12 months (O'Leary, Vivian, & Malone, 1992). Less than 1 in 20 couples mention the occurrence of physical violence in a conjoint interview without direct therapist prompting (O'Leary et al., 1992). It is only by direct specific questions to each individual partner that one gets reasonably accurate rates of aggression. While the reported aggression for the majority of distressed couples is of a less severe form, and often does not present an immediate danger to partners, a significant minority of couples report aggression which presents a substantial risk of physical injury (O'Leary & Vivian, 1990). If any form of violence is detected, there may be a need to establish a safety plan.

It is important to get a precise behavioral description of any violence that may be occurring. Beware of the use of emotive labels such as abuse or battering, which may mean different things to different people and which may lead clients not to report aggressive incidents. I often seek to normalize the occurrence of aggression and anger within relationships in order to increase the chance of accurate reporting of aggression. Consider the following statement: "Often when people have the sort of relationship problems you have described there is anger between the partners. This anger can spill over to aggression with pushing, slapping, shoving and the like. Have you ever made physical contact with your partner during an argument? Has your partner ever made physical contact with you?" If there is a report of any sort of incident of violence it is important to assess the number of times it has occurred, when the most recent occurrence was, and the exact nature of the violence. Establish whether there were injuries resulting from any of the incidents.

In addition to overt acts of violence there can be covert acts of aggression and intimidation. Ask whether there have been verbal threats or physical intimidation (e.g., raising of a hand, object, or weapon in a threatening gesture). It also is important to ask the following: "Has anything happened that made you feel scared or intimidated by your partner?" Examples of such intimidation include preventing access to money, following the partner, checking up on where he or she is, attempting to prevent contact with other people, and coercive sexual practices such as pressuring the person to engage in sexual acts against his or her will. If violence is reported in the relationship, a careful assessment of the nature of the violence and the threat it may pose to the safety of the victim needs to become the priority for the session.

Even when asked explicitly about relationship aggression in individual interviews, a substantial number of people do not report aggression that is occurring in their relationship (O'Leary et al., 1992). Self-report inventories such as the Conflict Tactics Scale (Revised) (Straus, Hamby, Boney-McCoy, & Sugarman, 1996) are more sensitive to detection of violence (O'Leary et al., 1992). In Chapter 5 I describe the use of that instrument, and later in this chapter I provide details on how to respond to violence when it is detected.

TIME USE

I am keen to understand the couple's usual routine, to understand how they spend their time. To access this I ask something along the lines of: "Can you describe a typical week for me, who is around at what times, and what activities are done with whom." It is important to get a sense of the behavioral ecology of the couple. Most of us are creatures of habit and follow common patterns of when we get up, whom we eat breakfast with, when we leave for work, when we get home, and so forth. Getting a description of this information can then be used to estimate how many hours a week the couple is together, how much of their time together is with children or other people, and how much couple time there is. I am interested in establishing how many hours are spent at work and at other activities. Some couples make their lives so busy they seem not to have time for a relationship. In dual-worker families with children to care for, making time to relate can be a major challenge, and the therapist needs to have some understanding of the lifestyle the couple has built together.

Having a balance of couple and individual positive activities is an important element in most satisfying couple relationships (Halford, 1999). In exploring time use I routinely ask whether the couple has regular activities they do together that are fun. I also ask about the last time the couple went out on a date. That is, when did they last go out together as a couple without other people being with them. I also try to establish whether the partners have regular positive activities that they do independently.

SUPPORT

Mutual support is an important element of satisfying relationships. It is helpful to ask a question such as the following: "In what ways does your partner support you?" This question can be followed up with another: "In what other ways would you like your partner to support you?" Exploring how the interviewee supports his or her partner also is important.

SEX

Some people are uncomfortable raising this issue with the therapist. I often acknowledge this in posing a question about sexuality. For example, I might ask something like this: "Sex is important, but some people find it a little hard to talk about. Can you tell me about what your sex life with [partner's name] is like?" If the client looks uncomfortable, I usually comment on this and normalize the response. In assessing sexual functioning it is useful to establish how often the couple typically has sex and how the partners feel about the frequency and quality of sex. If either partner has difficulties with sexual interest or arousal or achieving orgasm, this also is important to know. Very low frequency of sex, or total abstinence, may indicate a specific sexual dysfunction or low levels of positive affect within the relationship (Spence, 1997).

RELATIONSHIP BELIEFS AND EXPECTATIONS

The process of asking questions about the key areas listed in Table 4.5 is not just seeking information on content areas. The question asking can begin to establish how the client thinks about his or her relationship. I usually pose a question such as "How did the problems in your relationship develop?" toward the end of the individual interview. This assesses the client's implicit theory about his or her relationship problems directly. (It may also lead to useful information being disclosed on the external stresses affecting the couple's relationship.) Other questions also tap into the partners' beliefs about their relationship. For example, listen to how the client describes communication processes between him or her and the spouse. Does the client make spouse-blaming, hostile statements, or does he or she focus on interactive relationship descriptions? Also, listen carefully to how the client responds to the question on external stresses. If there is a long pause and the person is unable to generate any comment on the role of external factors, it is unlikely that he or she has seriously considered this aspect of their relationship functioning.

COMMITMENT AND SEPARATION

An issue that needs routine screening is each partner's current feelings about separation and divorce. In a substantial minority of presenting couples one partner has already decided to leave the relationship. When that determination is clear, therapy at that point may focus on helping the individual to explain his or her decision to the partner, helping one or both partners to cope with their feelings about separation or mediating between the partners to arrange a mutually acceptable separation agreement. More commonly, one or both partners are ambivalent about the relationship. In these cases assessment helps partners determine whether they wish to attempt to improve their relationship.

Thoughts about separation and divorce can be difficult for some people to acknowledge overtly. I try to normalize these thoughts with an introduction something like the following: "When people have problems that you have described in your relationship, many consider whether the relationship should continue. What thoughts do you have about the future of the relationship?" I also try to establish whether the couple has a history of relationship separation. Some partners find it hard to acknowledge that separations have occurred. They describe being apart for weeks, unclear as to whether the relationship would continue, and yet state that they have never separated from their partner. It can be useful to pose the following question: "Have you ever left the house after an argument not clear on whether you would come back?"

EXTERNAL STRESS

The term "external stress" in Table 4.5 refers to anything external to the couple which has an impact on their relationship. For most people, factors such as the nature of their jobs, other hobbies and interests, and extended family and friends all influence their relationship. I would often pose a question along the lines of the following: "Stresses external to the couple often affect relationships, like money, work, or extended family. Are there any stresses that you think affect your relationship?"

INDIVIDUAL PROBLEMS

Screening each partner for individual psychological difficulties also is important. In approximately one-half of all couples who present for couple therapy the women score in the depressed range on the Beck Depression Inventory (Beach et al., 1990), and in approximately 40% of couples the men are drinking alcohol excessively (Halford & Osgarby, 1993). It is important that the therapist knows of any individual pharmacotherapy or psychotherapy partners may be receiving. I routinely ask whether either partner is currently receiving, or has ever received, psychiatric or psychological treatment. I also pose the following question: "Is there anything about you or your partner as individuals which you think contributes to your relationship problems?"

CLOSING THE INDIVIDUAL INTERVIEW

All the areas identified in Table 4.5 cannot be covered in an initial individual consultation of 25 minutes. Typically, completing the gathering of this data extends into the second and possibly third session. I do try to allow the individual as much freedom as possible to tell me his or her perceptions of the relationship and its problems in the initial individual interview. However, it is important that the individual interviews do not extend too far beyond their allotted time. If that occurs the total session may become so long that fatigue undermines the value of the session. Alternatively, one partner may get substantially less time in the individual interview, and this may leave that partner feeling alienated from the process.

Toward the end of the individual consultation I explicitly state the need to wind up this part of the session and then briefly summarize the key issues that the individual has highlighted for me. I then usually pose a question in the following form: "Clearly I cannot understand everything that is important to know about you and your relationship in just 25 minutes, but I am wondering if there is anything else that you believe is very important for me to know right now?" This question is intended to underscore to the person that there may be important information that I have overlooked but which can be gathered at a later time. At the same time, it is intended to allow the person to raise issues that he or she thinks are important for me to know at that point.

On completion of the individual interview I aim to have an initial idea of this partner's most pressing concerns. I need to have established if he or she is physically safe in the relationship, and if he or she is not, to have established a safety plan. A safety plan might involve leaving the relationship, or having prepared means to leave should further violence seem imminent or actually occur. I want to have established some empathy with his or her feelings about the relationship and to have built an initial working relationship with the person.

Final Conjoint Phase: Leaving the Session with a Clear Product

The final phase of the initial session is a conjoint interview with three key therapist tasks: (1) to summarize the key concerns of the couple and establish sufficient common ground between the partners to proceed to a second session, (2) to assign further assessment tasks to be completed between sessions, and (3) to help the couple commit to being active in couple therapy. After discussing each of these tasks in further detail, I want to discuss how to structure conjoint interviews so that they are constructive and avoid destructive conflict.

SUMMARIZING KEY CONCERNS AND ESTABLISHING SUFFICIENT COMMON GROUND

In the final conjoint phase of the initial session I summarize the key concerns that have been identified by each individual partner. In doing this I go beyond simply restating in the clients' own words their concerns and attempt to reframe those concerns with a greater relationship focus. For example, in a recent intake interview I did with a stepfamily, both partners mentioned concerns about parenting issues. Specifically the man reported that he felt he was not given a legitimate role in parenting his wife's daughter. He felt resentful that the daughter did not take him seriously in his own home and felt that his wife did not back him up when he made disciplinary statements. In contrast, the woman reported that she felt that the husband was intrusive in his interactions with the daughter and overcontrolling. I expressed this concern to the two of them as follows: "Both of you mentioned concerns about the relationship between John and Emily's daughter. You both described how it's been difficult for you to reach an agreement on what role John should play in parenting. This seems to be something that we need to reach a mutually acceptable agreement on." The essence of this reframe is to take the two perspectives and describe them in a way in which the couple can jointly own the problem.

Table 4.6 presents examples of pairs of individual complaints that spouses might make about their relationship and relationship-focused reframes of those same issues. Two elements are noteworthy. First, the reframes are aimed at defining the common ground in seemingly different views of what are the problems. Second, many of the relational reframes focus on the positive aspect of the problems. It should be noted that the secret of effective use of these relational reframes is the same as the secret of great humor: timing. A reframe used when empathy with the individual perspective is established can be an effective, supportive challenge to a self-defeating perspective. A reframe without this prior condition can be seen as trivializing or missing the problem.

In doing this closing conjoint phase of the first session it is important for the therapist to highlight common ground for the couple. This common ground should emphasize both the positive aspects of the relationship which the partners have identified, or which the therapist has observed during the initial session, and the common areas of concern. At the end of Chapter 5 I discuss in more detail how to reframe common challenges in the initial presentation so they become a shared concern.

Occasionally there is no common ground in the concerns that couples

TABLE 4.6. Individual Partner-Blaming Problems and Relationship-Focused Reframes of those Problems

Problem focus	Relational reframe
"She never wants to spend time with me." "He resents me having any interest of my own."	As a couple you have not found a balance of independent and couple time which you both can live with.
"She thinks he spends too much time with his family of origin." "He thinks she is cold and distant from his parents and sibs."	Time with extended family is an area you disagree about; as yet you have not worked out how to accommodate to each other's needs in this area.
"She is never interested in sex." "He pressures me to have sex."	The two of you differ in the frequency that you desire sex.
"He's unemotional." "She's irrational."	You two are very different in how you react to things; the emotional and rational side of each of you could complement one another, but you have not yet found a way to make that work for you.
"She has no interest in anything that I like."	Finding interests that excite both of you has proved quite difficult so far; you have not yet found ways of creating new interests that engage both of you.
"We fight all the time, and we do not know why."	You care deeply about what happens in your relationship, and so you both become very passionate about discussions. Harnessing that passion to produce positive outcomes is eluding you at this stage.

state. Under these circumstances it is not wise to proceed directly to couple therapy as it is described in this book. However, it may be that the therapist can still help the partners to clarify some individual problems. Couple therapy sometimes can proceed after that phase of therapy. For example, one wife felt that the only relationship problem was that the man drank too heavily. The man disagreed that his drinking was excessive and felt the major problem for the couple was his wife's "obsession about alcohol." He attributed his wife's concerns about his drinking to her relatively recent involvement with a local church group whose members were strongly in favor of abstinence from alcohol. At the end of the first session both partners were adamant that the other person had to change. Under these circumstances, doing a general assessment of the relationship seemed inappropriate. Instead, it was agreed that I would meet twice with the man to do a careful assessment of his drinking and then feed back to the couple the results of that assessment.

ASSIGNING FURTHER ASSESSMENT TASKS

Toward the end of the session I underscore the importance of assessment and my intention to continue assessment and then to provide a feedback session on the results of that assessment. I usually then provide the couple with further assessment tasks to do during the week. These tasks typically include the filling out of appropriate self-report inventories, which were described earlier in Table 4.4.

The assessment tasks I ask the couple to complete between sessions 1 and 2 are selected on the basis of three key considerations. First, in this early phase of therapy I am trying to get an overview of the relationship issues that most frequently are a source of concern to couples. Therefore, in addition to finishing the DAS and ACQ if they are incomplete, I typically ask partners to complete the Marital Status Inventory (MSI; Weiss & Cerreto, 1990) and the DASS (Lovibond & Lovibond, 1995) between the first and second sessions. The MSI assesses steps taken toward separation and divorce and provides convergent evidence with the partners' verbal reports on dissolution potential within the relationship. The DASS is a 21-item inventory providing scores on anxiety, depression, and stress. It provides evidence on the presence of individual psychopathology or extreme distress in either partner.

A second consideration in selecting assessment tasks for couples to complete is the key relationship concerns identified in the individual and conjoint interviews. For example, if alcohol consumption in one partner was identified as an issue, I might ask the couple to complete the Alcohol Use Disorders Identification Test (AUDIT; Saunders, Aasland, Babor, de La Fuente, & Grant, 1993). This is a 12-item screening instrument designed to quantify the level of drinking problems.

The third consideration is the likelihood that the couple will complete the assigned tasks. There is a risk that if too many tasks are assigned; then the couple perceives therapy as an additional burden rather than a source of relief from their relationship problems. Having the couple complete the DAS and ACQ during the initial session allows the therapist to assess the level of reading and writing skills of the partners. Partners who successfully complete both inventories in 25 minutes are likely to find completing other inventories less time-consuming than people who do not complete the inventories.

DEVELOPING COMMITMENT TO BEING ACTIVE IN THERAPY

The things that occur in the therapy session are only important to the extent that they bring about change in the day-to-day adaptive processes of the couple. The assignments between sessions are the crucial attempts to help the couple try new ways of relating. By the end of the first session I want to establish an expectation for the couple that they will work at their relationship between sessions. I might introduce the importance of between-session tasks as follows:

> "The approach I take to couple therapy focuses upon you trying to change how you relate on a day-to-day basis. To help you experiment with new ways of relating, I will suggest various tasks between sessions. This speeds up what we can get through.
>
> I suggest you each fill in a couple of forms for me between now and the next session. Let me tell you what they are about. If, after I explain them, you do not think that filling them in is a good idea, please tell me. It could be I am off track, and if so it is important I know that. Or it could be that I just have not explained why I think the forms are important well enough. Again, it is good if I know that. I will ask you to do things quite often, and I really want to make sure that, right from the start, you can tell me honestly if what I am suggesting makes sense to you. I will check whenever I suggest something whether you are willing to try my suggestion. If you don't want to try it I would like to talk about that. If you agree, I would ask that you make the effort and get it done. Couple therapy is quite a bit of effort; but I think that if you put in the effort you will find it very rewarding. OK?"

The foregoing statement is specifically designed to encourage the clients to give feedback to the therapist. At the same time it is meant to promote positive expectations for completion of therapeutic tasks. As assessments assigned for completion between the first and second sessions usually are the first assigned tasks, it is important to maximize the chance that the tasks are completed and are found useful by the couple. To that end it is helpful to explain clearly the purpose of the assessment instruments being given to the couple. The couple should be given the opportunity to ask any questions about exactly what is required. It also is important to check that both partners perceive the assigned task(s) as relevant to their needs. As a check on the commitment to being active in therapy I ask each partner to make a clear statement that he or she is prepared to complete the tasks. In the final part of the initial session the therapist should seek to summarize the agreements which have been reached between the couple and the therapist at the end of that session. A typical closing summary from an initial intake interview might go something like the one that follows.

"Well, I have spoken to you individually, and we tried to summarize all that material back together now. I think we all understand that some key concerns that the two of you have are about your ability to manage conflict effectively, arguments often seem to get out of hand. In addition, both of you have described how you don't spend much quality time together. That, since the birth of your children you have spent less time together that's fun, and that this has significantly eroded your relationship. John and Andrea, you both highlighted that you have considerable commitment to try to make this relationship work. This is both because each of you has a considerable amount of time and relationship history together, and you are also concerned about what a separation might do to your children. It's clear that there are still some very strong positive feelings between the two of you. I noted throughout the session that at different times you smiled and looked at each other in a special way, and each of you has mentioned how much the other person means to them.

"We have agreed that over the next week each of you is going to keep the self-monitoring diary to try to track the good, and not so good, things that happen between the two of you. I have also asked you to fill out a form looking at the way that you manage conflict. In the next session I want to collect the forms from you, ask some more questions to fill in the gaps, and review your diaries with you. I hope that in either the third or fourth sessions, depending on how far we get, I will be able to summarize that information and feed it back to you.

"I also understand that each of you has some ambivalence about the relationship. On the one hand you would like it to work, but there have been a lot of things that have gone wrong in the last few months, and you are not sure if the damage can be repaired. One of our goals in discussing the assessment data would be to look at what would be needed in order to make the relationship more how each of you would like it, and how realistic it seems to each of you that you will be able to produce that change."

In general, determining the goals and the process of therapy occurs across a number of sessions. A crucial function of the initial session is to decide whether there will be a second interview. A second interview is useful if the partners are still open to the possibility of rebuilding their relationship, and if some common ground can be found in their perceptions of the relationship problems in the first session. I would not conduct a second conjoint interview if either partner has expressed a clear intention of permanently leaving the relationship, unless the couple requests mediation for their separation.

Structuring Successful Conjoint Interviews

A conjoint interview is not a particularly efficient or reliable method of gathering data. Information that is collected conjointly seems to be less reliable than do data that are collected by individual interview or self-report inventories (Haynes et al., 1981). In fact, if the sole purpose of conjoint interviews were to collect factual information, then conjoint interviews might be entirely replaced by individual interviews or the use of various self-report inventories. However, conjoint interviews are important in at least three ways. First, conjoint sessions allow the therapist to build a shared understanding with the couple by summarizing concerns raised in individual interviews or self-report measures. Second, they allow the therapist to explore positive aspects of the couple's relationship that distressed partners often overlook. Third, conjoint sessions allow the therapist to observe the partners interact.

Building a Shared Understanding of Relationship Problems

Building a shared understanding of relationship problems with both partners can be difficult in the conjoint interview given that the distressed partners often express concerns in hostile and critical forms. Individual interviews in which empathy is established separately with each partner often help, as this can allow the therapist and individual to develop ways of expressing relationship concerns that are likely to be acceptable to both partners. The therapist can promote positive expression of relationship concerns through individual interviews in numerous ways.

First, the therapist can promote use of descriptions of behavior and responses to that behavior in place of pejorative labels. For example, phrases such as "She is too emotional" or "He is a drunk" can be followed up with questions on exactly what behaviors occur and how the person feels in response to that behavior. This might lead to a more specific statement such as "When your wife gets upset and cries, you feel really uncomfortable, and do not know how to react." If the individual agrees that this as an accurate summary of the concern, the therapist or client can reflect the concern in these specific behavioral terms in a conjoint session.

Second, many relationship concerns reflect positive motives. For example, a complaint that a spouse does not express feelings usually reflects a desire to relate better to that spouse, and a complaint about excessive drinking usually reflects concern about the effect of the drinking on the health of the spouse and the relationship. The therapist can draw out these positive motives in the individual interviews (e.g., such questions as "If your partner did express feelings more, how would that be helpful for you?" or "What worries you most about the drinking?"). Once the positive motives underlying concerns are identified, the statements of concern in the individual and conjoint sessions can incorporate these aspects of the problem. For example, the desire to have greater partner expression of feelings might be introduced by "Understanding how John feels is really important to you, so. . . . "

Several strategies can be used in the conjoint sessions that also help to develop a shared understanding of relationship problems. One useful strategy to increase the likelihood of one partner's reports about relationship problems being interpreted constructively by the spouse is to emphasize the emotions being expressed rather than criticism or attacks on the spouse. Second, the therapist needs to ensure that the reflection places ownership of the feeling with the client. Consider the following discussion between the therapist and Nancy.

NANCY: I hate it when Andre leaves after an argument, it's so stupid. He feels I am disposable, he is so focused on his needs, he's so selfish . . . he thinks I only need a bit of attention every now and then . . . so I get a pat on the head. I am not really part, not central to his life.

THERAPIST: So, when Andre leaves you feel unimportant, unloved by him?

In the reflection the therapist leaves out the attack against Andre and the pejorative attributions made about him. Instead the therapist focuses on the feeling being expressed. Emotion-focused therapy (EFT; Greenberg & Johnson, 1988) distinguishes between primary and secondary emotions. Secondary emotions are described as "hot" emotions such as anger and disgust. Primary emotions are "cooler" emotions such as fear and a sense of vulnerability or potential loss. In the foregoing reflection the therapist reflects the primary emotion of a fear of not being loved rather than the secondary emotion of anger. It is often easier for spouses to empathize with this focus on primary emotions than with the secondary emotion of anger toward them. Thus the therapist is being empathic, but selectively empathic to emotion, and in particular primary emotion. In a subsequent conjoint interview with Andre and Nancy, Nancy's concerns were expressed in terms of this primary emotion.

In conjoint interviews several related strategies help to focus couples on constructive ways of expressing their relationship concerns. One strategy is to reframe relationship complaints in terms of relationship processes. For example, suppose one partner complains about lack of shared time together and the other partner complains of being pressured to spend all her free time together as a couple, without any individual space. This pair of complaints can be reflected thus: "As a couple you find it hard to agree on the balance of time together and independent time. Neither of you is happy with the current balance."

Another useful strategy in conjoint sessions that promotes couple's ability to work together in describing negative aspects of the relationship is the "universal truth" (Weiss & Halford, 1996). The universal truth relies on posing seemingly unchallengeable truths and presuming the couple will attempt to answer conjointly, focusing on their relationship successes and identifying their relationship failures. For example, the therapist can state: "All couples need to be able to resolve conflict effectively. In what ways do you two do that?" Other examples of universal truths include the following: all couples need to show affection to each other, to introduce novelty into their relationship, to accommodate to differences in personality between partners, to do fun things together, to sort out parenting responsibilities, to manage their time to have a balance of independent and couple activities, or to make their sex lives interesting. Posing challenges in the form of universal truths to couples in the initial phase of therapy also allows the therapist to assess the partners' openness to new ways of looking at their problems.

Often use of the foregoing strategies does allow couples to start to explore their relationship problems conjointly in a constructive manner. However, one must be careful about overgeneralizing observed interaction within therapy to other settings. The sudden shift a couple might show from a partner blaming to a conjoint focus in response to the challenge of a universal truth does not mean the couple's way of thinking or behaving in response to each other has shifted at home. However, these initial observations of interaction do allow the therapist to evaluate the ability of couples to collaborate in defining their relationship problems. This is an important step toward having the partners self-appraise their personal contributions to these problems and ultimately to self-direct change to address these problems.

Exploring Positive Aspects of the Relationship

Many distressed couples find that their problems and conflict dominate their experience of their relationship. In the context of couple therapy many distressed couples focus all their attention on the negativity in the relationship and seek only to reduce that level of negativity. An inordinate focus on negativity is unfortunate for several reasons. First, reviewing and discussing the relationship only in terms of problems can be discouraging for the couple. The motivation to enhance the relationship, or even to remain in the relationship, can be severely undermined. On the other hand, helping the partners focus on the good aspects of their relationship often strengthens the sense of commitment to change. Second, a relationship may become more tolerable by reducing negativity, but that really does not make for a great relationship. People rarely report that they see a great relationship as one in which there are few problems and little conflict. Rather, most couples seek positive relationship attributes such as intimacy, companionship, support, and shared positive times. For couple therapy to help develop strong, positive relationships, it needs to address how to strengthen positive aspects of the couple relationship.

The therapist needs to prompt attention to positive aspects of the couple relationship, and to explore the importance of positivity with the couple. This can be done in many ways. For example, I usually ask the couple in the second or third session to describe the development of their relationship. This exploration is focused on what attracted the partners to each other, what led them to become committed to their spouse, and what the major positive qualities are that have led them to stay in the relationship over time. In the selection of self-report inventories, self-monitoring, and behavioral observation tasks I choose procedures that assess positive aspects of the relationship and review these in conjoint sessions. For example, I routinely ask the couple to do a positive reminiscence task in which they talk about positive times in the relationship. (Chapter 5 provides more detail on how to do these procedures.)

Given the negative biases in distressed partners' recall of relationship interaction (Osgarby & Halford, 2000b), seemingly neutral questions often solicit a list of negative experiences. Perhaps the most crucial example of this is a question many therapists ask at the beginning of sessions along the lines of the following: "How has the last week been?" Distressed partners typically respond with a predominance of negative comments about the partner and the relationship and ignore positive aspects of the relationship (Osgarby & Halford, 2000b). For that reason, I explicitly state that I need to know about both the good and bad things that happen in the relationship. When reviewing a couple's week I would say something like the following. "I am wondering about the good and bad things for you two in the last week. Let's start with the positives, what have been the best things about what has been happening for you two in the last week?"

Exploring the positive aspects of the relationship in the conjoint interviews helps to shift the partners' relationship self-appraisals. The common problem of distressed partners focusing only on the negative is challenged by providing a balance of attention to relationship positives. Over time, if the process is working, neutral questions such as "How has your week been?" should elicit a balanced report of relationship positives and relationship problems.

Observing Couple Interaction

The presence of both partners in the room allows the therapist to observe couple interaction directly. It is important that the therapist provide therapeutic tasks that allow assessment of relevant interaction. For example, I often pose couples a conjoint question such as the following: "What do the two of you see as the major changes you need to make to let you have the relationship you want?" My interest in posing such a question is rather less on the specific content of the answer and rather more on the process by which the couple jointly attempts to answer the question. For example, do the two partners look to each other and give each person an opportunity to respond? Is there any evidence of interpersonal warmth in the way that they interact?

The therapy setting clearly is different from the settings in which couples normally interact, such as in their home. Settings influence how couples interact (Halford et al., 1992), and it is a mistake to assume that what the therapist observes in the therapy setting necessarily reflects couple interaction in other settings. However, it is possible from observations in the therapy setting to develop hypotheses about couple interaction that can be explored with the couple. For example, when I posed the question in the previous paragraph to one couple the two partners looked at each other, then the woman began a detailed description of the changes she thought the man needed to make. As she spoke, the man looked out the window and sighed. I asked the couple to pause, described what each of them was doing, and asked them if this pattern ever happened at home. Both partners agreed that the woman did much more of the talking when they were discussing their relationship, and that she often felt frustrated by his relative silence. They also agreed that the man tended to withdraw and feel criticized by his partner's talk. The process of observing couple interaction and exploring this with the couple assists self-appraisal of the relationship. It prompts the partners to attend to their patterns of interaction as those patterns are occurring.

When Assessment Reveals Relationship Crises

There are a variety of common crises that can have a dramatic impact on relationships. Some crises reflect chronic disorganized, chaotic, and ineffective coping patterns. Other times a single event precipitates a crisis. For example, one of the most common events precipitating a crisis within relationships is the discovery of an affair. For the therapist, responding to crises often poses particular challenges in managing effective therapy.

General Crises

Some people seem to live their lives in a state of continual crisis, and difficulties in their relationship seem to reflect these more general problems. For example, when Dave and Samantha presented to me they were in the midst of multiple crises. They had three children under 6 years of age, they had little money, Dave had recently lost his job, and they were living in a trailer park in a 16-foot-long, single-room trailer. About once a month Dave would go on a drinking binge and disappear for 2 to 3 days at a time. Samantha felt overwhelmed by parenting, her 3-year-old son was throwing lots of tantrums, and she had lost her temper and hit him on two occasions in the past few weeks. Samantha had developed a habit of spending money on a credit card and had run up a debt of over $5,000, and they had no money to pay that debt or to buy food. The immediate precipitant for the presentation had occurred 2 days previously when Dave had arrived home after a drinking binge that had lasted 3 days. Samantha and Dave had gotten into a loud, vicious argument, the children had been crying, and the owner of the trailer park had threatened to evict them. They also received a demand notice from a debt collection agency for the money owed on credit cards.

On presentation Dave and Samantha were both extremely haggard looking and reported having slept little for the last 2 nights. After I had written down the key points in their presenting problems, it was clear that this was a crisis intervention. The couple rapidly listed a seemingly endless number of pressing concerns that needed attention, including ensuring the safety of their children, trying to ensure they had somewhere to live, and making sure they had enough food on the table for them and their children. Other important issues were to reassess their finances and develop a means of controlling their spiral into poverty, developing parenting skills, and controlling Dave's drinking. They also mentioned the need to decide whether they were to stay together and possibly rebuild their relationship.

In common with many approaches to crisis management, I talked through with Dave and Samantha what the most important immediate things to do were. We agreed that providing the children with a comfortable and safe environment was the first step. It was agreed that Samantha was to ask her mother to have the children stay with her for the next week. Dave contracted not to drink any alcohol for the next week and to review his drinking and set more long-term goals in the next session. Samantha agreed to cut her credit card in half so she would not run up any more debts. They also agreed that having a few days together without the children would enable them to get some sleep, which might allow them to problem-solve other issues.

Dave and Samantha's presentation was extreme in that multiple things were going wrong for them at once. However, the general approach taken is illustrative of how I respond to crises. The first step is to provide empathic support for the stresses experienced and then to identify the most pressing issue. The focus must be on what needs immediate attention, and the first therapy session helps the partners to work out concrete steps to be taken to solve those problems, or at least to reduce the immediate impact of those pressing problems. These considerations take priority over the usual structure of the therapy.

Managing Disclosed Abuse or Violence

Once detected, spousal abuse is difficult to manage well, particularly if the abuse is severe and there is some present danger to a partner. Although I am keen to preserve an open relationship with both partners, I will compromise this view if I believe there is current danger to one person. Relationship violence usually has a particularly negative impact on women. While violence in couples seeking couple therapy often involves equal rates of male-to-female and female-to-male violence, women are much more likely than men to be physically injured (Cascardi et al., 1992). Furthermore, women are much more likely than men to report feeling psychologically intimidated and to have other negative psychological effects from relationship violence (Cascardi et al., 1992). Hence, in assessing the couple's problems it is important to attend to the potential gender differences in the meaning and consequences of violence within the relationship. In particular, if a male partner is reported by the woman to be threatening violence and has been violent before, the safety of the woman becomes the priority in the session.

In my experience, presentation for couple therapy when the male partner is extremely violent is unusual. I suspect that violent men generally are reluctant to seek relationship therapy. However, when significant violence is part of the presentation, it is important to develop a safety plan to protect the victim. On occasion I have seen couples in which the woman reports in an individual interview that she currently is fearful of her partner. Some women have realistic fears that their husband will seek physically to prevent them from leaving the relationship, or will seek reprisal after they leave. It is important to recognize that some males do escalate violence when their partners attempt to leave, and the therapist has a duty of care to minimize that risk. Let me illustrate how I handle that situation with an example of one woman who reported significant abuse by her partner.

THERAPIST: Noela, let's summarize what you've told me. Ray has beaten you up on three occasions in the last few months, once you were so badly bruised and cut up you had to go to hospital. He has threatened you many other times, and is frequently rude and verbally abusive toward you. I would guess that having all that happen, you must have thought about leaving. Have you?

NOELA: Are you sure he cannot hear us in here?

THERAPIST: I am sure. We specially designed the rooms so they are sound proof. See the heavy rubber liner around the frame? That stops sound leaking out. Are you scared of what might happen if he hears what you have to say?

NOELA: (*sobbing*) Yeah ... I am scared of him ... Last week he said he would find me if I ever left. I ... it's confusing ... I still love him in some ways. I would like it to work out with Ray, but I am ... so angry with him. ...

THERAPIST: Noela, given all you've said about what has happened to you, I think being afraid is smart. He has hurt you, he has threatened you, and he might well try to hurt you again if you let him know you are leaving. No one has the right to make you live in fear in your own home, to beat you. Do you want to leave?

NOELA: I want to be safe. I want not to be afraid any more. But I have nowhere to go ... my family is 1,000 miles away. And it's not just the physical stuff, I probably could bear a slap or two every now and then ... it's the names he calls me, how hateful he is. I feel unclean when he talks to me.

THERAPIST: Let me put a suggestion to you. I am writing a telephone number on this card. It is a 24-hour crisis care number. If you ring that at any time they will send a taxi to pick you up and take you to a shelter. They will provide you with legal advice, give you somewhere to stay till you work out what you want to do. Ray would not be able to find you; the addresses of the shelters are kept secret.

NOELA: But if I told him I was going he would explode ...

THERAPIST: You do not have to tell him. I think you are right, he might well get nasty if you say you are leaving. When he is at work you could ring these people up, pack up your things and you need never see him again if you don't want to.

NOELA: Hmmm. I am not sure I can just walk out, never see him ... we've been together 3 years.

THERAPIST: Of course it up to you how you do this. You could tell him before you go; though he might get nasty then. Or, you could ring him after you leave. If you wanted to continue with couple therapy, I would be open to that if Ray was.

NOELA: Do you think there is any hope for us?

THERAPIST: Noela, I really cannot be sure about that. Clearly, if it is to work between you two Ray has to learn to control his temper. He has to allow you to feel safe again. It might be that he would work hard at that if you were gone, or he might just refuse to have anything to do with therapy then. Let's write down and talk through your options.

In the transcript I illustrate trying to establish the current views of my client about the issue of leaving her partner. I attempt to reassure her that I think her evaluation of risk is realistic. Some people believe they are exaggerating the risks, though it is actually is more common for people to underestimate the danger from their partners. It may be necessary to discuss with them that partners can be violent in the face of threatened separation.

The provision of an emergency telephone number is an important step. Most cities in Western countries have domestic violence shelters. This provides an escape for women at any time if they need it. Even if the woman resolves not to leave in the immediate future, she may want to change her mind if there is another episode of violence. The numbers and suggestions about how to proceed allow her to get out at a time of her choosing. Some women may prefer when they leave to be with someone they know, though there is the real risk that the men will look for them there. A careful assessment of the risks needs to be taken. (For example, have you ever left before? Has he threatened to follow you? Does he check on your whereabouts when you are apart? Does the man have a gun or other weapon? Has he threatened or actually used that weapon? How frequent and severe was the violence in the past? What threats have been made? Would he be likely to know that you would go to that friend's house?) Ultimately the woman should leave the session with an agreed-on plan on how to leave if she chooses to leave.

The possibility of seeking a restraining order should be raised with the client if the danger seems severe, and then referral for legal advice is needed. Many legal jurisdictions within Western countries have stalking laws. That is, an individual can take out a complaint against someone who follows, harasses, or threatens him or her. Often courts will institute a restraining order preventing the person from approaching or making contact with the victim.

In the same session as the foregoing transcript, the therapist and Noela identified four options that Noela was willing to consider. The options were (1) to leave immediately without telling Ray and never contact him again, (2) to leave immediately and tell him later that she wanted Ray to go to individual therapy to control his anger, (3) to leave immediately and tell Ray later she wanted them to continue in couple therapy with a focus on anger management for Ray and Noela (Noela had reported that she often got angry and was verbally abusive toward Ray), or (4) to stay where she was and continue with couple therapy. Advantages and disadvantages of each option were discussed, and Noela opted not to leave at the time and continue with couple therapy. It was agreed that the therapist would raise the issue of violence with Ray in an individual interview with him. If he was open to anger control being a key focus of therapy, then couple therapy could proceed. It also was agreed that the therapist would not disclose to Ray that Noela had reported the occurrence of violence or that she was actively considering separation. It transpired that Ray did hit Noela again about 2 weeks later and she left the next morning. She terminated the relationship with Ray at that point.

Affairs

When the occurrence of an affair by one partner is reported to the therapist in confidence, I believe the therapist must respect that confidence. If the therapist breaches such a confidence it is likely to shatter the therapeutic relationship, which then is unlikely to be of benefit to anyone. If one partner confides to me that he or she had an affair in the past that the spouse does not know about, I would not feel the need to tell the other spouse. It has been my experience that disclosing about a past affair often is extremely distressing to the spouse and may have little positive benefit. However, it is important that the partner who had the affair works in a committed manner to enhance the relationship and does not engage in any extrarelationship affairs during the course of therapy.

If one partner reports currently having an affair that the spouse does not know about, I think that is an issue that has to be addressed before therapy proceeds. I think it is untenable for therapists to work with a couple when they are withholding such important information from one of the partners. In the individual interview with the partner having the affair I express the view that couple therapy is unlikely to work while the person is trying to maintain two relationships. I suggest that he or she end, or at least suspend, seeing the other person while therapy proceeds. If the person refuses to end or suspend the affair (this is rare in my experience), I decline to conduct conjoint therapy. I still do not report the affair to the spouse. However, I do say to the partner having the affair that I will tell the spouse that couple therapy will not be proceeding, and it will be up to the partner having the affair to explain to his or her spouse. I suggest that the couple talk about it later to give the partner who has decided to continue with the affair time to reflect on what he or she wishes to say to the spouse.

There has been limited research on the impact of affairs on committed relationships. The research that has been done suggests that the majority of people experience the discovery of an affair by their partner as a traumatic event (Glass & Wright, 1997). For some spouses the discovery of an affair immediately initiates termination of the relationship. Some people simply will not tolerate their partner having an extra relationship. In other instances, the relationship may be in a state of great crisis, and I have seen many couples who have presented for therapy at this point.

There has not been any systematic evaluation of the psychological interventions to help people recover from the discovery of infidelity. However, there have been a number of clinical reports of interventions, and these often provide useful guidelines for how to work with a couple when one of the partners has had an affair. Glass and Wright (1997) suggested a number of steps in rebuilding a relationship after the discovery of an affair. I have found them to be useful guidelines when working with couples. However, I add an initial step of crisis management that I will describe before discussing the Glass and Wright steps.

CRISIS MANAGEMENT AFTER AN AFFAIR

Some people have a traumatic reaction when they discover infidelity by their partner. For example, I have seen partners become extremely depressed, suffer rage outbursts, and have difficulty sleeping. This combination of events may lead a person to feel so severely distressed that he or she finds everyday functioning quite difficult. This severe stress reaction often makes it difficult for the person to engage in the usual problem-solving strategies associated with therapy. As is the case for general crises, the therapist may need to identify the most pressing problems and provide concrete steps for management. In some individuals the response to their discovery of the affair is so traumatic that it is similar to posttraumatic stress disorder. People may have recurrent intrusive images of their partner having sex with the other person, find it difficult to think of anything else, and report psychic numbing.

The factors that influence extreme responses to the discovery of an affair are multiple. It seems that people who have poor preexisting psychological adjustment, particularly with some susceptibility to anxiety disorders or depression, show more extreme responses to the discovery of infidelity. If the discovery of the infidelity is particularly graphic (e.g., walking in on one's partner having sex with someone else), it probably is more traumatic for an individual than simply having the affair described to him or her. Some people discover infidelity through the reports of a third person, such as a well-meaning friend or neighbor. For some individuals the sense that other people knew about the affair when they did not is particularly distressing. A final issue is the quality of the relationship itself prior to the discovery of the affair. If it has been a severely distressed relationship in which the person was contemplating separation, the discovery of an affair may not be a particularly difficult event to deal with. On the other hand, if the individual believed that the relationship was entirely satisfactory, the affair may shatter his or her assumptions and beliefs about a satisfying relationship, which can be very destabilizing.

ESTABLISHING SAFETY IN THE RELATIONSHIP

Once the most pressing crisis management has been attended to, the next step is to reestablish a climate of safety within the relationship. Often this involves some relationship psychoeducation describing some of the points I have made in the foregoing paragraphs about the impact of affairs on relationships. It is important to spell out the need to gradually reestablish trust and to point out that many couples overcome the effects of an affair.

An important part of the recovery process is breaking contact with the extrarelationship partner. This needs to be done clearly, so that the partners in the existing relationship both know that the other relationship has been terminated. To reassure the spouse that the extra partner is no longer being seen, one partner may need to agree to change his or her daily routines. For example, if the affair took place with someone at work, the partner may need to seriously consider changing jobs, or at least changing work routines within the job, so that there is no ongoing contact with the affair partner. Agreeing to make a public statement that the relationship is over, so that there can be no misunderstanding, is important.

Another element in this initial phase is to hear and validate the wounded partner's experience. This means allowing the spouse to express the pain and anger that often are felt and to have the offending spouse hear and accept the expression of those feelings.

EXPLORING THE AFFAIR

Some partners who have had an affair would prefer that it was simply put behind them. I have often had people express the desire that their partner would simply "forget about it." This can be particularly difficult for people to do. One important step that seems useful is to ensure that the person who had the affair has self-disclosed as completely as his or her spouse requires.

Exploring the affair needs to be done carefully. I find it useful to stress the importance of reestablishing trust by dissolving any secrets that have occurred. I suggest a ground rule that the spouse can ask any question he or she wishes about the affair and the partner agrees to answer the question completely and honestly. Affairs almost always involve some degree of deceiving one's partner. If trust is to be reestablished, any pretense or deception has to be overcome. I set up the session with Tanya and Paul in the following manner:

THERAPIST: It does seem important if you two are to reestablish your relationship, which each of you has said you want to do, that the trust is rebuilt. In order to have an affair, it is necessary, to some extent, to mislead your partner . . . to implicitly at least pretend that nothing much is going on when in fact you are having an affair with someone else. For that reason, I think that it is very important, Paul, that Tanya have the opportunity to find out anything that she feels that she needs to know about the affair that you had. Would you be willing to answer all of her questions in this session?

PAUL: I am worried about this, we have talked and talked about the affair. Tanya drives me crazy always wanting to know more details. I just feel like I will never escape from the affair.

THERAPIST: So, Paul, you feel that you have talked and talked and talked about this, and you are wondering if more talking will help. Tanya, do you feel that there are things about the affair that you really still need to know?

TANYA: I do. Paul has not told me the truth about what happened. He denied that it was going on when I started to feel that there was something wrong. When I found out that he had been spending a lot of time with this other woman, I actually asked him straight out and he denied it. Then he said that he did have feelings for her but that he hadn't actually had sex with her, and when I pushed him further then eventually after a few weeks he did admit that he had been having sex with her. Then he told me that he had stopped seeing her entirely, and then I walked around to a local cafe, and saw them having lunch together. So, I feel like he has just never really come clean with me. Given that he lied to me so much before, I find it really difficult to believe I can trust him now.

THERAPIST: So, the fact that Paul told you one thing, and then you found out something different had happened, and that you kept pushing and finding out more each time you pushed makes you feel it's difficult to trust Paul?

TANYA: Yes, it's very hard to trust.

THERAPIST: Paul, you have heard how Tanya says it is difficult for her to feel trust in you. I guess my sense is that if you really do open up to her about anything she might want to know, that would be a start. What do you think?

PAUL: Look, the affair was wrong. I'm sorry that I hurt Tanya. Really sorry. And if it will help to talk all of this out once and for all, fine. I didn't tell her all the stuff at the time, because I thought that . . . well the more that I told her the more that I thought she'd be hurt. . . . I didn't want to hurt her. Maybe I was wrong, wrong to protect her . . . that was just how I thought at the time.

THERAPIST: OK, so let me check. Paul are you willing to answer any of the questions that Tanya might ask you about the affair that you had? Any of the questions?

PAUL: Yes. I really want this to work with Tanya, and I will tell her whatever she needs to know. I think I have told her everything, but I am happy to go over anything.

THERAPIST: Excellent, thank you very much Paul. Tanya, just before we get to questions, I have a couple of suggestions for you.

TANYA: Suggestions?

THERAPIST: Yes. I think that you should feel free to ask any questions that you want. It is important that you feel anything that you need to know, you can find out. At the same time, I would caution you that there may be some things that you could ask but that may be unhelpful. In particular, it has been my experience that if people ask for very explicit details about sex, that is not always very helpful. Sometimes people will find images coming into their mind once the details are provided, and that really does not help. So, you might want to think about what is important. The other thing is that sometimes people really can't remember certain fine details. How often exactly you saw the person, if the affair had been going on for some time, can be difficult. Think for yourself. If I had asked you how often you'd seen Paul over the last month, it might be kind of difficult to piece together exactly how often. You might know it's most days except when he is traveling with work. But if you have to remember exactly whether he was there on a given Saturday, how much time you spent together the week before last, it might be difficult. My point is just that you may ask for levels of detail that sometimes the person can't answer. Any comments or reactions to what I have said?

TANYA: No, I accept what you say about the explicitness of the sex. All I want is that Paul tell me what he can generally remember, that would satisfy me.

At this point I then invited Tanya to pose any questions to Paul that she liked. An interesting thing happened in this particular case. Tanya reported that there were in fact no further questions she wished to ask him. She realized that it was the pressure that she had had to exert previously to elicit details that made her suspicious that Paul was being dishonest with her. Once Paul had genuinely stated a willingness to tell her whatever she needed to know, she was reassured that there were no other important things she needed to find out. This change often is crucial in my experience. The intent of exploring the details of the affair itself is to reestablish the trust between the partners—to remove the deceptions that allowed the affair to develop and continue.

COGNITIVE AND EMOTIONAL CHANGE ABOUT THE AFFAIR

In the process of exploring the events of the affair both partners are likely to bring up beliefs about the affair, and its meaning. Some of the cognitions about the affair may not be helpful. For example, the spouse having the affair may attribute blame to his or her partner for causing the affair. For example, some people assert that "she never gave me love" or "he was not interested in me sexually any more" as reasons for the affair. These blaming attributions do point to aspects of the relationship that may need attention. The therapist needs to reframe these areas of the relationship as goals for later therapy sessions.

For the partner whose spouse had an affair, the affair often raises a variety of difficult issues. Many people wonder whether they are inadequate as a spouse (e.g., "he would never have had the affair if I was a good wife"). Other people wonder whether their spouse is intrinsically untrustworthy and will repeat the affair. For most people the fact that their partner had an affair shatters many of their assumptions about their relationship. In the context of these confusing thoughts and feelings, the therapist needs to help each partner develop adaptive cognitions about the meaning and significance of the affair. The guided exploration process can be used to help the partner identify and challenge unhelpful cognitions.

Strong emotional responses to the discovery of an affair are usual. Sometimes the discussion of the affair and associated emotions, combined with identification and challenging of unhelpful cognitions, is sufficient to ease hurt and anger. Other times a more specific focus on changing negative affect is needed. One strategy I have found useful in this context is the notion of controlled affect expression. Controlled affect expression involves the distressed partner expressing his or her feelings within a specific controlled setting in which continued pain expression is not reinforced, and where escape from the feelings is prevented. The principle guiding my use of this procedure is extinction of negative affect through repeated expression of that affect in the absence of reinforcement. Many people find that the expression of the affect associated with an affair by their partner is painful. Often they begin to think and feel things about the affair and then switch off those thoughts and feelings. For example, partners may distract themselves by watching television, by doing something, by getting angry with the spouse, or by starting arguments. I believe this escape often negatively reinforces the affect and prevents extinction of the strong feelings.

To allow extinction of intense negative feelings I encourage the person to express those feelings. I try to structure the expression of feelings so that neither reinforcement nor escape is likely. This usually involves the individual expressing the feelings to me in the therapy session. I may have the spouse present, but in this case it is important that the spouse not respond to the affect expression by his or her partner. I also often get people to express their feelings privately without an audience (e.g., by writing a letter about what is experienced and then reading the letter to themselves repeatedly).

REBUILDING THE RELATIONSHIP

Sometimes one or other partner will not want to continue in the relationship. The sense of crisis and anger may abate; the partners may have forgiven each other for what has happened but still feel the relationship is not one they wish to continue. When this is the case, the therapist may still provide useful assistance to the couple by helping them learn from what has happened. That learning may strengthen them as individuals and perhaps allow them to enter subsequent relationships with fewer difficulties.

If the disclosure about the affair is successfully resolved and the couple wishes to continue together, often there is a need to attend more broadly to the relationship. Sometimes affairs occur in relationships because the relationship has significant difficulties. Poor communication, poor sex, and a lack of excitement and interest in the relationship can often make an affair much more attractive. It is important to consider, therefore, the circumstances under which the affair arose. Were there things that seemed to be missing from the relationship which need to be rebuilt? Such consideration then leads back to standard assessment for couple therapy.

5

Assessment, Part II:
Second and Any
Subsequent Sessions

This chapter begins with an overview of the content and structure of the second assessment session. If further assessment sessions are required, they can follow this same format. A review follows of how to interpret the initial assessment findings. Included is a description of additional assessment tasks that are useful with some couples. As mentioned in Chapter 4, a key task in assessment is to find common ground between the partners. Toward the end of this chapter I discuss common themes that emerge during assessment for couple therapy. I suggest how to manage the assessment process with those often challenging presentations. Finally, I describe how to determine when to conclude assessment.

Structure and Content of Second and Any Subsequent Assessment Sessions

Table 5.1 provides a summary of the structure of second and any subsequent assessment sessions. As outlined in the table, the second and subsequent assessment sessions almost always begin with a review of what has been covered so far and negotiation of an agenda. These sessions always end with negotiation of tasks to be completed between sessions. The main body of the

TABLE 5.1. Structure of Second and Any Subsequent Assessment Sessions

Content	Goals
Initial orientation	Review what has been covered thus far and negotiate session agenda
Further individual interviews	Gather further information not completed in Session 1
Conjoint sessions	Develop shared understanding of relationship
Review results of self-report assessments	
Summarize key relationship concerns	
Behavioral tasks	Observational assessment of couple interaction
Closure	Summarize progress to this point
Negotiate any assessment tasks to be completed before next session	

session is usually a combination of three different segments. First, the therapist conducts further individual consultations to complete discussion of the areas described in Table 4.5. While the therapist conducts individual consultations with one partner, the spouse usually completes additional self-report inventories (the specific inventories are described later in this chapter). Second, the therapist discusses with the couple the context and life events that may influence the couple's relationship and clarifies and summarizes issues raised in individual consultations and by completed assessment tasks. Third, the couple often does specific behavioral assessment tasks in session, such as a communication task. Between sessions the therapist needs to spend some time reviewing completed assessments.

As noted in Chapter 4, couples usually are asked to complete two self-report inventories in the first assessment session (the Dyadic Adjustment Scale and the Areas of Change Questionnaire), and further assessment tasks usually are suggested for completion between sessions. It is important to collect the completed inventories from the couple early in the session. I make a point of thanking the partners and restating how valuable the information from the inventories usually proves to be in couple therapy. (If the inventories were not completed I would follow the procedure described in Chapter 3 for responding to failure to complete agreed tasks.)

In session, I usually scan the inventories as I collect them. (I describe what to look for in each of the key assessment measures later in the chapter.) I note out loud any major issues that have been identified previously that also are evident in this assessment. I also note any new issues that have not yet been explored in sessions and then ask the partner(s) to say a little bit about their perspectives on this issue. (I make two exceptions to this process: If violence or affairs are first reported in assessment tasks, I explore these issues in individual consultations.)

Across the course of assessment the proportion of sessions spent in individual consultations usually decreases once individual concerns have been explored. The proportion of time spent in conjoint consultations usually increases as the couple work together to define a shared understanding of the relationship problems. The shift from individual to conjoint consultation occurs more quickly if the partners describe their relationship concerns in nonhostile terms and are able to recognize the contribution of their own behavior, context, and life events to their relationship.

Initial Orientation and Negotiation of Agenda

In self-regulatory couple therapy (SRCT) the second and subsequent assessment sessions begin with negotiation of the agenda for that session. Typically this negotiation starts with a brief summary of what was covered in the first session and a check on whether the partners agree that the summary accurately reflects what has been covered so far. Then the therapist offers some suggestions about what to cover. The partners are asked whether the suggested agenda items are acceptable to them and whether there are other issues they want to discuss in the session. All this usually takes only 2 or 3 minutes, but it is an important step in promoting active collaboration between the couple and the therapist.

In determining the session agenda to be suggested to the couple I consider four issues. First, those relationship problems that seem most pressing to the couple need to be acknowledged early in therapy. Second, the process of the session should have some focus on assessment tasks that address positive relationship processes (e.g., the relationship history review or the positive reminiscence task described later in this chapter). Third, the assessment process needs to address all the areas set out in Table 4.1. Those areas not yet assessed in session 1 need attention in session 2. Fourth, assessment needs to balance attention to the needs of both partners.

In conducting an assessment I try to use a variety of methods with the partners, which helps to anticipate which self-change strategies may be most useful. People vary in their responses to different assessment methods. For example, some people report that self-monitoring is really helpful in clarifying what is going on in their relationship. Other people find the process of monitoring tedious and do not see the information gained as all that valuable. In having couples complete the various tasks, the therapist can use the response of the partners to the assessment tasks to guide suggestions about how to achieve partners' self-change goals (see Chapter 6 on feedback and negotiation for a discussion of this process).

Individual Interviews

In the second and any subsequent assessment sessions one function of individual consultations is to complete assessment of areas that initially are best done individually (e.g., violence, affairs, and thoughts about separation). A second function is to reframe individual concerns that the partners currently express in hostile terms and to attempt to develop empathic ways of describing these concerns that are less attacking on the partner. (This is of particular importance if the therapist finds partners continuing to be hostile toward each other in conjoint sessions.) The strategies described in Chapter 4 for achieving these ends continue to be used throughout therapy. Specifically, the therapist prompts use of behavioral descriptions of problems rather than pejorative labels, prompts attention to the positive motives that often underlie negative behavior, selectively summarizes concerns to focus those concerns more on feelings and less on attacking, and reframes individual concerns in terms of relationship processes.

Conjoint Interviews

Conjoint consultations are the place in which the therapist can work with the couple to develop a positive shared understanding of their relationship. This understanding should promote self-change. As noted previously, distressed partners often attribute relationship problems to stable characteristics of their partner. One important role of the therapist in conjoint sessions is to explore with the partners the role of context and life events in shaping their relationship interactions. This process achieves two purposes. First, it often reduces the blaming and anger attached to negative interaction. For example, a perceived lack of support from one's spouse that is attributed to a conscious, selfish choice by the spouse often is associated with anger and hostility. However, if the couple comes to see that they provide limited support for each other, and that this occurs in the context of demanding jobs combined with a transition to parenthood, the problem may be associated with collaborative efforts to reduce stress or enhance support. Exploration of context and life events can be achieved in many ways. Two useful methods described later in this chapter are exploring hypotheses generated from the couple's biographical data and discussing the couple's relationship history.

Conjoint consultations also are the means for the therapist to explore issues identified in individual consultations and completed assessment tasks. For example, in a second session with a couple I collected the Areas of Change Questionnaire (ACQ) from each of them. (They had not completed these in the first session and took the forms home to complete.) I began a discussion with the wife, Beth, as follows.

> "Beth, I notice that you believe you need to go out with Marcus more, which seems to be what you were saying last week about having more quality time together. You also feel you need to show more appreciation for what he does well. Tell me a bit about what is important to you about showing appreciation."

Some partners are unable to explore the identified issues constructively in the conjoint session; they resort to hostility and anger in their descriptions of the problems. In such instances it is necessary to explore the issues first in individual consultations and then to summarize and review those issues in the conjoint session.

Completion and Review of Behavioral Tasks in Session

As noted in Chapter 4, having couples complete behavioral tasks in session allows the therapist to observe the couple interacting, and reviewing the process helps develop a shared understanding of the couple's interactional processes. Later in this chapter I describe the details of how to conduct several behavioral assessment tasks, what to look for when observing these tasks, and how to structure the review so that the focus is on process not content.

Closure: Couple Tasks between Sessions

I almost always ask couples to complete additional tasks after the second and subsequent assessment sessions. It is important to leave time at the end of the session to negotiate the tasks couples will undertake. Typically, when there are about 10 minutes left in the session I mention the amount of time remaining; then I say that I want to summarize where we are up to and work out what the couple can do between sessions. In the summary I identify the key points we explored about the nature of their relationship and its problems and check whether they agree with that summary. Assuming assessment is not yet complete, the suggested tasks involve further assessment. As described in Chapter 4, it is important that the therapist explain carefully the rationale for suggested assessment tasks and check that the partners understand what is being suggested and that they agree the tasks are useful.

Interpreting Core Assessment Tasks

Reviewing Relationship Context and Life Events

Distressed couples rarely attend sufficiently to the context or life events that influence their relationship, and unfortunately, there are few measures of these aspects of couple relationships. However, it is possible to assess these important elements of the couple's relationship within conjoint interviews. This is done by discussing ideas generated from the couple's biographical data and by reviewing their relationship history.

REVIEWING BIOGRAPHICAL DATA

The most important thing to do with gathered information is to use it. Many clinicians begin their intake assessment process by asking individuals basic biographical information such as their age, years married, whether they have been married before, the number and ages of any children, their address, and employment. The therapist can generate important clinical hypotheses about the impact of context and life events on the couple's relationship from this basic demographic data.

Couples have a series of developmental tasks that are somewhat predictable across the course of a relationship. For example, in the early phases of a relationship typically there is the initial attraction followed by increasing intimacy, commitment, and the transition to marriage or living together. These processes often mean reductions in contact with parents and family of origin to create the time for the couple relationship. Living together involves the definition of roles and development of a shared lifestyle, including the sharing of money and other resources. The transition to parenthood typically involves a loss in disposable income for the couple, changes in roles, particularly for the woman, and changes in lifestyle and activities. Other major transitions include relocation, changes in employment, major changes in health, and changes relating to children growing up, such as the children becoming less dependent on their parents and leaving home.

In evaluating biographical data it is useful to relate the couple's biographical data to the common developmental processes of couples. Consider the age at which the couple got together, previous relationship experiences they may have had at that time, the impact of family and work responsibilities, and the couple's financial position. From these data the therapist can develop hypotheses about the influences that are having an impact on the couple. For example, consider the following scenario: Germaine is a 34-year-old former teacher who is now home full time looking after children, and Tony is a 33-year-old medical specialist. They have been married for 10 years, and have three children ages 5, 3, and 1. They live in an outer suburban area of a large city on a 1-acre small farm. They moved to this city about 6 months ago from another city approximately 1,000 miles away. What hypotheses might we generate in response to this biographical data?

Knowing that the couple has only recently moved to this city, it is likely that they do not know many people. Germaine, being at home full time, is relatively isolated and may have a relatively small or nonexistent social support network. Tony, being recently arrived and in a fairly high-pressure profession, probably is working hard to establish his practice. Based on no other information, I would hypothesize in this case that it is likely that Germaine feels isolated and has a high need for support from Tony. In contrast, I would suggest that Tony is probably getting his adult company needs met outside the home but feels very conscious of the need to develop his earning power. We might guess that in having these traditional gender roles, there might be conflict between the two partners in terms of the amount of contact that they feel they need to have together and the level of supportiveness shown by Tony toward Germaine. On the basis of the biographical information alone, one could not conclude that this is an inevitable conflict. But, on the basis of baseline rates of occurrence, this is quite a plausible hypothesis.

Consider a somewhat different scenario. Ray is 52 and works as a delivery van driver, Margaret is 51 and works as a librarian. They have been married for approximately 3 years, and it is the second marriage for each of them. Margaret's 21-year-old son, Robert, lives with them, and both Margaret and Ray have other grown-up children who are married and living away. Margaret's first husband left her after 3 years of marriage, and Margaret raised her three children as a lone parent. Ray's wife died 4 years ago, and she had always adopted a traditional homemaker role.

Again, based on the baseline rates of occurrence, one might hypothesize that this couple could have difficulties in adjusting to each other's expectations about their relationship. Margaret lived without a male partner for a very long time and maintained a role as a single parent raising her three children. Ray, on the other hand, is used to having a partner who fulfills a traditional role. In this instance Ray was complaining that Margaret was not being "a real wife," by which he meant she was not fulfilling traditional female roles. Margaret, on the other hand, felt that Ray really wanted "a slave rather than a wife." Furthermore, as one might expect, Ray found it difficult to share a household with another adult male. Margaret's son, Robert, did not see the need to accommodate his lifestyle with the arrival of this new person (Ray).

When hypotheses about the nature of presenting problems and the influence of context and life events are developed, they are explored with the couple in conjoint interviews. For example, in the case of Margaret and Ray I posed a universal truth to the couple in this way: "All couples who enter a new relationship later in their life are challenged by how to accommodate to each other. There often are long established habits each person brings to the relationship. How have you two dealt with this challenge?" The aim with this question was to prompt attention to the processes of accommodation each partner needed to make in order to develop the relationship. I also asked about how Margaret and Ray supported each other in developing a relationship between Ray and Robert. The overall goal was to explore the hypotheses derived from the biographical data and to do so in a manner that encouraged a useful, shared perspective on their relationship.

REVIEWING RELATIONSHIP HISTORY

Reviewing the couple's relationship history in a conjoint interview serves several functions. First, it gathers further data about the context and life events that shape the couple's relationship, thereby supplementing the biographical data. Second, for distressed couples that tend to focus selectively on the negative aspects of their relationship, it is an opportunity to review positive aspects of the relationship. In reviewing a couple's relationship history, many couple therapists access positive relationship intimacy by focusing on having partners describe the positive things that attracted them to each other (e.g., Jacobson & Margolin, 1979). The process of stating the positive aspects of the relationship in a conjoint interview often generates positive affect in the session and prevents therapy from becoming a place where the couple focuses only on their problems. Third, it ensures that therapists attend to positive aspects of couples' relationships, and this should be reflected in the summaries therapists reflect back to the couple. The attention to positivity, intimacy, and history together in therapy seems to motivate partners to work on their relationship.

I usually begin such a discussion by highlighting the importance of knowing the context in which the current relationship difficulties developed and understanding more about the couple's relationship. Few couples object to this as an unreasonable process. It might begin something as follows: "I want to understand more about your relationship, and how it has developed. In particular, I would like to know more about how you two got to know each other. Can you tell me about when the two of you first met?"

As the couple talks about how they first met, I probe each partner using such questions as "What first attracted you to your partner?," "As the relationship became more serious, what were the qualities of your partner that made you feel this person was special?," and "What was it that led you to want to marry, or live with, this person?" I reflect and draw out from the partners the importance of these positive attributes of their partner and the relationship. For example, if someone mentioned that her partner was a good listener I might respond: "So he really listened to you. What was it that was important about being listened to by him?" The intent with each of these questions is to draw out the intimate bond, the "glue," that keeps the couple together. Sometimes I seek information about this bond more directly by asking a question such as the following: "You have had a lot of difficulties in your relationship, as you have described, and yet you still choose to be with your spouse. What is it that is so special about this person and this relationship for you?"

Self-Report Inventories

Effective use of couple assessment sessions requires the therapist to do some preparation for sessions. A key task is to score and interpret self-report inventories that the couple completes. (I describe how to do this in the next section of this chapter.) I find it useful to compare the assessment data with the areas identified in Table 4.1 to check whether I have missed any areas. Sometimes this leads to the selection of supplementary assessment tasks to assess areas identified as important.

RELATIONSHIP SATISFACTION

An important area to assess early in couple therapy is each partner's relationship satisfaction. Relationship satisfaction refers to the overall positive or negative valence that the partners feel about their relationship and has been variously referred to as relationship satisfaction, relationship adjustment, and relationship feelings. There has been considerable debate in the literature about whether these different terms refer to different constructs and about the interrelationship between these different constructs (e.g., Heyman et al., 1994). Whatever the terms or constructs used, it seems that all of the different measures that have been developed thus far are strongly interrelated (Gottman, 1994).

One of the first measures given to partners in session 1 is the most widely used measure of relationship satisfaction, the Dyadic Adjustment Scale (DAS; Spanier, 1976). The DAS was designed to provide a series of subscale scores on various domains. However, in a number of studies the factor structure of the scale has not been replicated. In most factor-analytic studies of the scale, up to 80% of the variance in the total scale can be attributed to the single item in which partners rate their overall evaluation of the relationship (Sharpley & Cross, 1982). Based on this finding I use only the total score in assessment. It has become conventional, based on the original normative data provided by Spanier (1976), to use a total score below 100 as indicative of relationship distress. The standard deviation on the DAS is approximately 17 points. The population mean is around 115, making a score of 100 approximately 1 standard deviation below the mean. From this it can be seen that scores of 80 or lower are 2 standard deviations below the mean of the population, indicating severe distress.

The DAS total provides an overall index of severity of distress, which can assist the therapist to reflect more accurately to couples their level of dissatisfaction. For example, a score of 100 or more might lead to a summary beginning with "You are overall quite happy in the relationship, but you want to strengthen the relationship by. . . . " In contrast, a score of 80 or less is likely to be reflected by a summary beginning: "You are very unhappy in the relationship at the moment. . . . " Substantial discrepancy (approximately 12 points or more) between the DAS totals for the partners is important information. If distress is extreme in one partner (a score of 70 or less), that person may either be extremely angry and hostile, reflecting his or her distress, or may be withdrawn, reflecting having given up on the relationship. If only one partner is distressed, the nondistressed partner may be hard to engage in therapy if he or she sees little need for change, and particular attention may need to be focused in assessment on the potential benefits of therapy for the nondistressed partner.

In using any self-report inventory to assess a couple's relationship, it is important to follow up on how couples complete the inventories. Many of the early questions on the DAS relate to areas of disagreement between the partners. If any of those areas have not been previously identified in an interview, I would ask the partners to elaborate. For example, both partners of a couple I saw recently indicated that they disagreed at least frequently on religious matters. On probing further, it turned out that the wife, Maria, was a devoted Catholic and wished to attend church on a weekly basis. The husband, Ted, saw this as a load of "religious bunkum" and did not want to either have to attend church himself or have his children attend church. Maria saw his steadfast refusal to support her religious beliefs as trivializing her opinions. This turned out to be a central issue in the relationship but one they had not identified in individual or conjoint interviews.

A number of later questions on the DAS relate to the occurrence of positive things in the relationship, such as working on projects together, having interesting conversations, and so forth. Again, if these issues have not been discussed previously, the responses to the DAS can be reviewed as means of exploring these aspects of the relationship. The DAS has an item relating to the level of commitment to improving the relationship. This item can help assess the extent to which couple therapy might be useful. I always ask partners what they mean by the answers that they have given on this question. For example, if someone has indicated that he is willing to do "his fair share," then I would ask him what he sees his fair share as being. If someone indicated that she felt she had "done all that she can do," I want to probe what this means. It may mean that they now feel powerless to do further things but would be willing to consider whether other actions might benefit the relationship.

SEPARATION POTENTIAL

A concept related to global relationship satisfaction is thoughts about terminating the relationship. The Marital Status Inventory (MSI) is a 14-item true/false scale assessing steps taken toward relationship dissolution and divorce, with higher scores reflecting more steps taken. In general, scores of 4 or more are seen as indicating high levels of risk for separation. Scores of 7 or more indicate that couple therapy may not be helpful, as at least one partner is seriously engaged in the process of separation.

There can be discrepancies between the verbal reports of partners on their thoughts of separation and their scores on the MSI. Sometimes these discrepancies reflect that the person's thoughts about separation are volatile. For example, it is not uncommon for distressed partners to think and talk about a high commitment to the relationship after a good day and then suddenly to change to thoughts and talk of ending the relationship in response to an argument or other negative relationship event. Whatever the source of such a discrepancy between verbal report and the MSI, it does suggest that further exploration of the issue of dissolution potential is needed.

Combinations of high DAS and high MSI or low DAS and low MSI are worthy of exploration. Clarification of the source of the seeming paradox of either contemplating ending a satisfying relationship or not ending a very distressed relationship can be important. A high DAS combined with a high MSI may reflect very high (perhaps unrealistic) expectations of the relationship, low commitment to the relationship, or both. Low commitment to a satisfying relationship may reflect a lack of realistic appraisal of the costs of separation and divorce, a value system that attaches limited significance to the relationship, or the existence of another relationship. A low DAS with a low MSI may reflect very low expectations of the relationship. This can occur in people who have low self-esteem or who are depressed and view themselves as unlikely or unworthy to get a better relationship. High commitment to a distressed relationship also can reflect an unrealistically negative view of separation.

DESIRED CHANGE

A key element of assessing couple relationships from a self-regulatory perspective is to assess the changes that each partner wants to make in the way that he or she interacts with the other partner. The ACQ was first developed by Weiss and Perry (1983a). This instrument lists 34 fairly specific behaviors which are common sources of difficulty within relationships. The individuals are asked to rate from −3 "*do much less*," through 0 "*do not change*," to +3 "*do much more*" the extent to which they want their partner to change the frequency of the listed behaviors. The original instrument has been modified by a number of authors and is scored in a number of different ways. Weiss and

Perry (1983a) defined two subscales: In the first, partners rate how much they want their spouses to change each of the specified behaviors; in the second, they rate how much they believe their spouses want them to change. Weiss and Perry used quite a complex scoring system where the behavior changes requested by one person are compared with the perceptions the spouse has of what is expected of him or her.

The version I prefer is the form revised by Weiss and Halford (1996). The revised ACQ includes the first subscale in its original form. The instructions for the second subscale have been changed so that partners rate how much they think they personally need to change the frequency of the specified behaviors. One useful scoring system is the sum of the absolute scores on each of these subscales. These sums reflect the total amount of behavior change requested of the partner, and the total amount of behavior change believed to be desirable for self. Higher scores represent greater requested change, which in turn reflects lower levels of satisfaction with the status quo.

There is an additional score than can be derived from the ACQ that I find useful. One can calculate the ratio of requested partner change to self-change by dividing the sum of the absolute scores of the first subscale by the sum of the absolute scores of the second subscale. If the resultant ratio is greater than 1, the person is requesting more change of his or her partner than the person is rating as desirable for him- or herself. In terms of self-regulation, this is indicative of a partner-blaming perspective. If the ratio is approximately 1, the partner has a balanced view of the amount of behavior change required of him- or herself versus his or her partner. A ratio substantially below 1 indicates that the person is advocating substantially more change for him- or herself than for his or her spouse. This may indicate excessive self-blame, which sometimes is associated with depression.

Reviewing the completed ACQ forms of each partner helps to build empathy with the partners' positions and to identify areas that most need change. Usually I would review the completed forms between sessions and mark the behaviors for which most change is requested. Often it is helpful to review with the individual partners the behaviors for which they are requesting the most change and to check my understanding of the issues. Consider the following brief interchange in the second session.

THERAPIST: Roger, I notice you mentioned you wanted Shona to show more appreciation for what you do well. Are there particular things you do which you feel she does not show appreciation for?

ROGER: Yeah, Shona feels I am not doing enough of the running around after the kids. There is a lot to do, sports and stuff, and I admit she does more than half. But I do try to contribute. She says to me "hell, that's nothing . . . I do it all the time," and she does. But I try, it's real busy at work, but I try to pull my weight with the kids . . . she just seems to think I do nothing.

THERAPIST: OK, so when you do put in for the kids, you feel Shona dismisses that . . . says it's not enough.

In the foregoing interchange Roger identified two important themes. First is the equity of the sharing of child responsibilities, for which Roger acknowledges that his partner, Shona, carries more of the burden. Second is Roger's view that he is trying to make a contribution to the parenting but that Shona does not appreciate his contribution. The therapist attempts to develop a clearer understanding of Roger's perspective and to demonstrate empathy with that position. In a subsequent session it may be useful to explore the issue of sharing household responsibilities and Roger's desire for approval by Shona for what he contributes.

Often reviewing behavior change requests identifies themes in the items requested. For example, a number of the ACQ items relate to communication, a number relate to the quantity and quality of shared couple time together, other items relate to reduction of conflict, and others relate to household management issues. When partners are asking for a lot of change within a particular domain, it identifies the domain as a key area of relationship concern.

COMMUNICATION AND CONFLICT MANAGEMENT

The Communication Patterns Questionnaire (CPQ; Christensen, 1988) is a 23-item self-report inventory. People rate on 9-point scales how frequently different patterns of communicating occur when they are discussing conflict topics with their spouse. The patterns assessed include mutual constructive discussion, one partner approaching and trying to discuss an issue while the spouse withdraws, mutual criticism and hostility, and mutual avoidance of issues. Although people rarely use the constructs assessed in the CPQ spontaneously to describe their communication, partners show quite high agreement on their level of endorsement of different patterns applying to their relationship (Christensen, 1988). Moreover, their ratings show good convergent validity with observational ratings of their communication patterns (Christensen, 1988). The CPQ is a useful way of assessing these patterns in couples and of introducing the ideas of the patterns to the partners.

AGGRESSION AND VIOLENCE

As noted earlier, approximately 70% of distressed couples have engaged in at least one act of physical aggression in the last 12 months, but less than 5% of distressed couples nominate aggression as a problem in the relationship (O'Leary et al., 1992). Even if asked specifically in a joint interview about the occurrence of aggression within the relationship, less than 30% of couples report aggression in this context. However, if each individual partner is asked to indicate the occurrence of aggression on the Conflict Tactics Scale—Revised (CTS-R; Straus et al., 1996), then approximately 70% of couples will report the presence of physical aggression (O'Leary, et al., 1992). Given the potentially serious consequences of physical violence in relationships (Cascardi et al., 1992), I recommend using the CTS-R routinely in assessment of couples presenting with relationship problems. Usually I administer the CTS-R during the second session and quickly scan the partners' responses during the session. In this way, if I detect aggression I am able to respond to it immediately.

The CTS-R (Straus et al., 1996) is a simple behavioral checklist, and each partner is individually asked to indicate whether specific behaviors have occurred in the last 12 months within their relationship. For example, in one item respondents are asked to indicate whether or not they pushed or slapped their partner in the last year, or if their partner has pushed or slapped them. Respondents also indicate approximately how often those behaviors occurred in the last 12 months. The scale measures psychological aggression, physical assault, sexual coercion, and injury occurring between the partners.

In the event that aggression in the relationship is detected via report on the CTS-R, it is important that it is discussed in an individual consultation with the partner reporting the aggression. Aggression by a man often is associated with fear by the woman, and one source of fear can be a realistic appraisal that the man will become aggressive if the woman mentions the violence (Holtzworth-Munroe, Smutzler, Bates, & Sandin, 1997). I respond to aggression detected via the CTS-R in the same manner as described in Chapter 4 for responding to aggression detected in individual interviews.

Behavioral Tasks

One of the best ways to assess couple communication is by observation. Several communication tasks are useful when observing couple communication, and I routinely use two: a problem-solving and a positive-reminiscence task. I want to describe how to conduct each of these tasks and then how to interpret observations when couples undertake the tasks.

While the couple undertakes a communication task such as the problem-solving or a positive-reminiscence discussions it is best for the therapist to exit the room. The presence of a therapist often leads the couple to talk to the therapist rather than to each other. The interaction between the partners can be followed through either a one-way screen or video. If therapists do not have access to those resources within their current clinical setting, they would be wise to attempt to set up these facilities, but in the meantime, they can approximate these arrangements by removing themselves from the visual field of the couples. Therapists can sit on the very far side of the room and turn the couples' chairs to face each other to minimize distraction. Although this helps, in my experience the interactions are still not the same as when the therapist is absent from the room.

PROBLEM-SOLVING TASK

The problem-solving task has been widely used by couple researchers and therapists and focuses on having the couple discuss an issue that is currently a problem in the relationship in order to observe their conflict management (Weiss & Heyman, 1997). Essentially this task involves the couple identifying an area of current disagreement in the relationship and discussing that area for 10 to 15 minutes. If partners cannot readily identify a topic area, I suggest one of the areas requested for change on the ACQ. Sometimes it is instructive to have the couple have two discussions: one on a topic where the man wants the woman to change and one on a topic where the woman wants the man to change. As noted previously, often the person seeking change will engage in criticisms and other approach behaviors. The spouse being requested to change sometimes withdraws in response to that approach. It can be helpful to establish if, within a given couple, one partner generally approaches and the other generally withdraws, or if these roles change as a function of who is seeking change.

Before beginning the discussion I usually give the couple a set of instructions something like the following:

"The purpose of the discussion you are about to have is to see how you normally talk about issues. You do not need to try and do anything special, just talk about this as you normally would. This may feel a little strange to you at first, talking in this setting, but most couples rapidly forget about the surroundings and just talk to each other as they normally would. I will leave you alone for about ten minutes to discuss this issue. At the end of ten minutes I'm going to ask you to do something fairly difficult, which is to stop talking about the issue. It is very important that you do stop talking. The point of this task is not to solve the particular problem, but to see how you two go about talking about it. After I ask you to stop talking we will discuss how you talk to each other."

As you can see, I place heavy emphasis on the importance of establishing instructional control over the couple before they begin the discussion. This is important. Some couples are almost reflexive in escalating conflict and find it difficult to stop arguments. If this degree of verbal structuring fails to halt the couple's argument then a large amount of structure may be necessary in therapy for the couple to control destructive conflict.

POSITIVE REMINISCENCE

A second useful communication task is the positive-reminiscence task. This task was developed in collaboration with my colleague Sue Osgarby (Osgarby & Halford, 2000a). In essence, it taps into the extent to which couples are able to experience positive intimacy through communication. I briefly speak to the partners individually and ask them each to think back to a time when they felt particularly close and positive toward their partner. I ask two or three questions of them, trying to elicit why this was an important event to them, and paraphrasing the affect to prime the person to describe this event. I then ask the couple to sit down together for about 10 minutes and I give them the following instructional set: "I have asked each of you individually about a time when you felt particularly close or positive toward your partner. I'm going to leave you alone for 10 to 15 minutes, and I want each of you to talk to the other about the particular time and events that you identified when talking to me. You do not need to talk about this in any particular way, but just talk about what each of you remembers, and felt, on the occasions that you have identified."

OBSERVING BEHAVIOR DURING COMMUNICATION TASKS

Considerable time is spent training observers how to code interactions such as problem-solving and positive-reminiscence tasks. Achieving adequate reliability for observational research often takes considerable time and skill. However, it is possible to use simplified observational assessments to derive useful clinical information. Table 5.2 lists a series of basic communication behaviors with their definitions. I watch for these behaviors as I observe couple discussions on the closed-circuit video. To record my observations, I take a blank sheet of paper and create two columns. I then jot down the responses being used by each partner. I am interested to observe a series of things about the interaction, including the balance of listening and speaking, the rates of different behaviors being demonstrated, and the patterns of couple interaction.

At a fundamental level there are two major functions of communication: sending and receiving, usually called speaking and listening. I look at and listen to each partner and note the amount of time each spends sending and receiving. Good communication generally requires that both partners send and receive. Obvious imbalances in talk time, when one partner does most of the talking, often reflect problems in communication. High rates of negative speaking and listening often are obvious in distressed couples. Deficits in positive listening and speaking are less obvious than excesses of negativity but also are important to observe. For example, watch how often partners ask their spouse in a positive, interested manner to expand on their perspective.

In addition to the base rates of behavior, it is important to attend to the

TABLE 5.2. Communication Behaviors

Function	Valence	Responses	Definitions
Listen	Positive	Attend	Look, nod, turn toward, verbal encouragers
		Accept	Paraphrase, ask open questions, positive feedback
		Agree	Simple agreement such as "yes"
	Negative	Withdraw	Look away, not respond, state desire to stop talking
		Negate	Immediate "no," disagreement
		Justify	Deny responsibility, explain away negative behavior
Speak	Positive	Describe	Neutral statement of event, issue
		Self-disclose	Revealing statement of own feelings or preference
		Suggest	Propose positive action or solution
	Negative	Criticize	Blaming, condemning negative statement
		Negative suggest	Coercive command, demand to cease doing something

patterns of interaction that occur. In particular, I look at the extent to which when one partner sends, the other actively listens in a positive way. It is common in distressed couples for people to respond to sending by their partner either by engaging in further sending themselves or by negative listening, such as immediately disagreeing or providing negative solutions. It is also helpful to consider the interactions in terms of the extent to which one sees the negative patterns defined in Table 5.3, such as demand–withdraw, mutual avoidance, and mutual negative escalation. The positive patterns of mutual engagement and meshing are typical of satisfied couples.

Overall, similar communication skills are evident in the problem-solving and positive-reminiscence tasks. However, within the positive-reminiscence task, it is expected that the therapist will see much more positive affect than in the problem-solving task. The extent to which partners demonstrate positive affect and responsiveness to positivity expressed by the other gives a sense of how much emotional closeness these two people are able to exhibit toward each other. A pattern of interaction which is particularly important from our own research (Osgarby & Halford, 2000a) is the extent to which meshing is exhibited in the positive-reminiscence task. Meshing refers to a situation in which one partner is describing a particular feeling, experience, or event and the other person responds by further elaborating on that particular experience or event from his or her own point of view. The elaboration must be consistent

TABLE 5.3. Patterns of Couple Communication

Pattern	Description
Negative patterns	
Unbalanced interaction	One partner does a disproportionate amount of talking, often combined with that partner engaging in large amounts of speaking behaviors and spouse in little or no speaking, and only listening responses.
Approach–withdraw	One partner does majority of speaking, usually negative speaking such as criticisms and demands, while partner seeks to withdraw or close off discussion.
Mutual escalation	Each partner engages in negative speaking with low rates of listening; what listening does occur is mainly negative. Interactions tend to escalate both in volume and expressed negative affect.
Mutual avoidance	Partners are detached, neither sends very much, and there is minimal listening. Any issues raised are minimized, little obvious affect expression.
Positive patterns	
Mutual engagement	Each partner engages in balance of positive sending and receiving; overall affect is neutral or positive in problem solving and positive in positive reminiscence.
Meshing	One partner sends positively with a self-disclosure or description and the partner responds by sending a self-disclosure or description that is consistent in content and affect with the first response.

in content and affective tone to the first person's response. The effect when watching an interaction with high levels of meshing is that it looks as if the two partners are conjointly telling the story. They seem to have a sense of shared history and build on each other's reminiscences about events to develop a positive sense about the relationship as a whole. The absence of meshing may be indicative that the couple have difficulty accessing shared positive aspects of their history. Helping them access this history may be an important part of effective therapy with them.

COGNITIONS DURING COMMUNICATION TASKS

In addition to assessing the behaviors that couples exhibit during problem-solving and positive-reminiscence tasks, it can be useful to look at the cognitions couples have during these interaction tasks. One measure I have used in my research and clinical practice (Halford & Sanders, 1988b) is the thought-listing procedure. After an interaction, each partner is asked to complete a thought-listing form, which consists of a series of rectangular boxes down a page. Partners are instructed to write down all the thoughts that occurred to them during the interaction, one thought per box.

The thought-listing form enables assessment of a number of different dimensions of cognitions that individuals may experience during interaction. Common cognitions reported by couples who are distressed include negative attributions about the partner, which are reported thoughts that the spouse is to blame for negative aspects of the relationship (e.g., thoughts such as "I think he is so selfish to never come home on time."). Also common are negative expectancies, meaning statements that the interaction will get worse (e.g., thoughts such as "We never get anywhere with this, we may as well give up."). The thought-listing procedure provides the therapist with a window into the partners' subjective experience of the interaction.

REVIEWING BEHAVIORAL TASKS WITH THE COUPLE IN SESSION

Reviewing behavioral tasks in session primarily is intended to assist the couple and therapist to develop a shared understanding of the couple's interaction processes. To achieve that end, when I ask the couple to stop their discussion I usually remind them of that goal. I typically ask each partner to describe his or her current feelings and then I summarize what he or she tells me, as it is useful to empathize with their emotional experience of the interaction before exploring the interaction process. One challenge in reviewing behavioral tasks is to focus the partners on the process of interaction rather than on the content of their interaction. For example, if the partners are discussing a conflict topic there is the risk that the review process focuses on the topic rather than on how the couple went about trying to resolve the issue. Let me illustrate the process with a review of a problem-solving discussion between Jan and Neil on the topic of completion of household chores by their son, Dennis. The couple had become quite angry with each other during the discussion, so I was conscious of the possibility that they might revert to arguing unless the review was carefully structured.

THERAPIST: Jan, Neil, I want you to do something quite difficult now. I want you to stop talking about Dennis and his chores. Remember, we are trying to understand *how* you two talk through problems, we're not trying to solve the problem straight away. It looked as if both of you were feeling frustrated. Jan, how do you feel right now?

JAN: I am really frustrated, we just never get anywhere with this, Neil seems to want to let Dennis get away with . . .

THERAPIST: (*interrupting*) Jan, I can see you are frustrated. And you seem to be saying that whenever you talk about this issue, you are frustrated. Is that right?

JAN: Yeah. (*Sighs.*) I don't know, Dennis just does nothing . . .

THERAPIST: Jan I am going to stop you again. I know this is hard, but you keep slipping into talking about the issue. Let's focus on how you talk to each other, rather than what you say. What you are saying is that the current process frustrates you, and though you've talked about this issue before, it never gets anywhere. (*Pause. Jan nods.*) Neil, how did you feel?

NEIL: Angry, I feel Jan does not listen to me, she just keeps on and on.

THERAPIST: OK, OK, so you're angry and you feel you are not being listened to. Let's see if we can explore what happened. First can you tell me if what happened during the discussion here was what might happen at home?'

NEIL: Much the same, though we would be louder.

JAN: *Much* louder, and Neil might walk away, or switch on the TV.

THERAPIST: Right, so both of you say similar but louder, and Jan feels Neil would end it, walk off or flick on the TV. Neil, do you agree you might end it that way?

NEIL: Uh huh, it gets too much for me. I worry Dennis will hear us, and he gets upset. I hate that.

THERAPIST: OK. So both of you get angry and frustrated at home, more so than here. Then Neil ends the discussion. I want to tell you a couple of things I noticed. No, let me first check with you guys what you think someone else would notice about this. Who talked the most?

JAN: Me. Neil clams up when we argue.

THERAPIST: Neil, Jan thinks she talks most, would you agree?

NEIL: Definitely, I feel barraged by her . . . I just don't see the point . . .

JAN: Well I have to do something if you just go dumb.

THERAPIST: You two are really still mad with each other aren't you? It seems that what happens really gets to each of you, and you find it really hard to let it go. There's something really interesting here, in what happens. You respond to the frustration quite differently. Jan, it seems you respond to being frustrated by talking, trying to get this out in the open. (*She nods.*) Neil, you try to stop the talk because it seems pointless to you. Is that right?

NEIL: Absolutely.

THERAPIST: I am sorry you had another frustrating talk. But there are some important things that come from this: (1) Jan talks more than Neil, and she feels frustrated he is not talking more; (2) Neil feels overwhelmed by Jan and angry she does not listen to him; (3) Neil tries to end what he sees as a pointless process, and this frustrates Jan; (4) at the end of the process you are both angry and it hasn't gotten you anywhere.

This example illustrates several important points. First, many distressed couples do find it difficult to deescalate negativity and focus on the process of their interaction. (In a subsequent assessment session with Jan and Neil I reviewed further the discussion they had, and we discussed the importance of being able to deescalate.) Sometimes the therapist can structure the review so that useful ideas about process emerge. In other instances it is better to work with individual partners to debrief them on the content, then focus on process, and then bring the partners together to review process. The therapist needs to be monitoring the reactions of each partner to determine what is most likely to be productive. For example, in this session with Jan and Neil I remember considering reverting to individual debriefing. After I had interrupted both partners to prevent further negative escalation and done a summary to refocus back to process, I was concerned that their attention was still on their anger and the issue itself. However, at that point they each started to engage with the process ideas I was putting to them, so I continued.

A second issue illustrated by the transcript is the need to limit the review to just a few key points. In this case the review focused on the imbalance of talk time, the withdrawal by Neil, and the frustration experienced by both partners. Excessively complex formulations of interaction are unlikely to be remembered or to serve as useful self-appraisals to prompt change. A third issue is that the therapist is summarizing the process of interaction. Ultimately the goal is to have each partner self-appraise the process. To that end I ask partners to summarize what they remember of the process of the interaction. (This might be later in the same session or in a subsequent session.) I then help the partners to shape up their self-appraisal, if required.

Supplementary Assessment Tasks

The core assessment tasks assess most areas of relationship concern that couples present. However, in the course of conducting the individual and conjoint interviews, and conducting the other core assessment procedures, sometimes relationship issues become evident that are not adequately assessed with the core measures. In such cases it can be useful to add one or more supplementary assessment tasks. One area that is a reasonably common couple complaint but is not assessed in depth with the core assessment tasks is the current and desired range of couples' shared positive activities. Other examples include unrealistic expectations and standards partners hold about their relationship (e.g., "if he really loved me, he would want to spend all his time with me," or "we should never argue"); difficulties with sex; work–family conflict; individual problems such as depression, anxiety, or alcohol abuse; work–family problems; and parenting issues. In the section that follows I describe a range of self-report inventories that assess these areas.

One difficulty that some couples have in interviews is being specific about the problems they perceive in their relationship. Complaints can be framed in vague terms, such as "She is demanding" or "He is distant," and the partners seem unable to be more specific about what the behavior is that is associated with this complaint. For such couples, self-monitoring the day-to-day occurrences in their relationship can be useful. A later section describes the use of self-monitoring in assessing couple relationships.

Self-Report Inventories

SHARED POSITIVE ACTIVITIES

An important element of relationship intimacy is shared positive activities. Distressed couples often spend less time with each other, and report fewer positive activities together than do nondistressed couples. If a couple's verbal reports suggest that lack of shared time is a problem but they have trouble specifying what they do currently or what they might like to do together, then administration of the Inventory of Rewarding Activities (IRA; Weiss & Perry, 1983a) is useful.

The IRA lists a large number of commonly occurring activities. Partners individually indicate whether they have engaged in these activities in the last 4 weeks, and if they did, with whom. Possible categories include with your spouse, with your spouse and other people, with people other than your spouse, and with spouse and children. Each partner indicates by a plus sign in appropriate columns the activities that they would like to engage in more often, and with whom they would like to engage in those activities. Completion of the IRA allows the therapist and the couple to assess the current patterns of time use and allows exploration with the partners of their degree of satisfaction with those patterns of time use. If the couple desires to change the balance of their individual and couple activities, a completed IRA often allows identification of specific activities that the couple want to increase.

EXPECTATIONS AND STANDARDS

The expectations and standards that individuals hold about relationships can often mediate relationship problems. Expectations refer to what someone *expects* to happen in his or her relationship and standards refer to what someone *believes* should happen in his or her relationship (Baucom, Epstein, Rankin, &

Burnett, 1996). When there seem to be extreme, or markedly different, standards being held about the relationship by the partners, administering a self-report inventory to explicate those standards can be useful. Baucom, Epstein, Rankin, and Burnett (1996) developed the Inventory of Specific Relationship Standards (ISRS). This inventory assesses the standards which partners believe relationships should meet, standards that vary in their degree of relationship focus. Three dimensions of relationship standards are assessed: boundaries, power, and investment. Boundaries refer to the degree of independent versus shared functioning that partners believe should exist in a relationship. A high relationship focus is associated with low boundaries, that is a preference for a high level of interdependence. Power standards refer to the processes of change and influence within the relationship. High relationship-focused power standards refer to a preference that relationships should involve mutual influence and shared control, while low relationship-focused power standards refer to a preference for exerting effort to induce compliance from a partner. Investment standards refer to the extent of contributions seen as desirable for each partner to make to the relationship. High relationship-focused investment involves a preference for large emotional and instrumental contributions from each partner to the relationship.

Baucom, Epstein, Rankin, and Burnett (1996) showed that relationship satisfaction was modestly associated with more relationship-focused standards, and relationship satisfaction was strongly associated with the extent that the relationship standards were perceived as being met. The ISRS is useful in helping identify the relationship aspirations of the partners and the areas in which they perceive their relationship as failing to meet those standards.

SEXUAL FUNCTIONING

Many couples with relationship distress report problems in their sexual relationship (Spence, 1997). For some couples a loss or lack of sexual interest may result from relationship distress, and the improvement of the general relationship may lead to improvement in the sexual relationship. For other couples, sexual problems may be more persistent and need attention in their own right. If sexual concerns are a strong element of the couple's presentation, then the use of a self-report inventory to assess this area is a good idea. The Derogatis Sexual Functioning Inventory (Derogatis, 1975) is a comprehensive self-report measure of sexual functioning that assesses the level of accurate information partners have about sex, the range of sexual behaviors they engage in, their individual levels of sexual interest, attitudes toward sex, sexual fantasies, body image, and sexual satisfaction. The sexual satisfaction scale consists of 10 items and serves as a useful brief screening measure for detection of sexual problems. The complete scale can be used to do a more thorough assessment of sexual problems.

INDIVIDUAL PROBLEMS

It is important for the couple therapist to know whether one or both of the partners has any significant individual problems and how those individual problems interact with the relationship problems. As advocated in Chapter 4, the assessment of prior psychological or psychiatric treatment within individual interviews provides some useful screening for more severe psychopathology, as does asking each partner if he or she believes either of them has difficulties that contribute to the relationship problems. In addition, it is useful to assess each partner for the presence of common psychological difficulties using self-report inventories. This may detect problems not evident from the interview or better operationalize the severity of problems detected at interview. Table 5.4 includes some useful self-report inventories for screening for individual psychopathology. As noted earlier, I routinely give partners the Depression, Anxiety, Stress Scale (DASS; Lovibond & Lovibond, 1995). The Alcohol Use Disorders Identification Test (AUDIT; Saunders et al., 1993) is also very helpful. This 12-item inventory gives a total score intended to detect alcohol problems. The DASS and AUDIT together provide a good screening assessment of the most common psychological disorders associated with relationship problems.

If significant stress, anxiety, depression, or alcohol abuse are detected in either of the presenting partners, then, in addition to assessing the problem itself, it is important to assess how the individual problem interacts with the relationship problems. To assess these interactive processes I often pose questions such as: "How does the problem show itself in ways you or your partner can see?" "How does your partner react to these specific behaviors?" "What are the effects of the pattern on each partner?" For example, I had the following discussion with a couple in which the man drank 15 to 20 standard drinks in binges occurring once a week or so:

THERAPIST: Ros, what do you notice about Terry after he has been drinking?

ROS: Terry is a depressed drunk. He mainly drinks at home, so I see what he has. When he drinks just one or two drinks he gets talkative, happy, a bit silly. Much of the time I don't mind that. I do get worried he will get tanked [intoxicated] if he starts drinking. But, after a lot of beer he gets morose . . . he talks about losing contact with his kids growing up [Terry had grown-up children from a previous marriage whom he did not see very often after that marriage broke up], how he has blown his life. After that he can get nasty, he gets a set on me, calls me names . . . really gets nasty . . . I (begins to weep) . . . it hurts . . .

TABLE 5.4. Supplementary Self-Report Inventories

Domain	Variable	Measure	Authors	Description
Couple adaptive processes	Shared positive activities	Inventory of Rewarding Activities	Weiss & Perry (1983a)	200-item measure of current and desired, shared, and independent activities.
	Beliefs and expectations	Inventory of Specific Relationship Standards	Baucom, Epstein, Rankin, & Burnett (1996)	60-item inventory assessing relationship standards of boundaries, investment, and power.
	Sexuality	Derogatis Sexual Functioning Inventory	Derogatis (1975); Derogatis & Melisaratos (1979)	254 items arranged into 10 subscales assessing a wide range of aspects of sexuality.
Individual characteristics	Individual psychopathology	Alcohol Use Disorders Identification Test (AUDIT)	Saunders, Aasland, Babor, de La Feunte, & Grant (1993)	12-item self-report measure for detection of alcohol problems.
		Khavari Alcohol Test	Khavari & Farber (1978)	14-item self- or partner-report measure of frequency, mean and maximum alcohol consumption.
Context	Work	Work–Family Conflict Scale	Thomas & Ganster (1995)	24-item self-report measure of perceived conflict between work and family roles.
	Parenting and child adjustment	Child Behavior Checklist	Achenbach & Edelbrock (1983)	118-item parent report or teacher report, comprehensive measure of child externalizing and internalizing disorders and social competence.
		Eyberg Child Behavior Inventory	Eyberg & Robinson (1983)	36-item parent-report measure of disruptive behavior in 2–16-year-old children.
		Parenting Scale	Arnold, O'Leary, Wolff, & Acker (1993)	30-item self-report of dysfunctional parenting practices.
		Parent Problem Checklist	Dadds & Powell (1991)	16-item scale of couple conflict over parenting.

THERAPIST: So he gets verbally nasty toward you. . . .

ROS: Uh huh.

THERAPIST: What sort of things does he say to you?

ROS: He calls me names, horrible names . . . calls me a whore . . . a f—ing pig.

THERAPIST: What do you do when he is calling you these names?

ROS: I try to get away, to leave him alone to sleep it off. But he follows me when he's drunk. Doesn't actually hit me, he's never done that . . . but he corners me and just rants and yells. I hate it, . . . and I hate him then.

THERAPIST: I think I would hate being treated like that too. Does this abuse occur only when he's been drinking?

ROS: Yeah. The weird thing is, he often doesn't remember in the morning. Reckons he can't recall saying any of those things to me.

THERAPIST: Ros what effect does this have on you, being abused like you describe?

ROS: It makes me feel dirty. I try to ignore him, tell myself he's drunk . . . he doesn't mean it, that it's not true that I'm hopeless. But you know when someone tells you over and over, year after year, that you're a bitch . . . hopeless . . . a whore . . . some of you starts to believe it. I get really down after a bad episode.

THERAPIST: Terry, are you aware of what happens between you and Ros when you drink?

TERRY: I know Ros gets shitty with me for drinking. I do hit it pretty hard some days. I know it's not doing me any good, or us. Thing is, Ros reckons I give her hell when I am full . . . can't say I remember it really.

THERAPIST: What do you remember, say, about when you first start drinking?

TERRY: Well often I have a beer after work after I get home. Ros is OK about that most days, but sometimes she gives me a hard time. Nags about not getting full . . . that makes me feel tense . . . Some days I think, bugger it, a man does a full day's work he's entitled to unwind in his own home . . . she's not telling me what to do. Then I have another drink. If I get on a roll I'll skip dinner and get stuck into the grog. If I have any more than 6 or 8 I wipe myself out, drink till I am out of it.

THERAPIST: Right, let's see what we have found out. There is this pattern where Terry will usually drink a few beers after work when he gets home. Ros is edgy about him drinking more, sometimes she will ask him not to drink any more.

ROS: Yeah, and some days he listens, backs off. But if he's tense, then he seems not to care . . . he just writes himself off.

THERAPIST: So, about once a week or so Terry drinks a lot of beer, and that's when you, Ros, say he gets verbally nasty . . . but Terry you say you cannot remember what happens once you get beyond a few drinks. What effect do you think this is having on the two of you Terry?

TERRY: It's one of the key reasons we're here. Ros said, before we came to you last week, that she was packing her bags . . . she was off. It was the night after I had tied one on [got drunk] . . . and this time she meant it, she packed her stuff. Scared the hell out of me that I might have blown the marriage. So I said to her, "Love, I want to fix this. Tell me what you want me to do, and I'll do it." She said come and see a therapist, so we made the call.

THERAPIST: So, the drinking is something you want to change, Terry?

TERRY: Yeah, I got to cut out the boozing, at least stop writing myself off.

The transcript illustrates how the couple was assisted to identify the patterns of interaction around Terry's drinking. Not all couples are able to report on these processes verbally, and they may need help with self-monitoring or direct observational assessments to identify the patterns. This initial assessment is not intended to solve the problem, just to assess the problems. At this point Terry has not explicitly acknowledged that his drinking and verbal abuse have hurt Ros, but as the therapist I noted to myself that this issue would need to be addressed at some point. I also hypothesized that we might need to address the issue of Terry's regrets about the loss of his children from his first marriage.

WORK–FAMILY CONFLICT

There are a variety of life roles outside the couple relationship that can have an impact on the relationship. Work is the life role that most often couples identify as interfering with relationships. Work affects relationships in a number of ways (Thompson, 1997). High work demands can be exhausting and interfere with relationship interactions or can limit relationship time (Thompson, 1997). Particular work demands such as shift work or work that requires absence from the family home for protracted periods (e.g., long-distance transport industry and military service personnel) have an impact on relationships. In the individual interview described in Chapter 4, I discussed assessing the usual weekly routine of the couple. If their reported work arrangements potentially seem relevant to the relationship problems, it can be useful to assess the work–relationship interface more extensively.

The Work–Family Conflict Scale (Thomas & Ganster, 1995) is a 24-item self-report inventory assessing perceived conflict between work and family roles. This scale is useful to establish specific domains in which conflict is experienced, such as not finding enough time for self, or children or partner activities, or work schedules interfering with couple activities. The Categories of Work–Home Role Conflict Scale (Wiersma, 1994) is a lengthy scale assessing both the areas of perceived work–family conflict and the current strategies being used to cope with those conflicts.

PARENTING

More than 90% of married couples in Western countries have children, and most who do have children begin to do so in the first 5 years of marriage (Houseknecht, 1987). There is a substantial association between couple relationship problems between partners and behavioral problems in the couple's children, with each set of problems often exacerbating the other (Sanders, Nicholson, & Floyd, 1997). Sometimes resolution of the couple relationship problems is aided dramatically by helping the partners to parent more effectively (Sanders, Markie-Dadds, & Nicholson, 1997). Consequently, assessing the parenting experience of couples is often important.

I routinely ask couples who have children what difficulties they have with their children's behavior. I deliberately pose this as a leading question; as a parent myself and as a family psychologist I find it hard to imagine being a parent with absolutely no difficulty ever with an offspring's behavior. If either of the partners seems to be expressing significant concern about their children, I would assess the child's behavior more carefully. Table 5.4 includes some useful self-report instruments for assessing parenting concerns. The Child Behavior Checklist (CBCL; Achenbach & Edelbrock, 1983) is a widely used instrument that provides a broad assessment of child behavior problems. Usually a parent or teacher reporting on the child completes the CBCL, but it also can be administered as a self-report measure by children once they reach about 12 years of age. The Eyberg Child Behavior Inventory (Eyberg & Robinson, 1983) is briefer and less comprehensive than the CBCL, but the Eyberg also is a useful general screening instrument.

If interview and assessment with the foregoing instruments suggest parenting concerns are significant, then a thorough assessment of the parenting practices of the couple is needed. Sanders and Dadds (1993) provide a very good description of how to do such an assessment. The Parenting Daily Checklist is a parent monitoring measure for child behavior problems that provides a precise assessment of the nature and frequency of child problems. The Parenting Scale assesses parenting behaviors, as distinct from child behaviors. The scale is based on a behavioral concept of positive parenting and assesses the use of maladaptive parenting behaviors such as coercion, lack of reinforcement of positive child behaviors, and so forth. The Parent Problem Checklist assesses the degree of conflict between the partners about parenting.

Self-Monitoring of Couple Relationships

Self-monitoring of day-to-day behavior is an important way in which to assess day-to-day couple interaction exchange. Weiss and Perry (1983b) developed the Spouse Observation Checklist (SOC) to assess behavior exchange on a daily basis. This instrument consists of a list of more than 400 fairly specific behaviors. On each day, each partner is asked to indicate whether or not the behavior occurred, and if it did occur, whether its occurrence was pleasing or displeasing. In addition, at the end of each day, each partner makes a rating of his or her global relationship satisfaction. The original intent with the SOC was to have partners map out the behavior exchanges that occurred on a daily basis and how these exchanges related to more global measures of relationship satisfaction. A significant disadvantage of this instrument is the amount of time that it takes for completion. Although it has been used successfully with many couples, in my experience it requires a great deal of commitment and time from the individual partners and I am not sure that the benefits of the data gathered warrant this commitment of time for most couples. However, for couples in which relationship complaints are vague, with limited ability to clearly specify problematic behaviors, the SOC may be useful. O'Leary (1987) presents an abbreviated SOC-type checklist consisting of just over 100 items. As for the SOC, each partner indicates on a daily basis whether the behavior occurs. Each behavior that occurs is rated for pleasantness or unpleasantness on a 9-point Likert-type rating scale. Although briefer than the SOC, the instrument still is quite time-consuming for people to complete.

One limitation of extensive behavioral checklists is that much of the information collected is not terribly helpful. Most people's lives have a fairly heavy concentration of mundane events that do not have a major impact on them or on their relationships. Having couples tediously record the minutia of their life, who spoke to whom, who did the dishes, who went and did a chore, and so forth, may not lead to a lot of valuable information. Often perceptions about relationships are shaped by low-frequency but high-emotional-impact events. For that reason Sue Osgarby and I developed the Marital Events Diary. This instrument is intended to provide some indication of the ongoing interchange between partners but to focus the information collected more on high-impact events.

Figure 5.1 shows a page from the Marital Events Diary (Osgarby & Halford, 2000b). At the end of each day each partner indicates, using half-hour blocks, how much time they spent together, the location and major activity during that half-hour block, and the degree of positivity or negativity of the affect during that half hour. Each partner also is asked to identify the most positive and the most negative interaction he or she had with the other partner during that 24-hour period. Each partner makes an event record for the interactions identified as most positive and most negative. As is shown in the fig-

FIGURE 5.1. The Marital Events Diary.

The purpose of this diary is to help you track what happens in your relationship day by day. There is an opening of two pages per day. Please do the following at the end of each day. On page 1 in the left column place a tick for each waking half hour, or part thereof, you spent with your partner. For each half hour with your partner record the symbols to indicate where you were and what you were doing. Then place a tick to rate overall how you felt in the interaction from "– –" very negative, through "0" neutral, to "+ +" very positive.

Location codes	Activity codes
BR = bedroom	HC = household chores
L= lounge	TV = watching TV
DR = dining room	PR = parenting
K = kitchen	RE = relaxing, reading
P = porch	TR = travel
C = car	TA = talking
Y = yard	
OT = other	

On page 2 circle the number that best describes your overall relationship satisfaction for the day. Then make an event record of the most positive and the most negative interaction you had with your partner for the day by filling in answers to the questions.

Page 1 of 2 for the day

Time	Together? (√)	Place	Activity	Affect rating – – – 0 + ++
6:30 A.M.				
7:00				
7:30				
8:00				
8:30				
9:00				
9:30				
10:00				
10:30				
11:00				
11:30				
12:00 P.M.				
12:30				
1:00				
1:30				
2:00				
2:30				
3:00				
3:30				
4:00				
4:30				
5:00				
5:30				
6:00				
6:30				

(continued)

7:00			
7:30			
8:00			
8:30			
9:00			
9:30			
10:00			
10:30			
11:00			
11:30			
12:00 A.M.			

Page 2 of 2 for the day

Overall relationship satisfaction for the day

1	2	3	4	5	6	7

Extremely
unhappy   Neutral   Extremely
happy

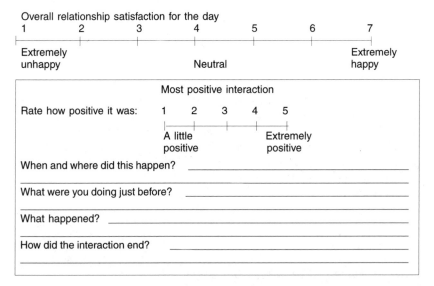

Most positive interaction

Rate how positive it was: 1   2   3   4   5

A little   Extremely
positive   positive

When and where did this happen? _____

What were you doing just before? _____

What happened? _____

How did the interaction end? _____

Most negative interaction

Rate how negative it was: 1   2   3   4   5

A little   Extremely
negative   negative

When and where did this happen? _____

What were you doing just before? _____

What happened? _____

How did the interaction end? _____

FIGURE 5.1. (*continued*)

ure, the individual partners indicate the time, the place, and major activity involved during the positive or stressful interaction. The degree of positive or negative affect elicited by that interaction also is rated. The intention is to try and find out where, when, and under what circumstances strongly positive or negative events occur in the relationship.

The intent with the Marital Events Diary is to help individuals identify relationship events that are affecting on them in major ways. Often distressed couples overlook positive relationship events and selectively attend to, and remember, negative relationship events. Making the positive relationship events salient is particularly important for developing a balanced view of a relationship. For example, I used the Marital Events Diary when I saw Toni and Russell. Each person had described how their relationship had deteriorated to the point where both felt that they did nothing together that was ever positive. Each asserted this quite strongly. I had each partner keep the Marital Events Diary for a week. We then reviewed each partner's diary individually on a day-by-day basis. The diaries identified a number of instances of positive interaction between the partners. It was noticeable that the events that were rated as most positive involved playing with one or other of their two daughters, who were 5 and 3 years of age. Interaction with their daughters provided fun and a sense of closeness in the relationship. The couple discussed with me the ways in which the birth of each of their daughters had changed their relationship. It was noticeable from their diaries, and from this discussion, that the partners had very little time together without their daughters. This eventually led to the identification of a specific goal for therapy: to attempt to change the balance of time so that there was some couple-only time as well as time with the children.

How to Manage Common Challenges in Couple Presentations

Couple therapy can be complex. The stress of relationship problems often leaves partners uncertain whether they wish to continue in their relationship. Each person may view the other as the problem and feel that the real change needs to be made by his or her partner. Either partner may have significant individual problems that interact with relationship problems. Past hurts may dominate one or both partner's views of the relationship and reduce motivation for change. A crisis, such as the discovery of an affair, may be so overwhelming that one or both partners find it hard to get through the day, let alone consider the future of their relationship. Actual or threatened violence can explode within some relationships. The couple therapist needs to respond constructively to the foregoing challenges, as these are common themes in couple's presentations. Next I describe the common themes in couple presentations and provide suggestions on how to respond to these challenges. Typically, the themes become evident early in therapy, and hence assessment needs to be conducted so as to manage these challenges.

The Relationship: To Be or Not to Be?

When clients first arrive at couple therapy, they can have a diversity of agendas. In most couples the future of the relationship is, at least to some degree, in question. In some couples one partner may already have decided to leave the relationship and may be entering therapy simply as a convenient way to break this news to the partner, or to provide some professional support to the partner once separation has occurred. (This was once explained to me by a woman as "Please look after him now, because I no longer want to."). While unusual, such a firm agenda precludes couple therapy, though it is possible that this presentation might lead to mediation for separation. A more common scenario arises when at least one partner is unsure either about his or her desire to be in the relationship, to be in therapy, or both.

Ambivalence about a relationship can result in a therapeutic stalemate. Most approaches to couple therapy require a fair degree of effort—effort that may seem difficult for the person to make when uncommitted to the relationship long term. On the other hand, if neither partner is willing to leave the relationship, the couple may feel stuck. In such instances the assessment process can be offered as a means to determine whether the partners wish to attempt change. In other words, the partners are not asked to commit to the relationship at this point, only to do an assessment to help them decide whether they wish to commit to the relationship. It is important to emphasize couple therapy as a choice that either partner may opt out of. If therapy is only partially engaged in, this often leads to resentment about the lack of effort from the other partner (and sometimes from the therapist as well). These issues were part of an initial interview with Meredith and Wayne. After meeting with each partner separately we all met together toward the end of the first session when the following interchange occurred.

THERAPIST: Let me, uh, summarize what each of you has told me. You agree that you have problems with communication, . . . with frequent arguments. You also agree that since the birth of your children, you have little time together as a couple. Together the arguments and lack of quality time have eroded the strength of your feeling for each other. Each of you has begun to wonder if the marriage can last . . . are unsure about whether to stay in therapy or not.

This is a real dilemma for each of you. On the one hand, you have been together a long time, and have two children together. At one time you were very much in love, and you still feel caring for the other. This makes it very hard for you to separate at this time. Yet, there has been a lot of hurt and pain in the last few years, and this makes it hard to know if things can work out between you. It seems you each find it hard to know what to do.

MEREDITH: I am not ready to give up yet, but . . . Oh, I don't know . . . (*starting to cry*).

WAYNE: Hmm, it's hard you know . . . when I found out about the affair I wanted to leave straight away. Now, well, I can't seem to decide to leave. I think about when we were happy.

THERAPIST: So, each of you feels stuck, unable to decide what to do. Try this idea for size. Let's do a couple more assessment sessions together. I will really try to understand your relationship. We will work hard together to find out what is causing the problems. In a week or two I will summarize all that you have told me and what we discover together. This will be like a formal report on your relationship. We then will talk about what goals you could work on if you decided to stay together, and how we would try to get to those goals in therapy. At that point you each will need to say, "OK, I will work on that," or "No, I don't want to do that." What do you think?

MEREDITH: So, the next couple of weeks is to decide? What if we are still not sure?

THERAPIST: In my experience the whole business of assessment helps most people to decide . . . at least if they at least want to give therapy a try. In the end it's up to each of you. If either of you wants to call it quits at any point, that's the end. Are you wanting to give assessment a try, or are you saying you would rather finish therapy tonight?

MEREDITH: No, I will do the assessment.

THERAPIST: Wayne?

WAYNE: Sure, why not. Ten years of marriage is worth weighing up before you give up.

At this point I went on to explain several different assessment instruments I wanted them to complete between sessions. I went to considerable lengths to emphasize the importance of completing the measures and checking that each partner agreed to complete the forms before the next session. The goal of this process is to engage the couple in deciding about the relationship.

"Fix Up My Partner So We Can Relate"

Often one or both partners blame their relationship problems primarily on the other person (Bradbury & Fincham, 1990). Sometimes this presentation is disguised in social niceties, such as "I know it takes two make a relationship, but . . ., " or "Neither of us is without fault, but . . . ." Often the "but" is silent but there if you listen for it. A key problem with partner blaming is that it is disempowering. By focusing on the partner's behavior, people miss the chance to change the thing over which they have most control: their own behavior. A key therapeutic question is whether each partner is willing and able to change a predominantly or exclusively partner-blaming focus to a conjoint focus within which the couple can work together. The initial interview provides a context within which the therapist can assess each partner's ability to identify aspects of his or her own behavior that may contribute to the relationship problems. Throughout the assessment process the therapist uses structured assessments that prompt attention to both the individual's own contribution to relationship difficulties and to interaction processes between the partners that are part of the relationship problems. Moreover, focusing on the contextual and life events that influence the couple can often serve to reduce blame and anger toward the partner. In most cases sensitive use of assessment will enable both partners to recognize that relationship problems are rarely attributable solely to one partner. However, in some instances even at the end of assessment one partner still blames the other for the relationship problems. In such instances relationship psychoeducation may be necessary to assist the partners to develop a broader and more helpful way of viewing their relationship. (Chapter 7 describes in detail the process of conducting relationship psychoeducation.)

Although many distressed partners inaccurately blame their spouse for their relationship problems, individual problems do contribute in a substantial manner to many couples' relationship problems. For example, alcohol abuse often antedates relationship problems and places severe stress on a relationship (Halford et al., 1999). The crucial issue for the therapist is not whether individual problems are relevant to the relationship but, rather, whether the individual functioning of the partners contraindicates couple therapy. If one partner is suicidal, rarely sober, or extremely depressed, then engagement in couple therapy focusing on relationship issues may be inappropriate, at least initially. However, if the two partners have a conjoint goal of changing an important aspect of one partner's behavior, an adapted form of couple therapy can be suitable. For example, O'Farrell and Rotunda (1997) describe use of conjoint contracts between spouses for use of Antabuse (disulfiram) to help heavy drinkers establish sobriety. In a similar manner I have contracted to conduct couple therapy contingent upon a partner diagnosed with bipolar disorder going back on lithium medication.

In summary, couple therapy is possible if the couple have at least some agreed-on goals. In couple therapy those goals often would be relationship focused (e.g., help us to communicate better) but could include conjoint efforts to change one partner's behavior (e.g., work together to help John cope better with his depression). The assessment process needs to explore these possibilities with the couple.

"I Can Never Forget . . . "

Some people present to therapy preoccupied by past hurts or pain in the relationship. The most common source of this preoccupation is the discovery of an affair, though any act seen as significant by a partner can be a source of intense distress. For example, in one couple I saw the wife, Bette, was very angry with her husband, Vernon, about his past gambling. Both partners reported that Vernon had a long history of gambling and that he had lost large amounts of money over a prolonged period. This problem had culminated 5 years ago in Vernon's stealing from his employer in a desperate effort to repay gambling debts. He had lost his job, the couple had lost their home to repay the debts, and Vernon narrowly avoided going to jail. The couple was now in their mid-50s, Vernon was unemployed, and they were suffering considerable economic hardship in living on Bette's part-time wage.

The issue in all couple therapy is whether the couple has shared relationship goals. In cases such as that of Vernon and Bette, where one partner is very angry about the past, that partner often finds it difficult to focus on the current and future relationship rather than issues of the past. The therapist needs to explore the impact of that past event on the aggrieved partner in individual consultation, to respond empathically to the hurt and anger, and then to establish if the person is able to refocus on the future. If that proves difficult, then additional relationship psychoeducation may be necessary to establish whether forgiving the partner can be achieved (see Chapter 7).

The Crisis

Couples who present in crisis are responding to events that overwhelm the capacity of one or both partners to cope. In my experience the most common events precipitating presentation for therapy with a sense of crisis are extreme conflict, particularly when associated with violence, or the discovery of an affair. However, many major life events can have an impact on couples and can elicit a sense of crisis, such as a death in the family, severe financial problems, or diagnosis of a life-threatening illness. I described responding to crises in some detail in Chapter 4. Here I simply want to reiterate that in response to a crisis, it usually is helpful to focus on what needs to be done immediately and to defer long-term decisions until the effects of the crisis have been brought under more control. The decision of whether or not couple therapy is appropriate often is deferred until the immediate crisis is resolved.

"We Need Help to Get This Right"

For most therapists the easiest and perhaps most rewarding presentations are couples committed to their relationship that wish to enrich or repair their relationship. The most common concerns that such couples initially identify at presentation, in approximate order of descending prevalence, are communication problems, conflict management, lack of affection or intimacy, lack of shared quality time, incompatibility, and sexual dissatisfaction. The best prognosis is for couples in which there are still significant positive feelings between the partners. In such couples, a collaborative approach to enhancing their relationship is often evident at presentation, and this makes the therapist's task much easier.

Concluding Assessment

If the therapist has completed the recommended steps in this and the preceding chapter, initial assessment should be complete. As a check for myself on whether assessment is adequately done, I find it useful to consider the following questions.

1. Can I list succinctly the key problem areas in the relationship as perceived by each partner?
2. Do both partners regard me as empathic with their distress and concerns about the relationship?
3. Can I define the core adaptive couple processes that seem to be the strengths and weaknesses of the relationship and the individual behaviors of the partners contributing to those processes?
4. Can I summarize any key individual characteristics evident in the partners that have an impact on their relationship?
5. Can I summarize key stressful events that impinge upon the partners and the relationship?
6. Do I understand the context of the development of the couple's relationship and its problems?

Ultimately the couple and the individual partners need to be understandable to the therapist. Specifically, the therapist needs to be empathic with how each partner experiences the relationship and to be able to suggest changes each partners might be willing to make in order to enhance the relationship. If I answer yes to questions (1) through (6), then I am hypothesizing that I understand the couple well enough to proceed to the treatment phase. This then raises the challenges of how to present my understanding to the couple and to determine whether we have a shared understanding. If we do have a shared understanding, we need to negotiate whether couple therapy is to proceed and, if so, what form it will take. Chapter 6 describes these steps.

6

Feedback and Negotiation

The assessment process should give the therapist and each partner of the couple an understanding of the relationship, including its key strengths, weaknesses, and what things need to change. The therapist will have formed a set of hypotheses, referred to as the working model, about the adaptive processes that constitute the relationship's strengths and problems and the crucial factors that influenced the development and maintenance of those processes. In the feedback process the therapist offers the hypotheses that form his or her working model and negotiates with the couple to form a shared model acceptable to both partners. Once a shared working model is agreed on, the therapist then negotiates with the couple on the potential goals for therapy and whether couple therapy will proceed. As described in Chapter 3, self-regulatory couple therapy (SRCT) has three major therapy structures: brief self-guided change, relationship psychoeducation, and therapist-guided change. If couple therapy is to proceed, the process of therapy is negotiated, which involves evaluating the viability of each of these options.

This chapter describes how to conduct the feedback and negotiation process. I begin with an overview of the process and then elaborates on preparation for the feedback session. Then I provide detail on how to conduct the feedback process, including negotiating the working model of the relationship. I then discuss negotiating the goals and structure of couple therapy. The final section addresses challenges in the feedback and negotiation process and how to address those challenges.

Overview of Feedback and Negotiation

With the therapist guiding the discussion, each partner negotiates a shared view of the relationship strengths and problems. This is done through a guided participation process that consists of five steps. The process begins by (1) establishing the agenda of the feedback session and (2) soliciting the partners' expectations of the assessment feedback. The majority of the time is spent with step 3: The therapist presents systematic feedback of the assessment results, and discusses these results with the couple. In step 4 the therapist summarizes the key strengths and weaknesses of the relationship and checks that this summary accurately reflects the views of the partners. In step 5 the therapist offers tentative hypotheses about the development and maintenance of the strengths and weaknesses of the relationship summarized in step 4. These relationship strengths and weaknesses, plus the hypotheses offered in step 5, form the therapist's working model of the relationship. Then the therapist checks the partner's agreement with the working model and negotiates any changes required to develop a shared working model of the relationship acceptable to both partners and the therapist. Table 6.1 summarizes the key elements of each of the five steps in the guided participation model.

Preparing the Feedback in Advance

Before presenting the results to the couple, the therapist first must identify the most important issues for making therapy work for that couple. Then the therapist must structure the assessment results so they are understandable to the couple. It is helpful to create in advance a list of descriptive points from each assessment measure. It is crucial to establish the broad areas of agreed relationship strengths and problems and to develop a sense of commitment to working on the problems. I aim to describe three or four key relationship strengths and three or four key relationship problems. A description of the relationship that is too complex is not all that helpful. Generally I expect to be able to discuss these key points in 20 to 30 minutes. Because the feedback session summarizes what has already been discussed, it is not necessary to cover every nuance of each relationship strength or problem.

Focusing on aspects of the relationship salient to the partners can be difficult if all the partners see are relationship problems. Restating a long list of relationship complaints is unlikely to build mutual effort toward relationship repair and enhancement. Almost all couples have experienced good times, though the positive intimate memories may feel distant. If the assessment process to this point has been done well, the therapist and the couple will be prepared for the therapist to prompt the partners in the feedback session to remember the positive aspects of the relationship history. This often sets up a

TABLE 6.1. The Guided Participation Process for Reviewing Assessment Findings: What to Cover

Step	Key points
1. Negotiate agenda.	Emphasize importance of reviewing key assessment findings, focusing on desired future change and need to develop agreed-on position.
2. Solicit couple's expectations of feedback.	Ask each partner to self-appraise the relationship, prompt and reinforce attention to both positive and negative aspects of the relationship, reinforce accurate self-appraisal.
3. Present results.	Focus on key findings, present data systematically measure by measure, balance presentation of positive and negative aspects of relationship, check partner agreement with descriptive data, discuss with partners.
4. Summarize key relationship strengths and weaknesses.	Provide summary of three or four key elements of positive aspects of relationship, and three or four key elements in the couple's adaptive processes that constitute the relationship problems. Check partners' agreement with summary and add other issues as required.
5. Negotiate shared working model of relationship.	Therapist relates relationship strengths and weaknesses to key individual, contextual, or life events hypothesized to influence onset and maintenance of relationship strengths and weaknesses. Therapist checks partners' agreement with working model and modifies working model as required.

desire to attempt to recapture the passion and positivity that once existed. The feedback of assessment results is an opportunity to draw on that desire to rekindle the past positivity.

Figure 6.1 provides an example of the notes I take into a feedback session. The notes highlight the core observations to make about the relationship and the exact data on which the observations are based. As is reflected in the notes, it is important to sustain a balance of attention both to positive aspects and to problems in the relationship. I am also trying to include the individual partners' perspectives as well as a relationship focus in the description of problem domains. The summary includes the key relationship strengths and problems to be covered and a few tentative hypotheses to offer within the initial working model. Finally, the figure illustrates four therapy goals to be suggested to the couple.

The use of notes is not intended to provide a rigid structure but a broad framework for systematic discussion of findings. The use of notes helps to keep the feedback descriptive, based on evidence, and not to offer premature interpretation. However, flexibility is necessary when using notes. For example, the content of the therapist's working model and suggested therapy goals

Amy and Tim: Feedback (Session No. 3), April 15

Interview data

Strengths

Strong history, bond together
Married 23 years, 3 grown-up children
Gone through tough times (e.g., Amy's mum's death), helped each other
Still enjoy going out, enjoy talking about lots of things (e.g., plant breeding hobby)

Problems

Arguments always a problem, gotten a lot worse in last 2 years
Affair by Tim 2 years ago hurt Amy, a lot of arguments since then, issue of Amy's
    jealousy when Tim away from her
Sex infrequent in last 5 to 10 years; Amy has never enjoyed sex that much,
    problems with orgasm for her

Dyadic Adjustment Scale

Amy 95, Tim 98; both mildly distressed, but both want to work on relationship
Major areas of disagreement identified by both as about sex, time apart, activities
    together
Both report kiss each other every day, often talk, do projects together
Sex infrequent

Areas of Change Questionnaire

Amy

Partner change: increase expression of feelings, increase time together, do more
    household chores
Self-change: more sex, less arguments, attend to physical appearance more, more
    affectionate

Tim

Partner change: argue less, have sex more often, go out more with others, be
    affectionate more
Self-change: express feelings more, have sex less, attend to household chores
    more

Overall

Neither requesting a lot of change; fine tuning
Agreement on needed changes

Communication Pattern Questionnaire

Both report Amy demands, Tim withdraws; has always been like that
Amy reports feeling Tim pulls away and won't talk to her about affair, thinks he may
    be hiding something
Tim reports despair that Amy keeps wanting to talk about affair, feels trapped

FIGURE 6.1. Example of notes for feedback session.

(*continued*)

Working model

Relationship strengths

23 years together
Mutual support
Fun together
Affection, love for each other

Weaknesses

Arguments (demand–withdraw)
The affair
Sex

Onset and maintenance

Less time together with children, work
Arguments always there, got worse
Distancing (Amy feels overworked, Tim neglected)
The affair

Possible goals

Reestablish trust, resolve affair
Manage negative jealousy, negotiate independence
Conflict management
Further assess sexual issues, work on enhancing sexual relationship

FIGURE 6.1. (*continued*)

often needs to be modified if the partners add extra, important information during the feedback process.

The feedback session needs to be focused on what is crucial and not to allow the process to get lost in detail. In the example in Figure 6.1, the notes do not cover the issue of what there was about Tim, or the relationship, which led to the affair. I did think that was important to explore at some point, but it was not necessary to understand that issue before beginning therapy. The notes simply reflect the key things that I believed, after the first two sessions, were crucial to making therapy work with these two people.

Step 1: Negotiating the Session Agenda

To optimize the opportunity for the couple and the therapist to be mutually collaborative, often it is useful to begin the feedback session by agreeing on the agenda and goals of that session. I try to tell each partner exactly what we are attempting to do together. The introduction might go something like this.

"Today is the feedback session. As we have discussed in previous sessions, today I want to talk with you about the results of the assessment work we have been doing together. I will go through each of the different assessments you have done, covering what you have told me in interviews, the results from the forms you have filled out for me, and the results of some of the tasks you have undertaken. It is very important that I really understand well the problems in the relationship, and if I get anything wrong I would really like you to tell me.

"The primary goal will be to see if we can reach a shared understanding amongst the three of us about the current strengths of your relationship and the problems that you have been experiencing. If we can achieve that, then we will focus on the goals you wish to set for therapy. I can then tell you about some of the ways in which we might work together to attain those goals. Finally, I will ask each of you whether you want to give couple therapy a try. Couple therapy does require a significant commitment of time and energy, and I am keen that you know exactly what it is that you commit to."

It is important to check with couples whether they agree with the proposed agenda or want to add anything. Sometimes an event has occurred which is seen as extremely important, and which would distract the couple from attending to the proposed agenda. For example, if the couple have had a large argument in the last day or so and are feeling very negative toward each other, the feedback session may be difficult to run effectively. The therapist may need to set aside the proposed agenda and deal with the immediate crisis of an argument.

Step 2: Soliciting the Partners' Expectations of the Feedback

Assuming that the couple agrees to the suggested session agenda, and this happens in the vast majority of occasions, I begin by asking the couple their expectations of the feedback. This serves several purposes. Most couples have formed views about their relationship difficulties through the process of assessment. If the appraisals the partners make are constructive, I allow them to self-define those relationship problems that they can. In other words, if the partners have developed the self-regulation skills of appraising their relationship, I prompt them to use those skills. It is important that the therapist reinforces the partners for their accurate appraisals. Let me illustrate with an example.

THERAPIST: Having completed the assessments, how do you two see the key relationship issues?

JOY: Should I go first, honey? (*Husband nods.*) Clive and I have had some terrible arguments over the last couple of years. We didn't used to. Somehow we seem to have got into a pattern of tearing strips off each other when we disagree. We're both stubborn . . . we just don't seem to be able to let go of an argument. I think we need to learn to fight fairer, . . . not to let little things blow up out of proportion.

THERAPIST: Clive, what do you think of that?

CLIVE: I agree. When we filled in that form about communication, I got to thinking about how we talk to each other. Both of us get pretty rude to each other. I gotta learn to keep my big mouth shut more of the time.

JOY: No, don't go quiet on me, love . . . I won't know it's you (*laughter from both partners*)

CLIVE: No, no, you're always telling me to say how I feel about things, so I won't go quiet. I just meant I want to be able to say . . . without getting into a fight.

THERAPIST: You seem each to be saying you want to be able to talk through disagreements without fighting or hurting each other. Is that right? (*both nod*)

THERAPIST: It's interesting that both of you came up with conflict management as a goal without my saying anything. How did you work out the problem?

CLIVE: Well we have been talking between sessions about what the forms and stuff meant to us. All due respect to you, but you don't need to be Einstein to work out some of the stuff we've been doing wrong. Coming to counseling just made me, and Joy, pay attention to what we need to do.

Some partners have particular concerns or fears about the therapist's feedback. The question "What do you expect me, as the therapist, to tell you?" often uncovers those fears. For example, I recently had a wife respond by saying, "You are going to tell us there is no hope for our relationship." Knowing that concern, I asked her why she believed I might say that to her. The comment reflected her pessimism about the future of the relationship.

Asking the couple to anticipate the therapist's feedback maximizes the chance for the partners to self-appraise their relationship. What the partners knew at the beginning of therapy may have changed because of the therapist-guided assessment process. The question also allows the therapist to identify any immediate concerns that may interfere with considering the relationship as a whole. The therapist can then add to the couple's perspective any additional points that are important.

Step 3: Presenting the Results of Assessment

Unless the couple accurately self-appraises all the important aspects of their relationship, the therapist next presents the results of the assessment. It is best to begin with descriptive comments based on evidence and to avoid interpretive comments that judge what has been observed or reported. The descriptive feedback focuses predominantly on the adaptive processes between the partners: the thoughts, feelings, and actions that make up the couple's interactions. For example, I usually hold up the actual form the partner filled in and summarize the key answers the partner made on that form. I do the same with the other partner, summarizing the key answers that the other partner made on that form. Through this process the therapist and the partners build up a set of agreed-on descriptions of the relationship strengths and problem areas before they attempt to interpret the meaning of these descriptions. Consider this example. Alison reported that she found John distant and unwilling to engage in regular pleasant activities with her. John reported that he felt pressured by Alison to spend more time with her. He resented what he saw as her denying him any independent activities or interests. The therapist presented this issue in the session as follows:

THERAPIST: On this form (*holding up Dyadic Adjustment Scale*) you both stated that you often disagreed about time spent together. Is that right?

JOHN: Absolutely, that's one of our regular fights.

THERAPIST: OK, it seems that it is often hard for you to agree on how much time you should spend together. Alison, you seem to experience this as John being unwilling to do things with you, and that you find hurtful. Is that right?

ALISON: I really don't understand why he wants to get away all the time. It seems like he doesn't care to spend time with me, that I'm boring or something.

THERAPIST: John, if I've understood your view, it's that Alison seems to want to restrict you doing things or seeing friends as an independent person.

JOHN: That's right. I think a healthy relationship needs each person to have some life of their own.

THERAPIST: OK, so do we agree that working out a balance of couple and individual time that works for both of you is important to do?
    (*Alison and John both nod assent*)

Here is another example in which I first present the data and then move to the inference about relationship functioning. In this case the data were based on observation of a problem-solving task completed 2 weeks before the feedback session.

THERAPIST: Remember that problem-solving task that I got you to do a couple of weeks back, where you talked about the issue of time together?

JOHN: Yeah, I do; we got into a fight in that room right down the hall.

THERAPIST: I would like to make a couple of observations about the way you two talked to each other that time . . . this is really going over what we discussed then, but I want to check we have a common understanding of what happened. One thing I noticed was a difference in the amount the two of you talked. Alison, you talked quite a lot more than John; you were relatively quiet John.

ALISON: That's often how we talk . . . John does not say much, which frustrates the hell out of me.

JOHN: I don't talk when I get barraged . . .

THERAPIST: Right, let's check what we agree on. When you talk stuff through generally Alison does more of the talking. John, you said in a an earlier session that you often feel pinned down by Alison, and get a feeling like you just have to get out of the situation?

JOHN: When Alison starts on me, I get worried we are going to argue. It never does any good. Seems hopeless going over the same stuff, so I sort of shut down. Often I go and play the guitar, just to mellow down a little.

THERAPIST: So you feel the need to escape?

JOHN: Yep.

ALISON: And that drives me crazy; we never finish anything.

THERAPIST: On several occasions you have said you want him to tell you more about how he thinks and feels. So it seems that there is this pattern. Alison will want to talk about an issue; she raises it. John feels pressured, and gets worried there is going to be a fight. Alison does more of the talking, John goes quiet. Both of you feel bad at this stage. Alison tries to deal with her frustration by talking more and trying to get John to talk. John copes by withdrawing, which tends to make you (*looking at Alison*) push more for you (*looking at John*) to talk. It leaves both of you feeling frustrated. Is that something like it?

JOHN: You got it.

THERAPIST: Alison?

ALISON: Yeah (*sighs*), I wonder if we can change this? We've been doing this all our marriage.

THERAPIST: So, this pattern is a long-standing habit. Habits can be hard to change, but in my experience many couples do change. Are you both wanting to try to find a new way to handle conflict, to try to change this pattern?

ALISON: I would love us to change.

THERAPIST: John?

JOHN: Sure, if we are to make this marriage work we gotta talk to each other better than we do now.

In presenting the evidence it is important to balance presentation of positive and negative aspects of the relationship. Excessive and unbroken attention to negatives can be discouraging, whereas overattention to positives may make a distressed couple feel the therapist has missed the extent of their distress. It also is important to balance attention to the two partners, so neither partner becomes disengaged during the session. To this end, it can be useful to alternate the presentation of issues that are of primary importance to each spouse. If the assessment process has accurately identified the thoughts, feelings, and actions that make up the couple's concerns, and each partner has received empathy from the therapist, this part of the feedback session usually proceeds with a high level of agreement to the issues presented by the therapist.

Step 4: Summarizing the Relationship Strengths and Weaknesses

On conclusion of presentation of the individual points, the therapist summarizes the key issues that the partners and therapist agree define the current relationship and its problems. I usually begin by stating my intent to summarize. I then restate three or four key positive aspects of the couple's life together, and then focus on the couple's problems. The therapist then checks if the partners agree with this summary, or if extra issues need to be considered. Extra issues are added as required, and a final summary is stated for partners to evaluate. Let me illustrate this process with an example from the case of Tim and Amy that was introduced previously.

THERAPIST: I want to try to summarize the important things we know at this point about your relationship. First, the relationship: There are lots of positives. You two have been together a long time, 23 years. You've raised three children together. You have supported each other through tough times. Amy, you mentioned Tim's support when your mum was dying, and Tim you mentioned when you were out of work. After all this time you still have fun together, you share your love of plant breeding, you both love the movies, you talk about lots of things. I've noticed how you smile at each other, the warmth in your voices, you both say you love each other.

But, on the other side, there are three key things you've mentioned that are real problems. First up, you argue lots, always have, but it's got a lot worse. We've described the Amy demands–Tim withdraws pattern you seem to get into. Second is the affair: the jealousy, arguments, the fact it happened just gets in the way of how you feel toward each other.

Third is sex. You aren't having sex together much, and when you do it's not very enjoyable for either of you.

Is that right? Have I captured the key elements of how you see things?

TIM: Yeah, that's pretty much it. I especially think we have to somehow put the affair behind us, let it go.

THERAPIST: So for you Tim getting past the affair is crucial. Amy, how do you see things?

AMY: Well Tim thinks I should forget it happened, but I can't. It did happen, it hurt, it still hurts, you can't just forget that your husband lied to you, sneaked out to see another woman . . .

THERAPIST: So Amy you are saying you can't just pretend this never happened. Tim did have an affair. But you seem to be agreeing that how you and Tim handle the fact that it happened is crucial. Is that true?

AMY: Well, I don't know how we get past something like this.

THERAPIST: Let's come back to what we are going to do in a little while. At this stage we seem to have agreement that managing the aftermath of the affair is important, that currently the effect of the affair on your relationship is very negative. Amy, I also mentioned the fighting and sex as issues. Do you have anything else that seems important to you that I have not mentioned?

AMY: Well, I feel Tim is not very open with me, you know he does not tell me his feelings. I want him to talk to me, not just about plants and the news, about him, me, us.

THERAPIST: So increasing talking about feelings, about how he really feels?

AMY: Uh huh.

THERAPIST: So we add increasing expressing feelings, to the arguments, the affair, and sex as key problems to address. Does that capture the most important problems? (*Both nod.*)

Step 5: Negotiating the Working Model of the Relationship

As noted earlier, the working model of the relationship consists of three parts: the key relationship strengths, the key weaknesses, and a set of hypotheses about the onset and maintenance of the problems. In step 4 the relationship strengths and weaknesses have been identified, in this final step the therapist negotiates with the couple to define a working model that incorporates hypotheses about the onset and maintenance of relationship problems. Specifically, the therapist summarizes the contextual factors, life events, and individual characteristics that the therapist hypothesizes have influenced the development and maintenance of the couple's difficulties. Sharing these hypotheses is intended to prime the partners to think about their relationship in terms of the range of influences on the relationship and to avoid the common trap of simplistic partner blaming for relationship problems. The therapist then asks the partners if they agree with the summary and negotiates until they feel the important elements of the relationship are represented in this working model of the relationship. Following is an example of negotiating a working model of the relationship again based on the case of Amy and Tim summarized in Figure 6.1.

THERAPIST: When we think about how things got to the point they have, I was struck by several things. You both mentioned that as you were raising your children you had less time together. You both were working full time, life was busy, there was less time together, and the time you did have sometimes was a chore rather than fun. There were few dates together. Arguments had always been a problem, but seemed to escalate, get worse.

Amy, you felt Tim left much of the parenting and household chores to you, you resented this and felt tired a lot. When Tim started to travel more with work, this threw even more of the load on you. Sex had never been great for you, but you really lost interest at that time. You just went through the motions of sex.

Tim, you mentioned that you felt Amy lost interest in you. You were aware she did not enjoy sex. The arguments really stressed you. When you started the new job 5 years ago there was travel, time away, and that time away sometimes seemed a relief. It seems like the business of life ate away at your time together, and things that had been minor problems, the sex and arguing got worse. Does that make sense to you?

AMY: Yeah, we sort of drifted apart over a long time.

THERAPIST: Tim?

TIM: It got to the point where I felt I wasn't welcome in the house you know. All the arguments, not feeling Amy was interested in me sexually—that was pretty tough, and she didn't want to talk about that.

THERAPIST: Then the affair happens. Things are wobbly before, and it gets really bad. Lots of angry words, hurt. You both wonder whether to leave, but hang in there because of the history. Two years go by and the fights continue, a real big argument ensues. Tim says he is leaving but cannot bring himself to make the final step of moving out. Julia [their eldest child] reads an article in the paper on couple therapy, you ring up and here you are.

AMY: Yeah, here we are. And I still don't know if we can make it work. Over 20 years together and we don't know if we want to be married.

THERAPIST: So, all the pain, what's happened means you really aren't sure you want to be together, but there are 23 years with quite a lot of good times. So, it's really hard to walk away. Now you both feel hurt, you are not having fun together, the arguments keep happening, and all that keeps the problems going. Tim, does that make sense to you?

TIM: Yes. I really regret the affair, I am sorry I hurt Amy. But sorry does not seem enough.

THERAPIST: So let's consider what might be enough to make this relationship one you both want to recommit to. Let's talk about what goals you might want to work on. But before that, Amy is what I said making sense to you?

AMY: Yes. Till now I have just focused on the affair, but things had been going down hill for quite a while. I can see that.

This summary illustrates several points about negotiating the working model. First, the working model is usually simple; complex prescriptions are too difficult for people to remember or work with. Second, discussing the model typically has high emotional significance to the partners. This is not just a rational review of data, and emotional responses need to be monitored by the therapist and responded to empathetically. Third, the working model is constructed to avoid excessive blame on either partner and is an acknowledgement that multiple factors usually contribute to the development of relationship problems. Fourth, if agreement about the working model is established then often most of the goals for therapy are implicitly defined in the working model. Finally, sometimes the partners' responses to the model guide the therapist as to likely priorities in negotiating therapy goals and structure. In the case of Amy and Tim the strength of each partner's emotional responses to the topic of the affair suggested that resolution of the affair and its effects would need to be addressed early in therapy.

Negotiating Relationship Goals and Therapy Structure

Once the therapist and partners have agreed on a working model of the relationship and its problems, it is time to negotiate the goals and structure of therapy. A key decision is whether to proceed to brief self-change, relationship psychoeducation, or therapist-guided change.

Defining Relationship Goals

Usually the agreed-on working model implicitly defines the relationship goals of the couple. For example, if difficulties in managing conflict are central to the working model, then developing better methods for managing conflict is a logical goal. Similarly, if quality time together as a couple is important, but lacking, then developing quality time becomes a relationship goal.

I begin goal setting by asking the partners to identify what the key goals are for improving their relationship. As this question follows on from the discussion of the working model, the couple often is able to define three or four key goals that they wish to work on to enhance their relationship. The most commonly identified relationship goals involve changing couple adaptive processes such as managing conflict better, enhancing quality time, improving communication, renegotiating roles, enhancing mutual support, increasing expressions of affection, and improving sex. The therapist should give positive feedback to the partners for successful goal setting. The therapist also uses questions and suggestions to help the partners define any goals the couple has omitted that flow from the working model. The therapist shapes up any vague goals (e.g., to be nicer to each other) to be more specific (e.g., to make requests for change of each other politely and to spend quality time together). The therapist then summarizes the defined goals and checks that the partners agree with the summary. Assuming that there is agreement between the partners and the therapist on the relationship goals, the next step is to determine the process for achieving those goals.

Negotiating Therapy Structure

Once relationship goals are defined, many couples can proceed directly to self-change, with minimal further input from the therapist. Self-regulated change is the ultimate goal of SRCT. Other couples have strong negative thoughts or feelings, or a lack of knowledge, that blocks their self-implementation of change. These couples need some sessions of relationship psychoeducation and then they may be able to implement self-change. Finally, some couples need to develop certain skills in order to implement their desired changes. For example, some partners may lack communication or affect regulation skills and need therapist guidance to develop these skills. Once these skills are developed, the couple can implement self-change.

Negotiating the structure of therapy begins by evaluating whether brief self-change is feasible. If self-change is judged not to be feasible, relationship psychoeducation usually is provided. The most extensive form of SRCT, therapist-guided change, is used only if neither self-change nor relationship psychoeducation is sufficient to produce self-change. Once the therapy goals are agreed on, I usually describe a couple of possible therapy structures to the couple. This introduction would go something like this:

> "I suggested that once we had established the goals of therapy, we would talk about how we can achieve those goals. In my experience once couples have a clear idea of how they want their relationship to change, they

often can make those changes with a small number of sessions with a therapist. Sometimes couples need more help from me. I suggest we talk through exactly who is going to attempt what changes. Then we can discuss what help you might need to make those changes."

Evaluating If Brief Self-Change Is Feasible

PREDICTORS OF RESPONSE TO BRIEF COUPLE THERAPY

Although there is no research that specifically looks at predictors of response to brief couple therapy, there are predictors of response to traditional couple therapy, as I reviewed in Chapter 2. As noted there, more severe problems at presentation, less positive affect expressed by the partners toward each other, and lower relationship focus (particularly by the male partner) all predict poor response to couple therapy. Based on such findings, I suggest that couples are most likely to benefit from brief couple therapy if they are suffering from mild to moderate, rather than severe, relationship distress. Mild to moderate relationship distress on the Dyadic Adjustment Scale would be a full-scale score of less than 100 but not less than 85. I would be reluctant to recommend brief couple therapy if either partner were suffering from an individual psychological disorder, if there were a history of physical aggression between the partners, or if there were little evidence of remaining positive affect between the partners. It is hard to imagine couples with such complications changing their behaviors easily. However, in traditional couple therapy these predictors account for only a modest proportion of variance in outcome. This does makes it difficult to rely solely on them to predict accurately whether brief couple therapy will be effective for a given couple.

I find it useful, when considering the option of brief therapy for a given couple, to reflect on their responses during assessment and feedback. Some couples commence therapy and remain focused on partner blame, are unable to appraise their relationship woes in terms of their interactions, and seem unable to identify goals for self-change. For some of these people couple therapy is not appropriate. If the couple have not successfully identified any shared relationship goals, then couple therapy usually cannot proceed. (More on what to do in this situation follows later in the chapter.) Other couples do identify some shared goals, but the goals are vague, or the couples are unable or unwilling to identify personal actions they can implement to achieve those goals. Often such couples need relationship psychoeducation to help them implement actions to achieve their goals.

Many distressed couples who present to me focus their in-session comments constructively. They comment on the adaptive processes between the couple, the influences that shape those processes, and the options for self-directed change. This focus may be evident from the beginning of therapy, or a shift to this focus may occur over the assessment and feedback sessions. In such cases, brief self-change therapy is an option that should be evaluated.

ASSESSING THE VIABILITY OF BRIEF COUPLE THERAPY

Given the absence of empirical data about predictors of response to brief couple therapy, I prefer to think of the viability of brief therapy as a hypothesis that the therapist and couple test together. The assessment and feedback sessions indicate whether the couple have self-appraisal skills and goal-setting skills. If brief therapy is a possibility, I begin to evaluate this possibility by asking a series of questions. The questions are designed to assess the partners' self-regulation skills in implementation and evaluation of self-change. Usually I begin with an open question probing how to implement change to achieve one of the agreed relationship goals such as: "What would you do to meet that goal?" I also follow up with a question on evaluation, such as "How would you know if what you were doing was working?"

It is important to ask each partner about the implementation and evaluation of self-change for each key relationship goal. Sometimes partners may not be able to respond initially, but the use of additional probes will help them structure the self-regulatory task. Table 6.2 lists the core self-regulation metaskills. Beside each skill is an example of a probe that may help a partner to clarify the various steps of self-directed change. I often do a series of these detailed probes if the person is unsuccessful in defining self-change goals from the initial open-ended questions. If this additional probing still does not allow the partners to formulate the implementation of their self-change, then brief couple therapy probably is not a viable option.

My work with Bill and Lorraine illustrates a high-level response to a self-regulation probe. They had identified four key goals in their relationship: to reduce the use of the pursue–withdraw pattern, which they used to manage conflict; to increase their quality fun time together as a couple; for Bill to make a bigger contribution to the household chores; and for Lorraine to increase her social activities outside the home. I asked Bill how he might implement a couple of the goals that had been identified in the first few sessions of couple therapy. I was looking to see if each partner could identify specific actions that he or she could personally take. The partner's personal goals also need to be relevant to the broad relationship goals that they had agreed to work on as a couple.

THERAPIST: Bill, one of the key goals you identified was to make a bigger contribution to the household chores. Have you thought about how you might go about doing that?

BILL: Umm, no . . . not really. If I think about this, what I would want is to

TABLE 6.2. Therapist Sample Questions to Prompt and Assess Self-Regulation

Domain	Skill	Question
Appraisal	Identification of key couple adaptive processes.	What do you see as the key strengths and weaknesses of your relationship?
	Identification of personal behavioral strength.	What is it that you do well?
	Identification of personal behavioral weakness.	What do you do that is not helpful?
	Identification of behavioral influences.	What influences you doing these behaviors in this way?
Goal setting	Specification of behavioral change.	What needs to change in your relationship? Can you be more precise about what needs to be different?
Implementation	Identification of means of self-change.	How would you go about making the change? What will you do and when?
Evaluation	Evaluation of implementation.	How would you know you had actually made the desired behavior change?
	Evaluation of effect.	How would you know if the changes that occur have the desired effect on your relationship?

work out with Lorraine what it would be most useful for me to pick up on. I would guess that if I did a bit more of the cooking and shopping, that would help most . . . that seems to be what she complains about the most. So . . . I guess I would offer to do those couple of things and then sit down and ask her if there is anything else she wants me to do. It's really not that hard.

THERAPIST: Excellent, Bill, it seems like you have got a pretty clear idea about some changes that you could make, and you have got a plan to ask Lorraine about what other things you might do. Are you wanting to go ahead and make these changes at this stage?

BILL: Yeah, I am. The main thing that I have learned from therapy thus far is that it is going to be largely up to each of us to do something if the relationship is to get better. I really want it to get better, so I want to do my bit.

THERAPIST: Great, Bill. I think if you carry through with these things you will notice a lot of improvement in your relationship. The more energy you put into this, the more you will gain. You also mentioned planning to alter the way in which you and Lorraine talk through things. Do you have ideas about what you can do about that?

BILL: Well, I think I have always had the view that . . . any form of disagreement is not a good idea. I can see that avoiding stuff has not been working well. The main thing I think . . . I need to do is simply hang in there and listen. If I make sure I am listening, and she knows that I am listening, I think that will do it. I also want to avoid interrupting. I often do talk over the top of her, you pointed that out after the communication session we had a couple of weeks ago, so I'd be keen to just hang in there, and listen, and see where it goes from there.

THERAPIST: Excellent, Bill. So we have two key things you are going to do: (1) Make a bigger contribution around the house with chores, you picked a couple of things you are going to change yourself and you are going to ask Lorraine about some other suggestions. (2) Hang in there and listen and eliminate that withdrawing from conflict. If you can do those two things consistently, that is really going to make a major difference. I will be very interested to find out how much difference making those changes makes to you and Lorraine. Lorraine, you have heard some of Bill's ideas, his goals for himself. What thoughts have you got about your goals?

LORRAINE: I was thinking a bit while Bill was talking. On the communication thing, I know that I get pretty stroppy [irritable] with him sometimes. If I just learn to say why I am unhappy and not get so critical or angry. So my thing is that I am going to try to be a bit less attacking. The other thing that is important to me is more fun together. Anytime when we do go out, it is generally Bill who sets it up. He books the restaurant. He orders tickets to the game. He lines up meeting friends. And then I feel we never do stuff that is what I really want to do. I need to take more responsibility for that stuff. And sometimes we just squander the weekend and don't do anything that is much fun. I don't fall into that trap any more. I will organize us to do some good stuff.

THERAPIST: Lorraine, that sounds wonderful. You have got an idea about improving the communication and also making sure that you have fun together. Are those two things that you want to do in the immediate future?

LORRAINE: Yeah they are. Neither of them involves lots and lots of effort, but I think they might really make a difference.

This couple's interaction illustrates high levels of self-regulation skills. Many couples, once they reach this point, are successful in implementing self-directed change. In the past, I have often gone to considerable pains to have couples spell out exactly where, when, and under what circumstances they will do exactly what to achieve these particular self-directed changes. However, in my more recent experience, I have found that such a high degree of specificity in goal setting is rarely required. Most people will fill in the gaps of detail adequately if they have commitment to the sorts of goals that Bill and Lorraine specified. In these circumstances I negotiate with the couple exactly how we will implement the brief self-change therapy process. Chapter 7 describes this process in detail.

Unfortunately, not all couples are able so early in the therapeutic process to self-implement change goals. Consider the following interaction that occurred with Trevor and Diane. They had identified having more expression of affection together as a key goal that each of them wanted to work on.

THERAPIST: Trevor, Diane, you have both said that greater expression of affection, of love to each other, is important. I am wondering what each of you might do to improve the expression of affection.

DIANE: Well Trevor has to behave civilly toward me more often, and then I'll be affectionate.

TREVOR: (*makes heavy sighing noise*) More civilized, that's what I'd like, more civilized behavior from Diane. Then affection would be fine.

THERAPIST: Trevor, I am wondering if there is anything that you feel you can do that would increase the expression of affection in the relationship?

TREVOR: I know how to be affectionate. I am happy to give Diane lots and lots of hugs, tell her that I love her. I can do all of that stuff. But I have to feel it. At the moment I just don't feel like it a lot of the time because of the way that she acts towards me.

DIANE: (*rolls her eyes*) The way that I act toward you . . .

THERAPIST: So, Trevor at this point you seem to be saying that you are waiting on Diane to change her behavior. Is that right?

TREVOR: Well it takes two to make a relationship, and I am unsure whether she really wants to make this work.

As the foregoing transcript illustrates, neither of the partners is offering to self-implement change goals. Their comments are focused largely on perceived negative behaviors by their partner and assertions about the need for the partner to change. This focus on reduction of negatives by the partner and an inability to focus on self-change suggest that the couple are unlikely to be able to make constructive changes in their relationship on their own at this point. In such cases relationship psychoeducation is undertaken.

Introducing Relationship Psychoeducation

Relationship psychoeducation is a process whereby couples are assisted to move from a general agreement on relationship goals to specific self-implemented change. As described in Chapter 3, the assumption is that partners who can agree on general relationship goals but cannot define self-implementation of change have one of two problems. First, they may have strong negative thoughts and feelings that interfere with self-implemented change. Often this is evident in repetitive arguments over one or two issues. Second, couples may lack the knowledge to define specific actions that will enhance their relationship. For example, couples may agree that they need to manage their money better, or better cope with work–family conflict, but may be unsure of how to attain these goals. If relationship psychoeducation is needed I introduce the idea of having further therapy sessions to explore the problem area(s) to attempt to determine how to produce change. For example, if strong negative thoughts and feelings seem to be blocking the couple I address that issue as follows.

> "It seems you are agreed on the goals you want, but you're stuck on how to make these changes. We've said that lack of affection between you is a topic that makes you both get angry; it seems this is really an important issue to both of you. I think we need to explore this area more and understand what makes it such a hot issue for you both. If you agree, I would like to have a couple of sessions together in which we get you to talk about this in depth. I will work with you to try and understand the thoughts and feelings you have about this. In my experience, once we understand what drives the feelings, then what to do about it falls into place. Would you be willing to give this a go?"

Assuming that the couple agree, the sessions of relationship psychoeducation then proceed. (Chapter 8 describes details of how to do relationship psychoeducation.) Therapist-guided change rarely is selected as the therapy of choice at the end of the feedback process. Therapist-guided change involves active skills training, and the need for this usually becomes evident when partners attempts at self-change are unsuccessful. (Chapter 7 describes how to determine if self-change is not proceeding satisfactorily, and Chapter 9 describes how to conduct therapist-guided SRCT.)

Managing Common Challenges in Feedback and Negotiation

Feedback and negotiation do not always proceed smoothly. Sometimes in the feedback process partners disagree, even argue, with each other. Other times, the feedback may be completed successfully but the couple either do not agree to shared relationship goals or they express ambivalence about the relationship goals. Yet another challenge is that some partners present in crisis such that one or both of them feels overwhelmed by stress. The effects of the crisis can interrupt the usual process of assessment and feedback. As noted in the introduction, couple therapy does not follow an invariant, recipe-like process. Therapy needs to be adjusted to the circumstances of the couple. In this section I address management of common challenges in the feedback and negotiation process.

Managing Common Challenges during Feedback

The art of doing a good assessment feedback session is to maintain sufficient structure to keep the couple focused on key relationship problems and their solutions but to allow sufficient flexibility so that the couple feels able to express their concerns and reservations. There are a number of ways in which the feedback process can go wrong. Table 6.3 identifies some of the most common problems and suggests ways to avoid or solve those problems.

As in all couple work, it is important that the therapist carefully monitor the reactions of each partner throughout the therapy session. It is desirable to maintain an appropriate balance of talk by each partner and to prevent either partner from withdrawing or overtalking during the session. For that reason, it is important to ensure that the discussion about a particular issue, with a particular partner, does not become unduly long and exclude the other partner.

It is also crucial for the therapist to recognize that the assessment feedback may implicate a particular partner as being at fault even though the therapist may not intend to blame the partner. If the therapist's comments illicit a sense of defensiveness in one of the clients, it can be quite unhelpful. To avoid this, it is useful for the therapist to focus on descriptive comments and to make all interpretations tentative. Also, it is important to recognize that therapists sometimes become defensive about their own interpretations, and to recognize that the assessment formulation at this point is simply a hypothesis. If one of the partners produces data that suggest that a different conceptualization might be useful, the therapist needs to be flexible in reformulating the nature of the problems.

After presenting each piece of assessment data, it is important that the therapist check whether the partners agree with what is being presented. As information is added, the therapist needs to summarize the key points and to check that the clients agree with that summary. In essence, the therapist is constantly seeking to build consensus about the nature of the problems through this process.

Managing Common Challenges When Negotiating Therapy Goals

AMBIVALENCE

Even when feedback is completed successfully some couples either express ambivalence about identified goals or do not even agree to shared relation-

TABLE 6.3. Common Problems in Discussing Assessment Findings

Problems	Possible solutions
1. Failure to establish goals of session clearly.	1. Negotiate an agenda, establish time limits etc.
2. Getting sidetracked by tangential issues.	2. Keep to agenda items, reschedule other business, use retrospective probes and transition probes to keep on track.
3. Being judgmental (e.g., by offering premature interpretations of the partners' behavior).	3. Present relevant descriptive data one at a time, before offering interpretations, select meaningful/ relevant examples to illustrate teaching points. Seek couple's views on your interpretations.
4. Being vague, overgeneralizing.	4. Be more specific, use clear examples.
5. Being too definitive or overgeneralizing from inadequate database.	5. Be more tentative, acknowledge possible alternative interpretations, look at future data collection tasks to test out alternative generated hypotheses about the problem.
6. Ignoring partners views, or becoming defensive when therapist's own views are challenged.	6. Encourage partners to present their own views of the problem. Reinforce them for mentioning their own ideas. Don't become defensive. Ask partners to be more specific, concrete, and to exemplify what they mean by statements. Point to existing data, or data that might be collected, to clarify disagreements.
7. Partners not understanding your interpretations or conclusions about the nature of the problem.	7. Don't use jargon, use more straightforward examples and vocabulary (role-play examples if necessary). Probe to determine partners' understanding of what you have said.
8. Partners becoming defensive (e.g., self-condemnation, upset, and angry).	8. Use summarizing, reflection, paraphrasing skills to identify source of partner concern. Be supportive. Challenge irrational assumptions by presenting alternative ways of conceptualizing the problem.
9. Using jargon.	9. Use everyday language. If you wish to teach a new concept, explain it clearly, exemplify it, and use it consistently.
10. The overtalkative partner.	10. Use agendas. Use interviewing strategies to get the partner back on track (e.g., closing-off summaries, transition probes, retrospective probes, interrupt partner, reschedule issue if it needs to be discussed).
11. The nonengaged partner.	11. Ask for partner's viewpoints/opinion. Reinforce partners for contributing, by summarizing their viewpoint, being attentive, etc.

ship goals. Many couples in which at least one partner initially felt ambivalent about the relationship will express more commitment to the process of change through the steps of assessment, feedback, and negotiation. However, some partners continue to express uncertainty about their commitment to the relationship or therapy. Self-change independent of the therapist is unlikely in this situation, and a useful strategy in the presence of such ambivalence is to propose that a small number of therapy sessions be undertaken with a built-in review process. This idea could be introduced in the form described next.

> "So, we have reached some agreement that your relationship would be better if you could manage conflict better, have more quality time together, and reach agreement on how you wish to approach parenting. However, it seems that each of you still has some uncertainties about whether therapy can change the relationship enough to make you want to stay together. At the same time, neither of you feels certain that you want to end the relationship. One possibility is for us to have three or four sessions, once per week, together. Each of you could give the relationship your best shot across that time; to agree to put some energy and some time in trying to improve the relationship. In three or four weeks then we would review how you think it's going. If things are not changing enough to make you feel optimistic about further improvements, then at that stage you could decide to cut your losses and end the relationship. On the other hand, it may be that you feel that things are moving in the right direction by that time, and it really is worth putting more time and energy into making the relationship work. What would you think about that?"

This strategy minimizes the response cost for the partners of continuing to work on their relationship. To this point many partners may have been seeing their choices as either ending the relationship immediately or having to accept things the way they are forever. This short-term therapy contract proposes another option in which partners work hard at improving their relationship, with a goal of seeing whether they want to remain together in a long-term committed relationship.

If the partners are clear on the self-implementation of their goals but ambivalent about whether to pursue those goals, then the sessions focus on self-change with regular therapy sessions to support that self-change. If the partners are both ambivalent about change and unclear on how to implement self-change, then relationship psychoeducation would be the focus in the contracted sessions.

LACK OF SHARED GOALS

It is rare for couples not to have at least some agreed therapy goals at the end of assessment and feedback. However, if an impasse is reached and the partners do not agree on relationship goals, couple therapy probably is not going to be effective. When there is no agreement, I offer the opinion that it is probably not worthwhile to proceed with therapy. I try to leave open the option of renegotiating to make therapy possible. For example, I might say something like the following:

> "We do not seem to have agreement about the nature of the problems, or how to proceed at this stage. In my experience unless the partners have broad agreement on what they are trying to achieve through therapy, then couple therapy rarely is helpful. But perhaps I have misunderstood what each of you is telling me. Do you two feel there are goals you both want to achieve?"

Sometimes couples respond to the possibility of not proceeding with therapy by generating suggested goals. Other times the couple seems defeated in their attempts to identify relationship goals. It is important for the therapist to avoid the trap of taking excessive responsibility for change. I would summarize where we have gotten to and ask the couple what they propose to do using words something like the following.

> "Well, you've told me you want to stay together [Or, " . . . you are not ready yet to separate," if that is more accurate]. As we have talked we have assessed the problems, but it seems you two can't agree on what goals you want in your relationship. What are each of you going to do?"

I listen to what the partners have to say. At this point they really have only three choices. One or both partners may decide to end the relationship, they can try to change the relationship, or they can retain the status quo. If they stay together the status quo is the default choice if the partners do not enact change. If their comments do not identify each of these three options, I point out the missed option(s) to the couple. Most commonly people do not mention the status quo. Exploring the likely outcomes of sustaining the status quo is often worth discussing. For example, the therapist can ask: "What do you think will happen to you two if you keep arguing the way you have been?" Often this discussion focuses on how the relationship would erode further and the eventual probability of separation would increase. Such a discussion can often lead couples to reexamine the possibility of agreeing to relationship goals.

If the couple still feels unable to formulate relationship goals but is expressing a keen desire to change their relationship, I offer other suggestions. I have suggested that couples go home and each write down the key relationship problems and the goals they have for the relationship. In a subsequent session we again attempt to negotiate some shared relationship goals based on their written self-appraisals. Alternatively, I also have suggested that we have one or more sessions of relationship psychoeducation during which we reexamine the relationship and its development and then return to attempting to formulate goals.

Let us assume our couple have been able to define their relationship goals and self-change looks as if it is a possibility. The next step is to work with the couple to help them define how they will implement self-change. Chapter 7 provides a detailed description of implementation of self-change.

7

Brief Self-Change

In the final part of the feedback and negotiation session the therapist assesses the couple's self-regulation skills. When each partner is able to accurately appraise his or her role in the relationship and the influences on the relationship (appraisal), agree on shared relationship goals (goal setting), and identify specific actions each can take to reach their goals (implementation), then brief self-change is possible. When this is the case, the final part of the feedback session is to negotiate the level of therapist support to be provided for the partners' change efforts. This means working out approximately how many review sessions will occur and with what timing. Brief self-change couple therapy usually has between one and three review sessions, and these are often the only sessions after the feedback and negotiation session. In review sessions the therapist discusses with the partners their implementation of self-change goals and helps them to evaluate the effects of self-change on the relationship. If the changes are successfully implemented, the therapist reinforces and seeks to maintain self-change efforts. If partners do not implement self-change successfully, the therapist helps the partners to diagnose and overcome the barriers to self-change. Once the couple has successfully implemented self-change, the final stage of self-regulatory couple therapy (SRCT) is to promote generalization and maintenance of relationship self-change.

Selecting brief self-change as the therapy structure really means that the therapist and the couple hypothesize that self-change is sufficient to achieve the couple's relationship goals. This hypothesis is tested in the implementation process. Many couples will implement self-change successfully with minimal further therapist intervention, and in such cases therapy concludes after a small number (often one or two) of review sessions. However, other couples may have less success with self-change. Sometimes additional review sessions are needed to prompt and reinforce partner's self-change and achieve relationship goals. In other instances self-change initially seemed feasible but is not effective. If self-change is unsuccessful, or only partially successful, then relationship psychoeducation or therapist-guided change is used to achieve the couple's goals. Some couples achieve most relationship goals with self-change but need some relationship psychoeducation or therapist-guided change sessions. Still other couples are relatively unsuccessful in brief therapy, and need more relationship psychoeducation or therapist-guided change sessions to achieve their relationship goals.

Table 7.1 summarizes the key therapeutic procedures that constitute the relationship psychoeducation and therapist-guided change components of SRCT. Table 7.1 describes the major goals of each procedure, as well as what is involved in the procedure. When self-guided change does not achieve the couple's desired goals, some combination of relationship psychoeducation and therapist-guided changes would be used to assist the couple. (Chapters 8 and 9 provide detailed descriptions of how to implement these procedures.)

As noted in Chapter 3, self-regulated change is the ultimate goal of all SRCT. Couples who need relationship psychoeducation or therapist-guided change move to self-change once the more therapist-intensive part of therapy is completed. Thus, all couples going through SRCT eventually undertake the self-change procedures described in this chapter. What characterizes brief self-change is that couples move straight to self-change from the feedback and negotiation session.

Implementing and Evaluating Self-Change

In brief self-change the therapist provides only as much structure and therapy contact as is necessary to promote self-change. Review sessions in brief self-change SRCT prompt and reinforce partners' implementation and evaluation of self-change attempts.

Negotiating Implementation

The therapist concludes the feedback and negotiation session by negotiating the implementation of self-change. I begin this negotiation by stating an intent to discuss what is to change by when and what other sessions may be needed. Then I ask the partners to nominate which changes they wish to implement and in what time frame. If the partners can nominate specific and appropriate self-change at that point, and many people can at this stage of therapy, I enthusiastically praise their success. Other people may need help to develop an ap-

TABLE 7.1. Therapeutic Procedures That Supplement Self-Guided Couple Change

Structure of couple therapy	Specific procedure	Goals of procedure	Content of procedure
Relationship psychoeducation (described in Chapter 8)	Guided discovery.	Develop couple's understanding of themes and influences on their relationship interactions.	Therapist uses questions and probes to explore the themes and influences on couple interaction.
	Cognitive affect reconstruction.	To assist partners to overcome high levels of negative affect.	Therapist explores with each partner the nature and subjective meaning of salient negative relationship events (usually conflict), and helps the couple develop a shared understanding of the negative events.
	Educational resource materials.	To develop partner's knowledge about adaptive couple interaction.	Guided reading, watching videotapes, and other educational materials are used to introduce new ideas to the couple and to assist them to develop the knowledge to find solutions for difficult relationship problems.
Therapist-guided change (described in Chapter 9).	Increasing positive day-to-day couple interactions.	Love days.	People identify specific positive acts to do for partner and to implement at negotiated times.
		Promoting rewarding activities.	The number, range, and frequency of positive couple and individual activities are reviewed and goals for change negotiated and implemented.
		Planned date.	Each partner negotiates to arrange a special couple activity.
		Promoting partner support.	Specific forms of partner support are reviewed and negotiated increases in support are implemented.
	Promoting better communication.	Self-regulation communication training.	Therapist gives intensive training in appraisal, goal setting, and implementation of change in communication.

(continued)

TABLE 7.1. (*continued*)

Structure of couple therapy	Specific procedure	Goals of procedure	Content of procedure
		The floor exercise.	Therapist separates the speaker and listener role and intensively coaches couple in effective communication.
		Pinpointing.	Therapist trains communication skills of specific expression of concerns.
		Enhancing emotional expressiveness.	Therapist coaches partners in recognition and labeling of emotion.
		Emotional exploration.	Therapist structures discussion of high-intimacy topics.
		Leveling and editing.	The concept of appropriate levels of self-disclosure are explored and changes in inappropriate expression negotiated.
	Conflict management.	Developing conflict management rules.	Possible relationship rules for managing conflict are discussed and implementation of selected rules is negotiated.
		Problem solving.	A structured means of resolving complex relationship problems is taught, and how this is to be used is negotiated.
		Managing negativity.	Cognitive and behavioral strategies for managing negativity before and after conflict are taught.
	Changing negative thoughts and feelings.	Contingency management of affect.	Contingencies maintaining negative affect are identified, and negotiated changes in contingencies are implemented.
		Rational self-analysis.	A self-regulatory means of identifying and changing negative cognitions that influence negative affect is taught and implemented.

propriate implementation plan. I encourage partners to identify two or three changes to implement. More changes than this tend to overwhelm partners with complexity.

It is important to ensure that people nominate specific changes that are related to their defined relationship goals. Vague statements of desired self-change (e.g., "I will be more positive") are probed by the therapist to promote specificity (e.g., "What exactly will you do to express this positivity?"). Self-change goals that are not clearly derived from stated relationship goals are probed for their association to those goals (e.g., "How would doing this improve the relationship?").

Once we identify the specific behaviors each partner wishes to implement, I ask partners to rate their self-efficacy for implementing each nominated self-change. Usually I ask people to nominate from 0 to 100 in terms of a percentage how certain they feel that they can carry out the desired change in the stated time. The estimates of efficacy can be very informative. Low rated self-efficacy (less than, say, 50%) suggests that there is something wrong in the proposed implementation process. Perhaps the person is still not really committed to the stated goals, or perhaps he or she lacks skills to implement the selected change. In this case relationship psychoeducation or therapist-guided change may be advisable before attempting self-change. Moderate self-efficacy (60–70%) suggests that self-change is worth a try, but the therapist may need to provide extra support to promote self-change. Scheduling a review session sooner rather than later might be a good idea. High-rated self-efficacy (more than say 80%) is the most common response if the goals are well defined and the process is proceeding well.

Review sessions should allow sufficient time for partners to implement change efforts but should not leave so much of a gap between contacts that the couple feels they are floundering. If partners have moderate- to high-rated self-efficacy for implementation of clearly defined goals, usually I suggest seeing them in 2 or 3 weeks' time. Doing follow-up just 1 week after the feedback and negotiation session seems to lead people to report they did not have time to implement the changes they intended. Also, as the focus becomes self-change, there seems to be a useful symbolism in reducing the frequency of sessions from the once a week typical during the assessment process to less frequent sessions. The timing of the first follow-up session does depend on the rated self-efficacy of implementing self-change, with less confidence leading to a shorter follow-up period.

Couples attempting self-change may need assistance before the scheduled follow-up appointment. I offer couples that report low self-efficacy but wish to attempt self-change the option of a telephone consultation to review progress. This is especially useful if there is a particular time at which they are trying to implement a change. The telephone call allows a review soon after the change attempt. For example, if one partner is to arrange a couple outing in the next 2 days, the therapist can ring and review how this task was undertaken. Telephone reviews also can be useful in work with couples that have difficulty attending face-to-face sessions. With some couples I have contracted to have regular weekly telephone contact over 5 or 6 weeks leading up to a review session.

An example of negotiating the implementation process is presented next. The couple, Mia and Chee, had identified reduction of conflict as their most important goal. Mia often withdrew during arguments, whereas Chee often was demanding, particularly when discussing money problems. Mia had decided to implement the self-change of active listening to Chee during discussions of money and trying to be more assertive. Chee had decided to implement being assertive rather than aggressive in his comments to Mia, and to listen and not interrupt Mia during their discussions.

THERAPIST: (*looking at Mia*) I want you to rate how confident you are in doing these things. Suppose 100% is "absolutely sure, I'll do this no matter what," and zero is "no chance at all." Let's call 70% "I expect to do this, but if something tough happened I might not be able to." What do you think the chance is of you being more assertive with Chee about your views on money if you talk about it this next week?

MIA: 100%, he's not getting away with it any more. (*Laughs.*) No, no, I find it hard you know. In my family the men always do the money, women do not do this. But, I want to. I think 70, maybe 80.

THERAPIST: OK, so the chances are pretty good. What about listening to Chee when he is talking? Where is that from 0 to 100?

MIA: That is 100. I found last week that I was listening much more. I just decided that I was not going to get upset, I would just listen, and it worked.

THERAPIST: Great, so you just sort of decided that this would not get to you, and you were able to make that work. Chee, what about you, from 0 to 100, what is the chance you will be assertive with Mia?

CHEE: That is tough. I get angry. I try to be more the reasonable husband, but this is new to me. I think 60 or 70%.

THERAPIST: What might get in the way?

CHEE: When I am angry, then I get rude, tell Mia off.

THERAPIST: Is there anything you can do to reduce being angry?

CHEE: Not sure.

THERAPIST: You remember last week you told me your dad told you to always treat your wife like a beautiful stranger you wanted to meet? That image stuck with me, of always being polite, respectful.

CHEE: Yeah, he used to say you must always woo your wife, all your life, every day. So I will think of Mia as the beautiful stranger I am wooing when we talk of money. (*Smiles.*) She is very beautiful.

THERAPIST: Wonderful. Each of you knows what you are trying to do, and it seems you are reasonably confident you can do those things. Remember you said you would set aside time tomorrow night to talk about your money hassles? I wonder how long you might need to have at least a couple of talks about money, and see how you go. What do you think?

MIA: Oh, a week or two.

THERAPIST: Maybe a week. OK, well how about we meet again in 2 weeks, just to make sure you have time to try these things out. How does that sound?

MIA: Fine.

THERAPIST: Chee?'

CHEE: That's cool with me.

THERAPIST: If things are going well when we meet again then we might only need that session plus maybe one more. If for some reason things are not working as well as we'd like we can throw in extra sessions if we need to. OK?

ANTICIPATING AND PREVENTING FAILURE TO CHANGE

Once it is agreed who is to do what by when, it is useful to discuss with couples things that might prevent them from implementing change. I usually ask couples: "What might go wrong and stop you from making these changes?" Any identified potential barriers to self-change can be discussed. The process of identifying potential barriers seems to reduce the frequency with which those barriers subsequently are cited as reasons for failing to carry out agreed-on changes.

A common reason for failure to implement change is an argument. If the couple do not mention this possibility, I do. We discuss how an argument affects feelings, and how an argument can lead to partners giving up on change, at least temporarily. I describe the importance of sustaining self-change efforts in the face of negative interactions, which inevitably occur in all relationships. I try to elicit an undertaking from the partners to persist with self-change efforts even if some negativity occurs in the relationship.

If partners express real doubts about their capacity to implement self-change, this doubt needs to be explored. Sometimes couples just need reassurance that the therapist will support them if they are unsuccessful in self-change. However, if the desired changes seem unlikely to be implemented, then the number of changes being attempted, or the time frame for change, may need adjustment. In some couples partners accurately evaluate low self-efficacy in implementing self-change, as they lack the skills to implement their nominated goals. If a skill deficit is suspected, having the partners attempt to enact the specified change in session can be useful. For example, Mia and Chee could be asked to begin their discussion of money in the session, attempting to self-implement change. If either partner were unable to demonstrate assertion in session, communication skills training to develop the partner's assertiveness may be necessary for implementation of self-change. This is an example of therapist-guided change being used to prepare the couple for self-change.

Evaluating Implementation

Typically brief SRCT consists of two or three review sessions. The primary goal of the review sessions is for the partners to self-evaluate implementation of their change efforts. In addition, the partners are assisted to develop further change goals as required, and to negotiate whatever further therapist assistance is required. The final session or two also focuses on the generalization and maintenance of change. (Details of how to promote generalization and maintenance of change are described later in this chapter.)

The structure of review sessions usually consists of an analysis of the couple's interactions in the period between sessions and specific consideration of the implementation of self-change goals identified in the previous session. Usually I begin a review session by asking the couple to describe the intervening period from the previous to the current session. If the descriptions are vague, or lack description of both positive and negative events, I probe first for positive things that occurred in the time period and then for any problems. In this process I am listening carefully to how the partners appraise their relationship. I note and reinforce helpful appraisals (e.g., recognizing the effects of stresses, recognizing positive changes, and describing difficulties in specific but not partner-blaming terms). I also provide feedback on less helpful appraisals and try to prompt attention to aspects of the appraisal that have been overlooked.

I ask each partner to describe the changes he or she intended to implement. Next, I ask each person if he or she actually implemented the self-change and what effects those changes had on the relationship. Two common themes emerge during this process. First, the partners often do not report their behavioral changes in as precise terms as the therapist may conceptualize those changes. The therapist can prompt the partners to describe specifically the changes they have made and the functional impact of those changes. Second, partners often need support to sustain their self-change efforts. I attempt to be highly supportive of change efforts, to praise the achievements people make, and to draw out the positive effects of successful change efforts. The follow-up session with Bill and Lorraine occurred 3 weeks after their feed-back and negotiation session, and it illustrates a typical follow-up review session.

THERAPIST: Welcome back. Tell me how things have been over the last few weeks between you two.

LORRAINE: Well, OK, better, I think. (*Looks at Bill.*) Don't you, love?

BILL: Yeah, better. Not perfect. But better.

THERAPIST: OK. So what are the best things that have happened between you two in the last 3 weeks?

BILL: We didn't fight. Not really. A couple of words here and there, but no real fights you know.

THERAPIST: Bill, are there particular things you did that helped to stop fights?

BILL: Not really. We just seem mellower with each other somehow. Maybe talking it through sort of cleared the air.

THERAPIST: Lorraine, do you agree, less fights?

LORRAINE: Definitely, I think we have been really trying to be, you know, just politer . . . be civil . . . we haven't . . . been tearing away at each other.

THERAPIST: That sounds a lot more comfortable. Any problems in the last few weeks?

BILL: Well, it's not been an argument or anything, but . . . well . . . sex is not happening.

THERAPIST: Bill, you have said that sex does not happen often enough in your view, and that has not changed. Lorraine, any comments?

LORRAINE: I know this is a problem for Bill, I just never have . . . you know been that interested.

THERAPIST: OK, the issue of sex sounds like something we need to work on. Let's come back to it. But first let's review the changes that have been occurring. Bill, what were the key things you were trying to change?

BILL: I wanted to listen to Lorraine when she was unhappy about something, and I did that, I think. Er, what do you think? (*Looks at Lorraine.*)

LORRAINE: You did, you really did. Remember when Joe rang about going away. You asked me if I wanted to go before you committed us, which is a new thing. When I said no you asked me why not, and you listened to the answer. Remember?

BILL: Yeah, I never realized you felt that way about Joe. He is pretty crude at times, but I didn't realize you hated being at his place.

LORRAINE: That's because you never asked before (*laughs*).

THERAPIST: Let me check what you are saying here. Bill, you did change the way you talk to Lorraine. Asking her views, and really listening. (*Bill nods.*) Lorraine, you found it really helpful to be asked and listened to, is that it?

LORRAINE: This was the first time for ages that we talked about something without us getting bogged down. Bill's mate Joe has a fishing shack up in the hills. Bill likes Joe, likes to go fishing, and I don't. We got into lots of fights about whether to go to Joe's. I never wanted to go, but I did want us to spend time together. Bill would get testy about staying home and not going to Joe's. I think us going out a bit more has meant I didn't care if Bill went alone to Joe's.

THERAPIST: So you have gone out more?

LORRAINE: Yeah, that was one of my goals. I set up some tickets to a show. We had a great time. I can't think of the last time I went and saw a live show. Real actors.

THERAPIST: Organizing outings was something you resolved to do. So you did it.

LORRAINE: I did. I feel like my anxiety is finally coming under control. I could never have rung up on the phone a year or two ago. But the thought of going to a show was enough.

THERAPIST: Good for you. And it's interesting that when you were going out together, having fun, the issue of Bill going to Joe's was less important.

The review session also can identify ongoing areas of discontent. Both partners report modest improvement, not a radical change to relationship bliss. As we continued, Bill again raised his concerns about the infrequency with which they had sex as a couple. This issue had been identified as a problem in the assessment but had been something both partners saw as a lesser priority in improving their relationship. In this case I saw the couple for a further three sessions at this point, and the sessions were focused on sexual enrichment.

RESPONDING TO FAILURE TO CHANGE

Sometimes partners do not implement the changes they intended. In such instances I use the procedure described in Chapter 3 for recovering from failure to complete agreed tasks. Specifically, I assess three things: If the partner understood and can actually do what was agreed, if his or her cognitions are positive toward implementation of self-change, and whether any environmental factors interfered with implementation.

I check the partner's understanding of the task by asking something like the following: "Let me check we were clear on the task. Can you tell me what you thought you were supposed to do?" If there is a lack of clarity in the partner's explanation, sometimes clarification of the change goal is sufficient to promote effective self-change. If the partner can accurately tell you what he or she was supposed to do, it is possible that failure to complete the agreed task reflects a skill deficit. For example, some people find it really difficult to express relationship concerns assertively; instead they become hostile. Asking the person to demonstrate what he or she is trying to do helps diagnose whether skill training is needed (which forms part of therapist-guided change).

Assuming the partner can describe and demonstrate the desired change, the therapist asks about the partner's thoughts and feelings about the task. It is important to frame a question that positively seeks the person's view about the self-change goals and does not elicit a defensive rationalization for the lack of change. The phrase "Why did you not do it?" is usually not helpful. On the other hand, a question such as "It is really important I know what you think about this proposed change. What do you *really* think about making this change?" often elicits a more honest response about perceptions of the potential benefits of change. If the partner does not perceive the proposed self-change as important, this is important information. Relationship psychoeducation may be needed to address negative thoughts or feelings about change. Alternatively, renegotiation of the relationship goals, or the means of achieving those goals, might be needed.

Even if change implementation is seen as valuable, sometimes self-change still does not occur. Environmental factors can interfere with the change, or at least not prompt the change. Sometimes providing extra structure to the implementation plan can help achieve self-change (e.g., being more explicit about exactly what is to be done when and even arranging reminders to prompt task completion). For example, rather than just agreeing to do the shopping, a particular time can be specified and a reminder written in a diary.

As noted earlier, a common occurrence is for couples to give up on change if they have an argument or other setback. Sometimes reaffirming the need for implementing change, especially in the face of negativity, is sufficient to prompt people to implement self-change. Other times the strength of negative affect is such that the couple may need relationship psychoeducation to assist them in identifying the source of these strong feelings before self-change can proceed. For example, if a couple revert to acrimonious argument in sessions, then relationship psychoeducation may be necessary,

In a review session with Jurgen and Rosie, Jurgen reported that he had not increased his share of household chores even though he had defined this as a key change he was going to implement. The following transcript illustrates how to respond to failure to complete agreed-on tasks.

THERAPIST: Jurgen, just let me check with you on this. What do you think doing more household chores would do for your relationship?

JURGEN: Well Rosie, she's unhappy about doing it all. You know, she has a point, there's a lot left to her . . . it's not really fair. I agree I should do more, but you know I get so tired after work .

THERAPIST: OK, so you agree that it's a good idea for you to do more around the house, that Rosie carries an unfair load. But you mentioned being tired . . .

JURGEN: A couple of days ago we had a fight about the dishes. I thought, uh, the dishes need doing, uh, they can wait, after some TV. Then, you know Rosie says, "Jurgen, aren't you ever going to do those dishes?" I forgot. I was going to bed. So I say, "I forgot. In the morning, I'll do them in the morning." She gets cross, and starts doing the dishes, banging things around. So I come back and want to wash them. She says, "No, it's too late, I already have them half done." We argue some more, then I say, "Fine, I won't do the dishes," and go to bed. Next day Rosie is still mad, so I sort of gave up then.

This transcript illustrates two important points described earlier. First, after Jurgen and Rosie argued, Jurgen felt discouraged about change and gave up on implementing his resolutions. In this case reminding Jurgen and Rosie of the importance of persisting with change was enough to lead to a strong statement by Jurgen that he wanted to contribute more around the house, that he knew this was important. A second point that emerged from this discussion was that Jurgen had made a somewhat vague self-change implementation plan. He had stated in the previous session only that he would do more household chores in the next week. As we talked about what he would do in the next week, I asked him what were the most important chores he could do to carry his weight and ease the burden on Rosie.

JURGEN: Umm, anything really I guess. Cooking, cleaning, washing. What ever. I'm not sure exactly what gets to Rosie most.

THERAPIST: How could you find out what would be most helpful?

JURGEN: Ah, I have a brilliant plan. (*laughing*) Rosie, my sweet but overworked partner, how may your Jurgen best ease your burden?

Rosie and Jurgen stated to talk about what tasks took the most time and what was most burdensome to each. After a while I paused them and asked them if they could negotiate after the session a sharing of chores that made sense to them both and then try to implement the arrangement. I suggested that they report back to me in the next session on the arrangement they had worked out and their implementation of that arrangement. This is an example of providing extra structure to enhance implementation of self-change.

Promoting Generalization and Maintenance of Change

SRCT is intended to empower partners to self-direct change in their relationship. The development of metacompetencies such as self-appraisal of relationship behavior, self-directed goal setting, and self-directed change efforts is intended to assist partners to sustain a satisfying relationship long term. However, like any set of skills, people do not necessarily generalize the use of self-regulation. For example, partners may successfully apply self-change to manage conflict over some topics but not other topics. Therapy needs actively to promote generalization.

Even if couples successfully generalize the effects of therapy when attending sessions, it may be difficult to maintain these effects. A variety of changes over time may lead to diminished satisfaction and functioning. Couples' interactions may be influenced by major stresses, such as ill health or financial problems. Other factors that have a major effect on couples include lifestyle changes produced by having children, having children grow up, partners changing jobs, and changes in leisure activities. These developmental changes may prevent the maintenance of therapy effects or may render interaction patterns acquired in therapy inappropriate. In such cases psychoeducation to develop knowledge, or therapist-guided change to acquire skills, may be needed to assist the couple.

The essence of SRCT is helping partners to self-regulate change in the way they behave, think, and feel toward each other in such naturalistic settings as their home. In that sense, generalization and maintenance of change are implicit parts of SRCT throughout therapy. However, in the last few sessions of therapy, generalization and maintenance become an explicit focus of therapy. In the following section I describe a range of strategies used throughout therapy, but particularly in the last few sessions, to promote generalization and maintenance.

Promoting Generalization

There have been a number of reviews of how to promote generalization of therapeutic effects (e.g., Edelstein, 1989; Stokes & Baer, 1977; Stokes &

Osnes, 1988). My intention here is to illustrate the application of those principles to SRCT.

THERAPY TASKS

Throughout this book I emphasize the importance of therapeutic tasks. Such tasks promote the application of changed modes of behaving, thinking, and feeling in the settings in which couples interact. The systematic reviewing of therapy tasks informs the therapist about the extent of application of therapeutic gains outside the therapy setting. It also prompts problem solving about difficulties in particular settings.

SIGNALED VERSUS UNSIGNALED INTERACTIONS

Most interactions in therapy are signaled whereas most interactions at home are not. By signaled I mean there is a clear antecedent to the interaction that cues partners to use self-regulation skills (e.g., the partners are asked by the therapist to discuss a particular issue). The very act of coming to therapy is a signal that interaction around key relationship issues is about to happen. On the other hand, most interactions with the spouse at home are unsignaled. That is, the interaction arises from the ongoing sequence of the events in the couple's lives, and there is no clear antecedent to elicit self-regulation of interaction. For example, conflict about parenting typically develops while one of the partners is engaged in parenting, and conflict about household chores typically develops while one partner is doing chores (Halford et al., 1992). Moreover, given the propensity of distressed couples to avoid discussion of difficult issues, most discussions about difficult issues occur as unsignaled interactions.

Signaled interactions can be increased at home by having couples contract to discuss issues at prearranged times, and even to agree on the topic beforehand. As the couple become more proficient at managing conflict, their avoidance of managing difficult issues in signaled interactions tends to decrease.

Unsignaled interactions still occur, and couples need to become more proficient at engaging in self-regulation efforts in unsignaled interactions. One means of promoting generalization of effective self-regulation to unsignaled interactions is to arrange, during therapy, for unsignaled interactions to occur outside therapy. For example, toward the end of therapy I often advise the couple to each raise an issue between sessions without warning the other and to raise it in a negative manner (e.g., by being very critical of the other person). The task of each of them is to respond constructively to this unsignaled interaction. The therapist reviews their handling of this task in a follow-up session.

TRAINING WITH SUFFICIENT EXAMPLES

Training with sufficient examples refers to having couples practice new skills across multiple problem areas and settings in order to have them generalize their new interaction patterns to a range of problematic interactions. For example, if a couple successfully applies self-regulation to manage conflict when discussing the issue of finance in a therapy session, the couple can be asked to apply the same processes to other conflict topics. Similarly, if the couple successfully resolve conflict under one set of circumstances (e.g., talking at home after dinner), it can be useful to ask them to apply the same strategies at a different time (e.g., talking on the weekend).

EXTRACTING GENERAL PRINCIPLES

Extracting and emphasizing the general principles underlying specific examples can promote generalization. This means highlighting for couples common elements in their difficulties and drawing out common means of managing those problems. For example, I saw a couple who exhibited a pervasive pattern of poor conflict management. They would escalate to mutual hostility and then one partner, usually the man, would withdraw and refuse to talk. The woman would give up on discussion for a while, then attempt to reengage in discussion, but negatively. For example, on one occasion she asked sarcastically: "Are you ever going to talk to me about our problems?" These negative comments would lead to the argument's recommencing, and again the man would withdraw. This cyclical pattern was highlighted to the couple, and they were asked to self-regulate means for overcoming the pattern. The partners developed a method of breaking this cycle. They resolved to state to the other when they thought the pattern was happening and to arrange a signaled interaction on the problem topic once the pattern was identified. In other words, this couple applied their self-regulation skills at the level of a pervasive pattern of conflict mismanagement in their relationship.

The discussion of general principles of self-regulation is not limited to problems in conflict resolution. One couple exhibited a pattern of making a lot of effort to increase mutually shared activities when their relationship was in trouble but would make little effort when no relationship problems were evident. The net effect was that the relationship would take repeated nosedives in quality, though the couple was unaware of the pattern of repeatedly reducing shared activities when things were good. The therapist highlighted the pattern, and time was spent on how the couple could maintain their shared positive activities. (Their solution was to schedule a monthly dinner at which they discussed the previous month's activities and formulated plans for future activities).

FADING THERAPIST STRUCTURING

Decreasing the therapist's structuring and increasing the partners' control over the process and content of sessions promote generalization. Initially the therapist may need to be fairly directive in making recommendations about change between sessions, in order to promote self-regulation to overcome overlearned habits. Over time therapy needs to be less structured by the therapist so that the prompts and consequences that elicit self-regulation are those that occur in the couple's day-to-day lives. In other words, the couple needs to be initiating evaluation of relationship functioning and self-change attempts and identifying solutions independent of therapy.

Therapists can fade their own structuring by prompting the couple to control therapy. In the last session or two I ask the couple to suggest the agenda and ask them how they would like to proceed to cover those items. I still offer suggestions if there is something important that is not being considered, but a key focus is evaluating the couple's capacity to engage in self-change with minimal therapist input.

MANAGING SETTINGS

High-risk settings are those in which the chance of negative or destructive couple interaction is high. For example, couples are more likely to have conflict if either has been stressed at work that day, or if there are distractions when discussing a difficult topic (Halford et al., 1992). Enhancement settings are those that increase the chance of positive couple interaction. Couple therapy needs to address how couples will manage high-risk settings and promote effective use of enhancement settings.

I usually ask couples to identify high-risk settings and ask how each partner currently manages these settings. For example, most couples with young children find late afternoon or early evening difficult times of day, and these times of day are associated with high frequencies of couple arguments (Halford et al., 1992). Often children are tired, there are multiple household responsibilities to be completed, and parents frequently are tired after work. Other examples of common high-risk settings include taking children on outings, discussing particular topics, and having certain people present (e.g., parents).

In discussing the frequent arguments a couple had in the late afternoons, the man described how he often thought about work problems while driving home. He arrived home feeling stressed and then felt the need for some quiet time. His wife described how she picked up the children from child care and usually was preparing a meal and keeping an eye on the children when her partner arrived home, and she wanted him to either cook or care for the children. They agreed that often they were terse or argued with each other at this time. The man identified a list of things he could do to reduce stress around the time he arrived home from work. The strategies were to walk slowly from his workplace to his car park and to attend to the day and his surroundings rather than rush, to play music in his car on the way home so he would not think about work and was more relaxed, to greet his partner and children warmly when he first got home, to take 5 minutes to change when he first got home, and to plan child-focused activities he could do with his children that would be relaxing. The woman also identified that either she or her partner could prepare double portions of a few meals and freeze the extra portions. Then if they had a particularly hard day, a meal could be prepared more easily.

The effective self-management of settings not only involves the partners recognizing the predictable stressful times in their relationship and planning ahead to manage those settings but also identifying enhancing settings and using those settings to promote good couple interaction. For example, the couple that was stressed late afternoon and early evening also tended to argue about child-care responsibilities at that time. In therapy we discussed the type of setting that would enhance talking constructively about sharing child-care responsibilities. The couple identified that talking in the evening after the children were in bed would be a good setting.

Promoting Maintenance

Maintenance refers to the persistence of the effects of therapy after the end of treatment. Sometimes when termination is gradual, defining the end of treatment is difficult. For example, if the therapist initially sees the couple on a weekly basis, then has monthly sessions, and finally a 6-month follow-up session, the time at which treatment is said to have been completed is somewhat arbitrary. Perhaps a better method to express the maintenance question is, To what extent do the partners self-regulate their adaptive processes after contact with the therapist is significantly reduced or stopped entirely?

Optimal couple therapy aims to improve current functioning and to reduce the chance of recurrence of problems. We would be justifiably dissatisfied if the effects of therapy disappeared as soon as therapy was terminated. However, a significant improvement in relationship functioning sustained over a period of years would seem a worthwhile achievement, even if permanent high relationship satisfaction is not achieved.

Systematic empirical research on the determinants of maintenance of couple therapy effects is sparse. Many couple therapists have suggested that booster sessions may help maintenance of effects (e.g., Beach et al., 1990; Stuart, 1980). Booster sessions refer to additional sessions occurring after the initial course of therapy, which are usually spaced at sessions further apart than during the regular course of therapy, and which focus particularly on the maintenance of gains achieved by the end of treatment.

Whisman (1990) reviewed the research on the effects of booster sessions across a number of different areas of clinical problems. He concluded that booster sessions were moderately successful in improving the maintenance of therapy gains. Successful booster sessions focused on clients self-reinforcing positive gains made over the course of therapy; identification of possible high-risk settings that might promote relapse, training people to cope with high-risk settings, and encouraging clients to interact in enhancement settings that promote maintenance.

REINFORCE THERAPY GAINS

Applying the general principles of Whisman (1990) to couple therapy suggests a number of strategies that can be used to maintain couple therapy effects. First, it is important that clients reinforce themselves for gains that they make. In review sessions I routinely ask couples about the efforts they have made to promote change and frame this positively. For example, I might ask: "You made numerous changes that have improved your relationship, even though you initially expressed some reservations about whether the relationship could improve. What has enabled you to sustain the effort required to improve things?" This question often prompts partners to attend to their own efforts and reinforces change efforts.

I routinely reassess couples' relationship functioning toward the end of therapy. Typically this involves completing one or two key self-report or self-monitoring measures used at the beginning of therapy, and possibly a behavioral task, at some point prior to the last session or two. Assessment of outcome toward the end of therapy identifies for the therapist and clients the degree of success of therapy. In those areas of relationship problems that have been improved, the assessment often reinforces the positive gains made. For example, if a couple reports substantially improved communication skills and relationship satisfaction, it is important to highlight these gains. Furthermore, it is important to emphasize the role of self-change in achieving these gains, and to prompt the couple to continue to self-regulate their relationship.

PLANNING RELATIONSHIP REVIEWS

It often is helpful for people to plan ahead to maintain self-regulation. For example, couples can schedule regular reviews of how they are going in their relationship. Regularly I ask couples to set aside a time on a weekly or fortnightly basis to discuss the positive aspects of their relationship over the last couple of weeks. Particular problem areas that had arisen also are discussed. The discussion is intended to prompt self-appraisal and self-directed goal setting. Prior to such a discussion, each partner can be encouraged to self-select goals for holding this discussion. For example, if the man in the couple has often had difficulty with active listening skills, there might be a specific self-instruction to actively listen and paraphrase his wife's comments. This regular scheduling of events with specific built-in antecedents is intended to help maintain the behavior changes achieved.

RELAPSE PREVENTION

An additional important maintenance strategy is to identify particular circumstances that may arise which might lead to relapse. Regularly toward the end of therapy I have couples fill out the Relationship and Life Stress Inventory presented in Figure 7.1. This inventory identifies situations that often are associated with relapse after the end of couple therapy. I have the couple fill out how likely they believe these events are to happen to them, and the probability that if such events did occur that they would cause relapse. The couple have a problem-solving discussion to identify what they could do should these situa-

The idea of this inventory is to assess how different life stresses may impact on your relationship with your partner. For each item, rate how likely as a percentage (0–100%) each event is to happen to you in the next 12 months. Then rate how much stress this would put on your relationship from 0—"no effect"—to 100—"devastating."

Event	Likelihood this will occur in next 12 months (0–100%)	Stress on relationship if it happened (0–100%)
1. An illness or injury that kept you in bed a week or more, or took you to hospital	_____	_____
2. A major change in your sleeping habits	_____	_____
3. A change to a new type of work	_____	_____
4. A change in your responsibilities at work:		
a. More responsibilities	_____	_____
b. Fewer responsibilities	_____	_____
c. Promotion	_____	_____
d. Transfer	_____	_____
5 Experiencing troubles at work:		
a. With your boss	_____	_____
b. With your coworkers	_____	_____
c. With people you supervise	_____	_____

FIGURE 7.1. Identifying future high-risk settings for relationship problems: Relationship and Life Stress Inventory.

(*continued*)

6. A change in residence: _____   _____
   a. A move within the same town or city   _____   _____
   b. A move to a different town, city, or state   _____   _____

7. A major change in your living conditions (home improvements or a decline in your home or neighborhood)   _____   _____

8. In-law problems   _____   _____

9. Spouse beginning or ceasing work outside the home   _____   _____

10. Woman becoming pregnant   _____   _____

11. Woman having a miscarriage or abortion   _____   _____

12. A major personal achievement   _____   _____

13. Sexual difficulties   _____   _____

14. Beginning or ceasing school or college   _____   _____

15. A change of school or college   _____   _____

16. A vacation   _____   _____

17. A change in your social activities (clubs, movies, visiting)   _____   _____

18. A minor violation of the law   _____   _____

19. A new, close, personal relationship   _____   _____

20. A "falling out" of a close personal relationship   _____   _____

21. Taking on a moderate purchase, such as TV, car, freezer, etc.   _____   _____

22. Taking on a major purchase or a mortgage loan, such as a home, business, property, etc.   _____   _____

23. Experiencing a foreclosure on a mortgage or loan   _____   _____

24. Experiencing a major change in finances   _____   _____
   a. Increased income   _____   _____
   b. Decreased income   _____   _____
   c. Credit rating difficulties   _____   _____

FIGURE 7.1. (*continued*)

tions arise. The rationale is to prepare people for the most likely events that might precipitate relapse. Getting people to have such discussions across several possible future high-risk settings enhances generalization of therapy effects to other possible high-risk situations that may develop in the future.

After an argument the risk of relapse is high. All couples are likely to have at least some negative interactions with their spouse. In some couples a very negative interaction can lead partners to give up on the relationship. I focus the couple on the possibility of arguments or other negative relationship events and ask them to consider how they will manage such events. Table 7.2 provides a list of possible suggestions for couples, which I often ask couples to review and consider. The purpose is to help partners to see negative exchanges as setbacks that need to be managed.

Some couples need more help later, and it is important to discuss the possibility of returning for further therapy. It is often difficult for couples to decide that problems have now gotten to a point where they should seek further help. It is useful to make explicit that this is a difficult decision, and to highlight how the couple may make such a decision in the future. The healthiness or positive aspect of seeking additional assistance when required should be emphasized. A slip in the quality of relationship functioning should be seen by the couple as a lapse rather than that they have destroyed all the progress they had previously made.

After assessment and feedback, brief self-change allows many couples to achieve their relationship goals. Other couples need relationship psychoeducation or therapist guided-change before self-change is possible. The next chapter describes relationship psychoeducation.

TABLE 7.2. Recovering from Setbacks and Destructive Arguments: A List of Suggestions

Leave some time and space, do not push things when people are upset.

Apologize to your partner for how you spoke to him or her.

Tell your partner that you love him or her, even when you argue.

Do a rational self-analysis of your anger, try to calm unhelpful hot feelings.

Identify a time and place where you can talk through the problems with your partner more calmly.

Do three nice things for your partner, even though you feel angry or hurt (being positive even when feeling negative is crucial to the repair process).

Tell your partner that you think you did not listen to him or her, and ask him or her to tell you again (seek first to understand, then to be understood).

Self-appraise your communication during the incident and identify self-change goals for future communication.

Write a note saying you are sorry there was an argument. Say how you will try to make the next conversation better.

Send flowers, a small gift.

8

Relationship Psychoeducation

"Relationship psychoeducation," as I use the term, is a guided process of interaction between the therapist and the couple in which the therapist helps the partners to integrate new ideas into their relationship schema. The term "relationship psychoeducation" is used because the process is a psychological integration of new ideas. It is not a process of gaining abstract, or emotionally neutral, knowledge. Rather, the goal of relationship psychoeducation is to gain personally relevant information, which often has high emotional impact and can be applied directly to one's own relationship.

Relationship psychoeducation is a means of developing self-regulation skills. As the partners develop understanding of their adaptive processes and the influences on those processes, they are better able to appraise the current relationship and set self-change goals. Through relationship psychoeducation, partners usually reduce partner-blaming attributions and develop more complete views of the development and maintenance of relationship problems. This more effective appraisal allows more appropriate goals to be set for self-directed change. In this sense relationship psychoeducation empowers the partners to self-regulate their relationship.

Relationship psychoeducation is used when the couple is unable to define self-change goals successfully. This failure usually reflects one of two barriers: lack of important knowledge or the effects of strong negative emotions and thoughts. Lack of knowledge is evident when the couple seem unable to formulate appropriate and mutually acceptable relationship goals. For example, I treated a couple that disagreed about the discipline of their child. One partner argued for physical punishment of a child; the other argued against it.

Neither partner was able to specify discipline procedures that seemed likely to be effective in managing the child's behavior. In that instance we had several sessions on effective parenting strategies. The most common expression of strong negative feelings is in repeated destructive conflict. If a couple report repeated arguments at home or burst into negativity in sessions, it is an indication to proceed to relationship psychoeducation.

The term "psychoeducation" is not used in couple therapy but is widely used in many areas of psychological intervention. For example, family psychoeducation is widely used in management of schizophrenia (Barrowclough & Tarrier, 1992; Halford & Hayes, 1991) and the process is interactive. Families are not lectured on schizophrenia, but, rather, are asked to share their experiences of living with their affected relative and are given guidance on how to relate those experiences to what is known about schizophrenia. The common element across psychoeducation approaches is the learning of personally relevant ideas by clients that enable them to change their behavior.

The content covered in relationship psychoeducation is based on the substantial empirical evidence on the common themes of interaction in distressed couples and the influences on those themes of interaction. Reviews of this evidence can be found in Fincham and Bradbury (1990) and Halford and Markman (1997). In this chapter I review the process, and then the content, of relationship psychoeducation.

Process of Relationship Psychoeducation

In Chapter 1 I outlined a model of the influences on couple relationship outcomes. Four factors were identified as important: the adaptive processes of the couple, stressful life events, individual characteristics, and the context in which the couple interact. The process of relationship psychoeducation has two main steps: identifying themes of couple adaptive processes and then looking for influences on these themes in the domains of contextual variables, life events, and individual characteristics.

Themes in adaptive processes refer to recurrent patterns of behavior, thoughts, and feelings that are of high salience to the couple. Often couples do not identify themes of interaction at initial presentation but, rather present a series of seemingly disconnected complaints. The identification of themes provides the therapist and partners with a summary construct by which to describe interaction patterns in the relationship. For example, one husband, Fred, began therapy with a series of complaints such as "She does not want to talk to me, go out with me, and is hostile when I express my feelings." The wife, Edith, started with the following view: "He is too dependent, he constantly wants to smother me, he resents any independent interests I have." After relationship psychoeducation they labeled their problems as follows: "We have different boundary preferences, one of us wants more closeness and the other wants more independence."

The influences on couple adaptive processes refer to the individual characteristics, life events, and context that have shaped the themes of couple adaptive processes. The exploration of influences in psychoeducation assists couples to understand the development of themes of couple interaction and to identify change options for addressing relationship problems. For example, identifying the impact of such influences as work, extended family, and prior learning experiences on couple interaction often allows partners to overcome partner-blaming attributions and to seek mutually acceptable changes to address relationship problems.

Guided Discovery

The most common process in relationship psychoeducation is one of guided discovery. Therapists use their knowledge of the research on couples to guide asking a series of questions that prompt identification of themes and influences on those themes. In the transcript that follows, the therapist and client have identified a theme in the relationship: the recurrent pattern by which George withdraws from conflict. The therapist then has George consider the influence of his family of origin on this theme of interaction via a series of questions. These questions focus on the role models to whom George was exposed and how they taught him about conflict. This line of questioning is selected deliberately, as a considerable volume of research shows that family-of-origin experiences have a significant impact on how people manage conflict in their adult relationships (e.g., Halford, Sanders, & Behrens, 2000; Sanders et al., 1999).

THERAPIST: George, it seems we agree that you tend to dodge conflict. You were saying that whenever Rachel raises things with you, particularly if she starts to get heated, you feel very uncomfortable. Is that right?

GEORGE: Yeah, yeah . . . it has always been that way for me. In my first marriage my wife always complained that I didn't talk to her, and Rachel is saying it as well.

THERAPIST: George, do you have any theory about what it is that has led you to be so uncomfortable with conflict?

GEORGE: No, it just seems to be the way that I have always been.

THERAPIST: Tell me about your parents, George. What do you remember about the way that they managed conflict?

GEORGE: I can't remember my parents ever arguing. It came as a real surprise when they separated when I was in my teens. I didn't know that they were even having problems. Mom used to get a bit worked up at times, but I never heard dad raise his voice.

THERAPIST: So, you never heard him raise his voice. What impression did you get about how he handled differences that must have occurred between him and your mother?

GEORGE: Well, dad never really spoke about anything. He was a very quiet guy. If ever there was any arguing going on between me and my brother, or anything like that, he'd always come out and tell us to quiet down. He seemed to get quite agitated if there was any form of shouting or yelling noise.

THERAPIST: This is just a guess George, and it may not fit. You never saw your father express any real anger. Like he kept it inside.

GEORGE: I didn't ever hear him express anger, I didn't ever hear him express anything much. He was a very withdrawn guy. Almost painfully shy, I guess.

THERAPIST: So your dad never really showed you what it is to be emotionally expressive. He didn't show you ways that you could talk about how you feel, or manage conflict.

GEORGE: No, no he never did. Everybody in our house was kind of withdrawn. I guess the message was something like don't argue and it will all be all right. Don't let things get out of control.

THERAPIST: Don't let things get out of control? Wonder what the connection is between that message and how you handle things now.

GEORGE: Well, I guess I never liked people arguing, I just don't know quite what to do, I don't know how to handle it. I get scared that things will get out of hand, that I'll lose my temper.

Rachel, the wife, was silent during this interaction. However, her presence is important. As George discovers possible explanations for his behavior, Rachel is sharing this process of guided discovery. As Rachel heard George describing his father, she came to see George's avoidance of conflict as an understandable result of his learning experiences. Her prior view was that George was avoiding her because he was not really committed to the relationship. This change in Rachel's cognitions was associated with considerable reduction in hurt and distress for her. As George and Rachel learned about each other and the themes in their interactions, these altered ways of viewing the relationship potentiated change.

This example of family-of-origin experience is not meant to imply that family-of-origin experiences universally are the most important influence on relationships. There is a wide range of factors that affect relationships, of which family of origin is one factor. Given that much of the exploration about the influences on partners is retrospective, it often is impossible to validate whether the identified influences on the partners actually had the impact that the couple and therapist come to believe. In one sense that does not matter very much; the goal of the process is to help the couple develop a shared understanding of the relationship that facilitates constructive self-directed change. To the extent that the ideas developed help the change process, these ideas are useful. The ideas developed in therapy will be most useful if they provide a framework that guides self-directed action across a broad range of relationship-functioning domains.

Cognitive-Affect Reconstruction

Cognitive-affect reconstruction is a structured form of guided exploration used to help couples that have difficulty with destructive conflict. As noted previously, strong negative emotions and thoughts often are evident in repeated destructive conflict, and this negativity can inhibit couples from defining relationship goals. When such repeated conflicts occur they often reflect important themes of the relationship problem. Cognitive-affect reconstruction assists partners in identifying the themes underlying destructive conflict and the influences on those themes.

Cognitive-affect reconstruction involves six steps.

1. The therapist identifies that destructive conflict is occurring and states the intention to use the procedure to explore the conflict.
2. The therapist explores the first partner's experience of the interaction while the other partner listens without interrupting.
3. The therapist summarizes the first partner's experience and prompts the listening partner to understand his or her spouse's experience.
4. The partners then switch roles; the partner whose experience initially was explored now listens without interruption while the therapist explores the other partner's experience.
5. The therapist summarizes the second partner's experience and prompts the now listening partner to understand his or her spouse's experience.
6. The therapist summarizes each partner's experience, drawing out the underlying themes of interaction and the influences on those themes.

Cognitive-affect reconstruction is similar to procedures described by Greenberg and Johnson (1988) within emotion-focused therapy, Snyder (1998) in insight-oriented couple therapy, and Jacobson and Christensen (1996) in integrative couple therapy. A common element to each of these procedures is helping couples to identify core feelings, thoughts, and behaviors that occur during high-intensity conflict (Halford, 1998). However, emotion-focused, insight-oriented, and integrative approaches emphasize historical and intrapersonal factors in understanding the source of couple's destructive conflict. In self-regulatory couple therapy (SRCT) these influences are seen as important, but life events and context also are explored as potential mediators of destructive couple conflict.

GOALS OF COGNITIVE-AFFECT RECONSTRUCTION

One characteristic of destructive conflict is intense negative emotions. Such intense negative affect reduces partners' attention to each other, focuses attention on threat, and reduces effective problem solving (Bradbury & Fincham, 1987). A key goal of cognitive-affect reconstruction is to provide a structure within which couples can explore the range of emotions and thoughts that each partner experiences during conflict. I use the term "range of emotions" because people often experience a diversity of specific affects across a heated discussion (Johnson & Greenberg, 1994). For example, many people report that they feel angry or resentful during conflict. But, across the course of cognitive-affect reconstruction I find that people also add a range of other emotions: emotions such as sadness, anxiety about being abandoned, fear of being disapproved of or not loved by the partner, an appreciation of strong shared concerns, and so forth.

A key goal of cognitive-affect reconstruction is to draw out cooler emotions. The first emotions of anger and resentment are what Greenberg and Johnson (1988) label "hot emotions." After destructive conflict, the hot emotions are the key emotions people feel. Cognitive-affect reconstruction often allows partners to describe the cooler negative emotions such as fear and hurt. These cooler emotions typically show the vulnerability many partners feel during conflict. These cooler, more vulnerable emotions usually are easier for spouses to empathize with, and an understanding of these emotions often precipitates change in how partners respond to conflict. For example, suppose a husband angrily denounces his wife for coming home late from work. The hot anger of the husband is quite likely to elicit anger from the wife ("How dare you talk to me like that!"), and possibly defensiveness ("and I am only an hour late, what is the big deal?"). On the other hand, arriving home late from work can be responded to with sadness ("I was hurt that you did not make a special effort to be with me, I worry that you do not enjoy time with me"). This cooler emotion often is easier to understand and elicits a more positive response from the spouse.

A second goal of cognitive-affect reconstruction is to help people identify the way in which their emotional arousal interacts with the emotional arousal of their partner. Usually this interaction of emotional states is reflected in the themes of couple adaptive processes that emerge. For example, the hot emotion of anger often elicits further anger, which leads to further negative escalation of anger. Furthermore, the hot emotion of anger often swamps the underlying cool emotions such as vulnerability.

Cognitive-affect reconstruction begins by having one partner describe his or her memory of behaviors that occurred at the beginning of the targeted interaction and then exploring the feelings associated with the interaction. Cognitive-affect reconstruction also involves identifying the particular cognitions that occur during the interaction. Combining the cognitions, affect, and behavior provides an integrated description of the interaction. By the end of the cognitive-affect reconstruction, I aim to develop in partners a broader understanding of their own and their partner's emotional experiences during conflict and how those emotional experiences develop and perpetuate destructive conflict. I use that new understanding to help the couple develop goals to change their management of conflict.

STRUCTURE

Table 8.1 summarizes the relatively simple basic structure of cognitive-affect reconstruction. First, I identify with the couple a conflict that seems to be important and that we should try to understand. I then explain the basic structure of cognitive-affect reconstruction. Essentially, I talk to each partner one at a time. While I am talking to one partner, I ask the other partner to remain quiet. I attempt to engage empathically with the partner to whom I am speaking, and to understand the key emotions that he or she experienced as the interaction developed. As the partner describes what was experienced, I draw out the underlying feelings and thoughts.

Once I think I have understood the emotional experiences of the first partner, I pause. I summarize and then ask the spouse to summarize in his or her own words what the first partner said. If I think he or she has reasonable understanding of the other person's perspective, I move to the second person and repeat the process. If there seems to be more to understand about the interaction I often go back to the first partner to explore his or her experience further. There can be multiple cycles of individual exploration with each partner. The cycling continues until each partner seems to feel understood and I think I understand the strength of each partner's emotional response. Then I draw together the two experiences, often reframing it into a more interactional way of viewing what has happened.

Let me illustrate the cognitive-affect reconstruction process with an example of the case of Nick and Giesla. They presented to me one evening with both partners glancing furtively at each other with much grimacing and sighing. The effect was one of them "looking daggers" at each other. The interaction then proceeded as follows.

TABLE 8.1. Structure of Cognitive-Affect Reconstruction

1. State intention to explore destructive conflict.
   - Explain rationale is to understand interaction.
   - Explain need for each person to be listened to in silence, one at a time.
   - Ask listener to be ready to summarize speaker's perspective.
2. Explore first partner's experience of interaction.
   - Ask about events, then probe for affect and cognitions.
   - Use empathy, vertical arrow to draw out underlying emotions.
   - Gently probe for "cooler" more vulnerable emotions.
3. Summarize and prompt each partner's summary.
   - Summarize and check validity of therapist understanding.
   - Get spouse to summarize first partner's experience; therapist prompts and shapes as required.
4. Explore second partner's experience of interaction.
   - Remind first partner of need to listen without interruption and that he or she will be asked to summarize at the end.
   - Then proceed as for first partner.
5. Summarize and prompt each partner's summary.
   - Summarize and check validity of therapist understanding.
   - Get spouse to summarize first partner's experience; therapist prompts and shapes as required.
6. Summarize partners' experience and underlying themes and influences.
   - Integrate summary of both partners' experience.
   - Identify themes of interaction.
   - Identify influences on interaction.

THERAPIST: Neither of you two looks very happy tonight, is there something that's worrying you?

GIESLA: We had an argument (*sighs*), again, because Nick never does what he says he will do.

NICK: Because Nick *never* does what he says he is going to do. (*sarcastic tone, sighs*)

THERAPIST: Nick. (*holding hand in stop signal toward Nick*) Giesla, I hear that you had an argument. It seems like it's aroused real strong feelings in each of you, and that each of you is feeling bruised. It seems to me that if an argument like this has happened, it's really important that we understand what has happened here. Am I right that this is something that has really upset the two of you?

NICK: Yeah, I was really pissed off.

GIESLA: You were pissed off . . .

THERAPIST: OK, OK. That answers the question. It seems to me that both of you are pretty cheesed off with each other. It's easy at this point for us to simply get into another slanging match [argument]. I want to avoid that, I want us to try and do something constructive about managing this conflict. But if I am going to achieve that, I really need the two of you to work with me on this. What I would like to do is this: I want to talk with each of you individually about your experience of this argument. I'll turn to one of you and when I am talking to that person I want the other person to be quiet. I want that person just to listen to what goes on, not to comment at all. After I have spoken and I seem to get an understanding of what happened for the first person, then I'll turn to the second person and talk to them. While I am talking to the second person I don't want the first person to say anything. It's very important that you let me talk to each of you individually, and don't interrupt. Giesla, how about I talk with you first. Nick, that means that I am going to ask you not to say anything while I talk to Giesla.

After I have finished talking with Giesla, Nick I'm going to ask you to summarize in your own words how Giesla experienced this argument. I am not going to ask you to agree with what she says, simply to show that you understand how she saw it. You may think that is the stupidest way in the world to view what happened, that really doesn't matter. What I am asking you to do is to show that you understand her perspective. Then I'll talk to you and I'll ask Giesla to summarize your perspective. Is that something you are willing to do?

NICK: So, I just shut up, and try to summarize what she says?

THERAPIST: That's exactly it, just listen, let her talk, don't interrupt. At the end summarize how she sees it, you don't have to agree, just summarize her view. OK, Giesla tell me about what happened.

GIESLA: Well, it was Friday morning. I've been trying to lose weight, as we have talked about in these sessions. I want to go to the gym, Nick keeps saying that he will come with me. I feel stupid going to the gym on my own, so it really is important for me to have some support from Nick on this. Well, he stalls, there's excuses, it drags on. Finally, early last week he promised Friday morning we'd make a start on this thing. Friday morning the alarm goes off, he groans, says he worked the late shift the night before, he's really not up for it. I said: "When are we ever going to do this?"

THERAPIST: OK, so losing weight is important, Nick's support for you is important, and there is this ongoing issue of when are you going to start going to the gym together. Eventually there is an agreement that it is Friday morning when it is all going to start, but when Friday morning comes, Nick doesn't want to do it.

GIESLA: Exactly, so I'm fed up. So I said to Nick: "When the hell are we going to go the gym? How long are you going to stall this thing?"

THERAPIST: So it sounds like you felt really frustrated by the fact that he was not carrying through with this, something that you thought he'd agreed to do?

GIESLA: He had agreed to do it. He often agrees to do stuff. He says things that would make him the most wonderful husband in the world, it's just that he never carries through.

THERAPIST: So when you get that sense that he's not carrying through on a promise to you, what effect does that have?

GIESLA: I got mad, I got really mad. I told him, Nick, you've promised me and you've promised me, but when you promise me you always let me down. You never come through for me.

THERAPIST: So you feel like he doesn't come through for you, he persistently doesn't come through for you. What does that mean to you?

GIESLA: Well ... well, I wonder why not. Does he not care about me? Here we are in therapy trying to do something about our relationship, and he won't even do a simple thing like go to the gym. I don't get it. He promises, but he doesn't do it. It just makes me mad.

THERAPIST: I hear that you are mad, you feel disappointed that he doesn't carry through. So what does it mean to you when he doesn't do things for you that you feel he's promised to do?

GIESLA: Well, he knows how much the weight thing means to me. I mean I know I'm not really obese or anything, but I just don't feel attractive. I put on this weight when I had the kids, and I never did get it off. I want to look after myself, I don't want to get old. When he won't help me with this, I really wonder if he cares what I look like. Does he care about how I feel about things?

THERAPIST: So, when he doesn't go to the gym it really makes you wonder whether he cares about your appearance, whether he cares about you.

GIESLA: I guess it does, (voice trembling) I wonder whether he's really committed to making things better, or whether he just hangs in with me because of the kids, but doesn't really care about me.

THERAPIST: So you wonder if he cares about you, or if he's just hanging in to be with the kids, and when you think about that possibility, how does that make you feel?

GIESLA: Sorta sick, really. I love Nick. The thought that he doesn't care about me, doesn't care about how I look, doesn't care about what I do, it ... (cries gently).

THERAPIST: So, Giesla, when Nick wouldn't go to the gym with you this was much more for you than just missing out on a workout. For you, here was

Nick not carrying through with something that you felt he promised to do. Because it was something that was important to you, something about how you feel about yourself physically, you interpreted this as meaning he doesn't care about me. Maybe he's just hanging in for the kids. And because you love him and care about him it makes you feel kinda sick, the idea that maybe things won't work out between the two of you. Is that it?

GIESLA: Yes, yes, that's what it is.

THERAPIST: (*turning to Nick*) Nick, like I said I'm not asking you to agree with Giesla's view. But what does she see and experience during the argument with you.

NICK: Well, she interprets me not going to the gym as meaning I don't care about her. But somehow I don't care what she looks like. That's just not true . . .

THERAPIST: Nick, you're starting to tell me how you feel about it, and in a moment, I really want to hear that. But just for now let's focus on Giesla. So when she thinks, rightly or wrongly, that she thinks that you don't care about her, what effect does that have on her?

NICK: Well she said that she feels sick, yes sick I think.

THERAPIST: So why does this have so much impact on her, why does she get sick?

NICK: Uh uh . . . I'm not sure why . . .

THERAPIST: She said that she loves you, and the idea that you don't love her really makes her feel sick.

NICK: Yeah, yeah she did say that.

In the next phase of the cognitive-affect reconstruction, I asked Nick about his experience of the interaction. He described how, when the alarm had gone off on the Friday morning, he really had been very tired. He had felt pressured and cajoled into agreeing to go to the gym in the first place. He described how he really loathes going to the gym. He sees gymnasiums as places where people get together in leotards and sweat, and he finds that very unpleasant. When Giesla had got so angry, he had found it particularly upsetting because she had accused him of never supporting her. He described how he had cut back on his work hours in order to help her with her studies and was doing a larger share of household chores and child-care responsibilities. He felt that all of that was dismissed, and that she really did not value what he did. It seemed to him that no matter how hard he tried, Giesla would never be satisfied with him, that she saw him as essentially a flawed and untrustworthy husband. When he felt like that, he seriously doubted Giesla's commitment to the relationship, and the thought that she might end the marriage was extremely upsetting to him.

As I explored with Nick his experience of the interaction, it also became clear that the pattern of interaction was one that was common to other conflicts this couple experienced. Often Giesla would attempt to talk to Nick about a problem; he would feel overwhelmed by her criticisms and would withdraw and try to terminate the interaction. As he pulled back and attempted to withdraw, Giesla interpreted this as further evidence that he was not committed or loving toward her. As Giesla approached Nick and tried to engage him in further conversation, Nick became even more overwhelmed by her list of criticisms and he felt even more inadequate and unloved. The therapist summarized the process in the following manner.

THERAPIST: So it seems like that there is a pattern of interaction that happens here where Giesla is raising what she's unhappy with. In this case it was that Nick was not going to the gym, and she felt let down. She expresses this, and Nick feels threatened by the criticisms. He never particularly wanted to go to the gym anyway, and so he tries to end the conversation. As he tries to withdraw you, Giesla, feel that he just is less and less committed to interacting with you, and this makes you feel scared. You try and raise it by talking more.

As Giesla tries to talk to you more, Nick, you feel here's another set of criticisms coming down on top of you and you just want to get away. You feel overwhelmed, and unhappy with what's going on. So, it seems that the argument was only in part about whether or not to go to the gym. But the reason why whether you went to the gym on Friday morning became so heated was because of what it meant to each of you. For you Giesla this was about the extent to which Nick loves you and feels committed to you. For you Nick it was the extent to which Giesla sees you as a fundamentally flawed person, and the extent to which she values the things that you are already trying to do to improve the relationship.

GIESLA: I didn't realize that Nick hated the gym so much. I don't want him to go to something that he just truly loathes. That's not part of it. I just wanted some support.

NICK: I'm happy to support you in lots of ways, I just don't want to go and heave metal around in a sweaty room. If you want to go for long walks, great. But not the gym.

After an interaction like this, often the need for people to get their partners to change dissipates. In this particular example, Giesla soon found someone else to accompany her to the gym and successfully managed to engage herself in a program of exercise. The struggle over the gym had become entrenched as unresolvable conflict because of the underlying meaning and emotions attached to the conflict.

The essence of cognitive-affect reconstruction is drawing out the underlying "cooler" emotions that often exist in destructive conflict and making these vulnerabilities and concerns accessible to the partners. In my experience partners usually expose their vulnerabilities if the therapy session feels safe to them. In other words, if therapy has been structured so that destructive conflict does not emerge in that setting, the partners often open up to each other. The therapist draws together this expressed "cooler" affect with the behavior and cognitions that accompany these emotions. Sometimes simply changing the way the couple experiences the conflict through cognitive-affect reconstruction produces a shift in the conflict, as in the case of Nick and Giesla.

For some couples, cognitive-affect reconstruction identifies a destructive pattern of conflict and the couple needs to behave differently to develop effective conflict management skills. Often at this point I shift to a self-regulated change process and ask the partners to self-define goals for change. For example, a couple worked with me that defined their interaction pattern as husband approach–wife withdraw, and they saw the need to change that pattern. I asked each partner to define self-change goals to achieve that goal. The woman identified her goal as engaging more effectively in discussion by using active listening and asking questions. The husband defined a goal of reducing the demand pressure of his approach by expressing concerns in a less critical manner.

Use of Educational Materials

Guided exploration and cognitive-affect exploration are the most common means of providing relationship psychoeducation. In addition, I use handouts, reading, and review of audiovisual materials to provide additional information to couples. For example, I often give clients the handout presented in Figure 8.1, which defines the core components of the model of relationships I described in Chapter 1. By sharing this model with the couple, I hope to encourage them to consider which factors are influencing the current relationship interaction. I then use the expertise and knowledge I have on relationships to help them elaborate further on the nature of their relationship difficulties.

The books *Living and Loving Together* by Montgomery and Evans (1989) and *We Can Work It Out* by Notarius and Markman (1993) both provide good overviews of common themes of dysfunctional couple interaction. Each book includes information about promoting intimacy, common difficulties in communication, and patterns of conflict management. Often getting couples to read particular sections of one of these books and then discussing the ideas in the therapy session can be helpful in identifying themes of distressed interaction.

The "big four" of couples' relationships

Research on couples has identified four main factors influencing how satisfied couples are with their relationships. These are the "big four" of relationships.

Couple adaptations: This refers to how couples adapt together to things going on in their lives. Couple adaptations include how the couple communicates, how they think about each other, and their feelings when together.

Life events: This refers to the major events in people's lives such as their job, their families, and their health.

Individual factors: This refers to the characteristics of each partner as an individual, and their capacities and vulnerabilities. These individual factors reflect the learning history the individual has.

Context: This refers to the background in which you live, your culture, your extended family, work, and friends.

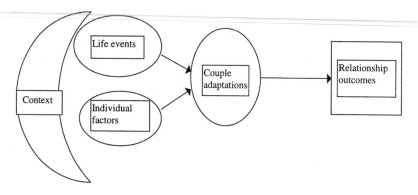

FIGURE 8.1. Handout for couples on a model of relationships.

Given that much relationship psychoeducation is focusing on couple interactions, audiotape and videotape materials can be helpful in relationship psychoeducation. For example, the videotape *Fighting for Your Marriage*, produced by Markman, Stanley, and Blumberg (1991) at the University of Denver, provides some very useful guides to dysfunctional communication. Similarly, the videotape and couple guidebook entitled *Couple Commitment and Relationship Enrichment* (Couple CARE) produced by our team at Griffith University (Halford, Moore, Wilson, & Farrugia, 2000) has demonstrations of effective and ineffective conflict management. The series of videotapes entitled *The Lovers' Guide* Parts 1 to 3 (Stanway, 1991, 1992, 1993) provides explicit and helpful advice on sexual enrichment for couples. I often ask couples to view particular sections of these videotapes and discuss them in subsequent sessions.

Common Themes in Distressed Relationships

A common element across empirically validated approaches to couple therapy is that they focus on themes of couple interaction (Halford, 1998). That is, within each of the self-regulatory, cognitive-behavioral, emotion-focused, and insight-oriented couple therapies, therapists try to identify underlying commonalities in repeated distressed relationship interactions. Within these different approaches to couple therapy, and from other research on relationships, a number of themes have been identified which correlate with relationship distress. In this section of the chapter I want to go through the most common of these themes. The typology of themes I am presenting is based largely on the work of Don Baucom and colleagues (Baucom, Epstein, Daiuto, et al., 1996), who proposed that there are three dominant areas in couples interaction themes: boundaries, power and control, and personal investment in the relationship.

Boundaries

Boundaries refer to the desired levels of closeness versus autonomy within a relationship. Low boundaries indicate a high level of desired intimacy and closeness; high boundaries indicate high desired autonomy and independence. Many different theoretical models of relationships include attention to boundaries but often use somewhat different terms to describe essentially the same idea. For example, Markman and Kraft (1989) refer to the closeness–distance dimension. Volker and Olson (1993) describe a circumplex model of relationships in which they label low boundaries as enmeshment and high boundaries as disengagement. Olson's model includes the assumption that intermediate boundaries are most adaptive for relationships, and his terms reflect the assumption that low or high boundaries are maladaptive. For me the term "boundary" avoids prior assumptions about what is adaptive, so I like that term.

I am unconvinced by the assertion by Olson and others that intermediate levels of boundaries are optimal for satisfying relationships. Couples vary enormously in their desired boundaries, and it seems to me that greater or lesser boundaries are not incompatible with a mutually satisfying relationship. Recent work by Baucom, Epstein, Daiuto, et al. (1996) supports this viewpoint. They showed that there was little association between absolute levels of boundaries and relationship satisfaction. However, the extent to which partners felt their desired levels of boundaries were met within the relationship correlated with satisfaction. Hannah, Halford, and Dadds (2000) replicated this finding that it was the extent to which the relationship met the partners' desired level of boundaries that predicted relationship satisfaction.

A number of writers about couple relationships suggest that differences between partners in their desired boundaries are associated with relationship distress (Christensen, 1988; Jacobson, 1989; Markman & Kraft, 1989). Often, repetitive patterns of interaction seem to reflect the theme of one partner seeking lower boundaries while the other seeks to maintain or strengthen boundaries. For example, the issue of boundaries often is evident when couples have conflict. The approach–withdraw pattern can be seen as a struggle over boundaries. The partner approaching seeks to engage the partner and lower boundaries, whereas the partner withdrawing seeks to disengage and maintain boundaries.

Power and Control

All couples need to make decisions, and many decisions that they make will have a substantial impact on both partners. Implicitly this means that couples need to develop ways to share influence or power within the relationship. There are a number of ways in which couples might distribute power and control within a relationship. Stuart (1980) provides a useful conceptualization for describing power within a relationship. Figure 8.2 is a diagram that depicts five options for decision making based on Stuart's (1980) concepts. The options are as follows: the man makes the decision without consultation with the woman, the man takes responsibility for the decision after consulting with the woman, the man and the woman jointly make the decision with mutual consultation, the woman takes primary responsibility after consulting with the man; or the woman makes the decision without consultation with the man. I use this diagram in couple therapy by having each partner place core areas of decision making in the area that reflects first the current mode of decision making within their relationship and then their preferred method of decision making within the relationship. By mapping out power and control within the relationship across specific domains, partners are able to identify where the problems in decision making exist.

Investment

Investment refers to the degree of commitment and effort each partner makes in the relationship. Investment often is thought to fall into two broad domains: emotional and instrumental investment. Emotional investment refers to the extent to which people are emotionally involved with their partner and sensitive to the emotional climate of the relationship. Instrumental investment refers to the extent to which people contribute to the required chores that form the basis of any relationship. These chores include tasks such as household maintenance, car maintenance, paying bills, and so forth.

Disagreement about household chores is a common area in instrumental

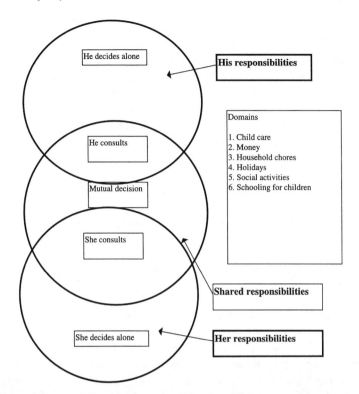

This is to help you define decision making in your relationship. Write the number code for each decision domain in the area that best describes how decisions are made now. Then write a second set of underlined numbers showing how you want decisions to be made in the future.

FIGURE 8.2. Power and decision making in relationships.

investment that creates difficulty in relationships. There is a large volume of research attesting that in two-career families, the women tend to do substantially more than half of all household chores (Goodnow & Bowes, 1994). This pattern often creates a source of considerable distress and resentment to women. Some men have little or no understanding of the amount of time basic household maintenance takes and may be relatively low in their investments in this aspect of their relationship. I have found that an important part of relationship psychoeducation is enhancing male understanding of the level of investment the male makes, and that his partner makes, in instrumental activities. For example, it can often be useful to get the male to monitor how many hours a week he spends on household chores versus how many hours his partner spends on household chores.

Influences on Themes of Couple Adaptive Processes

The common influences on couple adaptive processes in relationships fall under the headings of individual characteristics, life events, and contextual factors referred to in the model of couple relationships first introduced in Chapter 1. I explore with couples each of these possible influences on the themes of their couple adaptive processes. Exploring the influences on the development of identified relationship themes by itself sometimes leads to relationship change. As it becomes clearer how the themes developed, clients often see how the themes can be changed. For example, Martina and Malcolm presented with relationship problems that illustrate the value of identifying relationship themes and their influences. One of Malcolm' core complaints was Martina's lack of emotional expressiveness. Martina initially saw this as Malcolm being intrusive and demanding in their relationship. Over the initial phase of relationship psychoeducation the couple identified a recurrent pattern of Malcolm seeking more closeness and Martina withdrawing. That is, there was a difference in preferred boundaries. Martina identified a lack of self-disclosure as characteristic of her family of origin; she described her family as very achievement and career oriented. Discussions in her family tended to be very intellectual and goal focused. Discussions of career goals and achievements were particularly valued. Malcolm reported that his family was not at all career-minded. Both his mother and father were in the performing arts, and his parents and his sister all valued emotional expression and artistic pursuits above notions of career. Malcolm and Martina learned to identify their approach–withdraw interaction theme and the influences on the development of their respective boundary preferences that drove that interaction theme. A key relationship goal for this couple became to use the strengths of both emotional expression and goal-focused problem solving in their interactions.

Individual Characteristics

FAMILY-OF-ORIGIN EXPERIENCES

As noted earlier, there is substantial evidence that the family of origin has an important modeling role in the development of behaviors that influence couple relationships. We often learn things from our parents about intimacy, how to experience affection, how to manage conflict, and implicit standards about how relationships should be. Although many people try to avoid making the mistakes they feel their parents have made, often under emotional stress they fall back onto the means of interacting to which they have been exposed (Halford, Sanders, & Behrens, 2000; Sanders et al., 1999).

Parents in the family of origin are not the only source of influence in developing relationship behaviors and standards. For example, children exposed to high levels of interparental violence in the family of origin are more likely to be violent in their own relationships, but the effect of the family-of-origin experiences accounts for only a modest proportion of the variance (Widom, 1989). Only about 30% of the people exposed to severe family-of-origin violence will themselves be violent in their relationships. After being exposed to family-of-origin violence, having a good relationship with an adult who models nonviolent ways of resolving conflict reduces the likelihood of someone being violent (O'Leary, 1988). People need to learn to manage conflict nonviolently in intimate relationships. If the parents do not provide this modeling, it needs to be provided by someone else who is salient to the individual. Hence, it can be useful to explore the impact during childhood and adolescence of relationships with key figures other than parents.

When individuals hold firm, maladaptive assumptions about the way that relationships should be, this can often be an indication that family-of-origin experiences need to be explored. I often ask partners about the relationship between their mother and father and what they feel they learned about relationships from observing their mother and father interact.

PRIOR RELATIONSHIPS

Prior relationships have a substantial impact on the way partners interact in their current relationship (Furman & Flanagan, 1997). Sometimes prior relationships can have a positive effect on the current relationship, as when someone has learned intimacy skills through interacting with a valued partner. Other times, coercion or unpleasant breakups may characterize prior relationships, and this may exacerbate difficulties individuals already have with intimacy. For example, anxiety over abandonment may be severely exacerbated if a person repeatedly experienced relationships terminated against their wishes.

Prior relationships can be particularly important if one of the previous relationships involved high levels of commitment, such as a live-in relationship or prior marriage. Sometimes individuals ascribe the breakdown of a prior relationship purely to selecting the wrong partner. This may not be a particularly healthy way of reviewing prior relationships. In some instances individuals do pair with partners who did not suit them, and terminating the relationship is a good long-term resolution. However, most committed relationships break down because of a range of factors, not simply choice of partner. Individuals in second marriages often interact with their current partners in similar ways to their past interactions in the first marriage (Prado & Markman, 1998). Consequently, it often is useful to explore the experiences of partners in prior relationships and how unhelpful patterns can be avoided.

The case of Martha provides one example of the negative impact that prior relationships can have on a current relationship. Martha was upset about her current relationship and wondered whether she should break it off. Martha had been living with Keith for 2 years and previously had been married to Justin for 7 years. Martha described Keith as excessively emotionally expressive, which was very upsetting to her. This is a somewhat unusual complaint from a woman about a man, and so I explored with her what it was that she found upsetting about Keith's being expressive of feelings. In the course of this exploration we talked about her experiences in her marriage. Her ex-husband Justin was homosexual and had left her for another man. Justin was highly emotionally expressive and artistic. After exploration, we concluded that Martha associated high levels of emotional expressiveness by males with being homosexual. It seemed that when Keith was highly emotionally expressive it triggered a fear that he would abandon her. Once this became clearer, the therapeutic goal moved to helping her to appreciate Keith's strengths in emotional expressiveness.

ATTACHMENT STYLE

Attachment style is a generalized pattern of responding in intimate relationships that is thought to reflect prior experiences of intimate relationships and to be relatively stable over time (Feeney & Noller, 1996). Two important dimensions have been identified in adult attachment: anxiety over abandonment and comfort with closeness. Anxiety over abandonment refers to the extent of preoccupation and concern about the possibility that an intimate partner may be rejecting or may terminate the relationship. Comfort with closeness refers to the degree of subjective enjoyment versus distress that someone feels with intense emotional intimacy.

Some people have suggested that adult attachment is the central theme which influences intimate relationships (e.g., Johnson & Greenberg, 1995). Although I have reservations that it is universally the most important theme affecting relationships, high discomfort with closeness or anxiety about abandonment is dysfunctional in relationships (Feeney & Noller, 1996). Committing oneself to any intimate relationship involves a tangible risk that an individual will be abandoned. If people preoccupy themselves with this possibility, they may develop a variety of dysfunctional ways of responding to relationship difficulties. For example, high anxiety over abandonment is associated with attempts to control the partner (Skuja & Halford, 2000).

Johnson and Greenberg (1995) argue that severe conflict in relationships often results from unexpressed emotions relating to insecure attachment style. For example, the person who becomes extremely hostile with her partner when he arrives home from work may do so because she is anxious that this late arrival from work indicates a loss of interest in the relationship. In emotion-focused couple therapy, a variety of strategic questions and experiential techniques are used to bring concerns about abandonment, or discomfort with closeness, to conscious awareness. A similar process is described in insight-oriented couple therapy, again based on the idea that much of the conflict is the result of a hidden agenda about insecure attachment style. It is believed that by drawing out the person's sense of vulnerability as reflected in his or her attachment style, and making that vulnerability known to the partner, the couple will shift the way they think and feel about their relationship.

Recent work looking at changes within therapy sessions lends some support to the importance of attachment style in mediating changes in couple therapy. Johnson and Talitman (1997) found that couples who go through emotion-focused couple therapy change the way that they express themselves in sessions. They move from expressing hostility and anger to expressing vulnerability and concerns about discomfort with closeness or anxiety over abandonment. These changes often coincide with explorations about the individual themes underlying couple interaction, themes related to anxiety over abandonment or discomfort with closeness. In the context of relationship psychoeducation in SRCT I sometimes describe the notion of attachment style and explore how an insecure attachment style might relate to an individual's prior experiences (e.g., family-of-origin or prior relationships).

GENDER ROLES

Gender role expectations can create conflict within relationships. The most common difficulty arises when the man adheres to more traditional gender roles but the woman does not. Under these circumstances it can be useful to explore how that gender role expectation developed as a means of gently challenging unhelpful or rigid role definitions. For example, in Ben and Kathy's household, Ben made almost no contribution to the household chores. Kathy was resentful of Ben's lack of contribution. Both partners were working full time, and Kathy expressed the view that they each should do about half of the chores. Ben's perspective was that he did "help out" and that he did what was reasonable. Implicit in Ben's views seemed an assumption that the woman would take primary responsibility for household chores. However, if someone had directly challenged Ben with the view that he was holding on to traditional gender-role stereotypes, he would have disavowed it. In couples of the 21st century, gender-role stereotyping still exists, but it is often more subtle than that which existed a generation or two ago.

It can be useful to explore gender-role stereotypes by getting couples to look at the distribution of chores and responsibilities within their relationship. For example, Figure 8.3 lists common household and relationship maintenance tasks. Each partner is asked to identify which of these tasks is done by both partners approximately equally and which tasks one person takes primary

Item	Which partner typically does more?		
	Male	Female	Both
1. Balancing bank accounts			
2. Paying bills			
3. Budgeting			
4. Shopping/groceries			
5. Washing dishes			
6. Dusting/vacuuming			
7. Cleaning kitchen/bathroom			
8. Making beds			
9. Washing/ironing clothes			
10. Taking out garbage			
11. Organizing renovations			
12. Home repairs (handy work)			
13. Car repairs/changing tire			
14. Outside cleaning			
15. Mowing lawn			
16. Gardening			
17. Organizing "who does what"			
18. Driving car (when together)			
19. Organizing planned outings			
20. Organizing contact with male's family			
21. Organizing contact with female's family			
22. Organizing contact with friends			
23. Paying bill when out (e.g., meals)			
24. Organizing holidays			
25. Mending clothes			
26. Disciplining children			
27. Helping children with school work			
28. Playing with children			
29. Getting children to school/activities			

FIGURE 8.3. Relationship tasks.

responsibility for. Often people share more across gender-role barriers than in the past, yet many couples still adhere to fairly traditional gender-role divisions of labor. There are two key questions that often prime people to this adherence. If couples are asked who drove the last six times that they went out together, in the majority of cases it will be the male. It is not universally the case, but it is often the case. (Anyone who is skeptical about this and thinks his or her friends have transcended gender roles should think back on his or her own relationship and who drove in the last week or two. Then that person should ask some friends the same questions). If couples are asked who cooked meals when they ate at home over the last week or two, most often the answer will be that the woman cooked more meals than the man did.

It does not follow that couples must undergo gender-role reversals or have exactly 50/50 distribution of all household chores in order to have a successful relationship. However, it is clear that there have been considerable changes in role expectations for both genders. The most dramatic social change in gender roles has been the much greater participation in the paid work force of married women relative to a generation ago. Many women today have mothers who did not engage in paid work at all, or who worked many fewer hours than women now work. One effect of this change is that many women find it difficult to know how to balance work and family responsibilities. Work–family conflict is something that seems to be particularly stressful for women (Thompson, 1997). One difficulty for women is that they have not often been exposed to role models who successfully balanced these competing demands. Moreover, many women, despite their intellectual commitment to the importance of paid work, struggle with the idea that they should do all the things for their families that their mothers did in their families.

For men, having a partner who is in full-time paid employment has many advantages. The disposable income for the family is increased, and there is significant evidence that many men find it rewarding to have the extra intellectual and interpersonal stimulation of living with someone who has her own career (Thompson, 1997). At the same time, many men were raised in households on which their mother was a full-time household manager and their father undertook few household responsibilities. The modern man may espouse the importance of transcending traditional gender roles, but in practice many men leave the majority of household responsibilities to their partner. They implicitly often see these domains as being primarily the women's responsibility, and they "help out." Modern men often have had no role models who balanced work and family responsibilities.

Context

WORK

Work–family conflicts occur in a context, and it can be important to draw to the couple's attention the context within which their particular beliefs and behaviors exist. Some organizations have developed family-friendly work practices, such as providing child-care services, allowing some sick days per year to be used for family responsibilities, and providing some flexibility in the timing and setting of work. Companies that provide such family-friendly poli-cies develop greater employee loyalty and reduce costly losses of highly trained staff (Edgar, 1997). However, few work settings are sensitive to the family responsibilities of workers. In fact, there is often an implicit value in organizations that anyone who is serious about his or her career will be able to accommodate heavy work demands. Raising issues about the impact of work practices on family responsibilities is sometimes interpreted as indicative of slothfulness or lack of career focus (Edgar, 1997). In couples in which work–family conflict is a problem, it often is useful to explore with the partners the organizational context within which they work and the implicit and explicit messages received about how to manage family responsibilities.

The effects of work on family are multiple. All the foregoing examples can be described as role overload, which occurs when the person feels that he or she simply does not have the time to achieve all the tasks that his or her various roles entail. This seems to be a particular problem for women (Thompson, 1997). A second type of work–family conflict, which is subtler, is role overlap. This phe-nomenon occurs when people engage in behaviors at work that are often suc-cessful in achieving goals and then engage in those same behaviors at home. For example, Darren was very successful at business; he ran a large building supply firm. Darren had a reputation for being a tough businessperson who was de-manding of his workers but also an effective leader. His approach to running his large business empire was to be focused on tasks and conscious of using his time efficiently. He often arrived home after having spent 10 or 11 hours during the day in highly focused problem solving. When his partner, Adele, spoke to him about something that was concerning her, he would often apply the same skills he had used successfully at work to the family situation.

Adele found Darren's instant problem solving unhelpful and unsympa-thetic. Often she was seeking somebody who would simply listen to her and allow her to express how she felt. When we discussed the ways in which there was this role overlap, one of the therapy goals became to more clearly differ-entiate appropriate ways of behaving toward work colleagues versus appropri-ate ways of interacting with your partner.

FRIENDSHIPS

Friendships serve a number of important functions, which can support part-ners in relationships. We know that individuals who are socially isolated are more likely to suffer relationship problems (Weiss & Aved, 1978). Perhaps the availability of good friends prevents people from becoming overly reliant on their partner to meet all of their psychological needs.

At the same time, certain friendship networks may be destructive in terms of their impact on relationships. Julien, Markman, Léveillé, Chartrand,

and Bégin (1994) analyzed women talking with their best friends about difficulties in their relationship. They found that among women who were in distressed relationships, the interaction with their friends was often associated with mutual complaints about partners and negative comments about their relationships. In contrast, for people in a happy relationship, often the interactions about difficulties in the relationship prompted problem solving. This finding is open to a number of interpretations. One is that some friends may prompt and assist relationship difficulties being solved whereas others may prompt and assist attention to difficulties and increase the likelihood of separation.

It is striking that separation and divorce are not evenly distributed throughout the population of couples. Certain networks of friendships seem to support and reinforce relationships and seek to nurture relationships that are in distress. In other friendship networks, greater emphasis is placed on individual satisfaction, and divorce and separation are seen as more desirable ways of resolving relationship difficulties. This is not to suggest that people get divorced simply because their friends suggest it to them but, rather, that friendship networks may mediate the likelihood of separation, versus attempts to improve, distressed relationships.

EXTENDED FAMILY

Aside from the developmental effects of family-of-origin experiences, parents and other extended family provide an important context in which current couple interaction occurs. The role of extended family in couple relationships is subject to enormous variations. For example, Henry had been raised in a family of origin in which the extended family was highly valued. The grandfather in the family was seen as the head of the household. Henry saw respect and involvement with the extended family as normal. In contrast, Helen's family of origin had little contact with extended family. Helen perceived the heavy involvement of Henry's parents in the couple's relationship and childrearing decisions as intrusive. In the context of their conflict about the role of extended family I explored their experiences of extended family during childhood. By highlighting how their expectations about the role of extended family developed from their own experiences when growing up, the partners became more tolerant of each other's views and were able to negotiate about the role of extended family in their relationship.

CULTURE AND ETHNICITY

The goals of intimate relationships are, to a substantial degree, culturally defined. Most often people marry individuals who are similar to them in race, ethnicity, and culture. However, in many multicultural societies, cross-cultural marriages are common. Cross-cultural relationships have many potential strengths. Different cultures emphasize different elements of human experience and often the different cultures can complement each other (Jones & Chao, 1997). For example, in an interracial relationship between a Chinese Australian woman, Vivian, and her Anglo-Saxon partner, Richard, Richard made the observation to me about how much he had learned about the importance of family from Vivian. He highlighted how she liked to see her parents regularly, and how her parents were actively involved with their children. In contrast, Richard commented on the isolation he felt from his own parents, and how he had had very little contact with his grandparents before they died. At the same time there are special challenges in intercultural relationships, particularly the conflict that may arise from different relationship assumptions and standards. It often is necessary to explicate the core assumptions of each culture so that the couple can discuss where those assumptions differ.

Even within one ethnic tradition partners can vary substantially in the extent to which they identify with their particular ethnic background (Nesdale, Rooney, & Smith, 1997). Factors such as use of language at home, style of food eaten, attendance at ethnic community activities, religion, and style of dress have been used to quantify ethnic identification (Nesdale et al., 1997). Different strengths of ethnic identification can be a source of couple conflict. For example, Ricky and Maria were Italian Australians. Ricky did not speak Italian, preferred varieties of food other than traditional Italian style, and had given up on his Catholic upbringing. In contrast, Maria highly valued her Italian heritage, had repeatedly visited Italy, was a practicing Catholic, and spoke Italian. Maria was keen for their children to learn Italian, and to spend at least 12 months living in Italy, so that they would understand something of Italian culture. Ricky had been to Italy, and did not like it. These differences in the extent to which the Italian part of their identity was important to them led to a number of conflicts about major decisions to do with childrearing. By explicating the source of those differences, we were able to help them resolve it. Ricky talked about the oppressive nature of his experience of being raised as an Italian Australian child. He felt coerced into attempts to teach him Italian by his parents. He also reported that he had been subjected to considerable taunting by other children at school based on the fact that he was Italian. In contrast, Maria went to a school that was predominantly Italian Catholic. She strongly identified with her Italian roots and had been active in the Italian community for much of her adolescence. When they first met, Ricky had been very attracted to the exotic nature of her knowledge of Italy and her ability to speak Italian. Later, he found her identification with her Italian ancestry much more difficult to deal with.

Couples that marry across racial and ethnic lines, sometimes have to deal with significant prejudice. Consider Noel and Patricia. Noel was an indigenous Australian and Patricia was of Anglo-Saxon origin. Neither partner's parents approved of their marriage. Both sets of parents believed that Noel and Patricia were denying their respective ethnic identities, and sought to prevent the marriage before it occurred. Fortunately, Noel and Patricia had a circle of friends, which included both indigenous and Anglo-Australians, who were very positive about their relationship. Both Noel and Patricia commented on the positive effect their friends had in their transcending the beliefs of their parents.

Patricia experienced one particular difficulty with what she perceived as Noel's inconsistent behavior toward his relatives as opposed to hers. It is a common part of indigenous Australian culture to share material possessions with your extended family. Noel valued this approach to life and would often lend household goods, money, and other items to his extended family. On the other hand, he was resistant to doing this with Patricia's family, arguing that this was not part of his kinship network. Patricia felt that this was inconsistent and rejecting of her extended family. As the couple discussed these issues in therapy, Patricia came to understand how the traditional teachings of Noel's kin had influenced his thinking. Noel also came to understand how different Patricia's upbringing had been from his own in terms of perceptions of fairness in dealing with extended family. This greater understanding of each other reduced negative feelings about their different views on sharing with extended family.

Life Events

ENGAGING IN THE RELATIONSHIP

A number of common changes occur across the course of a long-term committed relationship, and many of these changes are somewhat predictable. The transition into being in a committed relationship is the first such change. In the beginning phase of relationships many people experience infatuation. Infatuation is that wonderful feeling of novelty, of being overwhelmed by your feelings for your partner. These feelings are fabulous at the time, but rarely do they persist consistently throughout a long-term committed relationship. For most people the intensity of initial passion is gradually replaced by a long-term deep commitment, but without the overwhelming nature of the initial infatuation.

For some people the excitement of novelty, the overwhelming nature of infatuation, is what they identify as being in love. When the relationship matures, and these initial intense feelings abate, some people feel disillusioned and disappointed with the new form of the relationship. Because the vast majority of people in committed relationships value fidelity and monogamy

(Australian Institute of Family Studies, 1997), there is some trade-off between the novelty of infatuation and long-term commitment. In essence, most people have to forgo some opportunities for novelty to make long-term committed relationships work. That trade-off can be addressed more directly. I have asked couples to imagine themselves on their 30th wedding anniversary. If the relationship were wonderful, what would they be saying to each other about those 30 years? Prompting partners to attend to the value of a sense of shared lives, of growing together, of working to do things together that are important to them as individuals and as a couple often increases the salience of the value of lifelong relationships.

TRANSITION TO PARENTHOOD

The majority of people who get married have children and do so in the first 4 or 5 years of marriage (McDonald, 1995). Many couples report that sharing parenthood is one of the most positive experiences of their lives (Belsky & Kelly, 1994). At the same time, transition to parenthood requires the couple to renegotiate many aspects of their relationship, particularly the sharing of household tasks and paid employment. There are substantial additional tasks, and there may be changes in work routines for one or both partners that necessitate such renegotiation. The transition to parenthood also increases the salience of gender-role beliefs about career and the sharing of work and family duties. If this has not been an issue until now, it can be a source of substantial disagreement.

The transition to parenthood typically involves some reduction in work hours by one of the parents, often the mother, or a substantial increase in the total workload for the partners, or some combination of both. Typically there is a loss of disposable income, associated both with the likely reduction in total number of hours worked plus the additional cost of caring for a child. Overall, the transition to parenthood often is associated with a move to more traditional gender roles, and the pressure to adopt these more traditional gender roles is often forced on the couple by social structures. For example, maternity leave is generally more widely available than paternity leave in most Western countries (Edgar, 1997). There also is usually a reduction in the time available to the couple for activities that they do just as a couple. Arranging for appropriate child care becomes an additional expense and task for couples to be able to go out together. When children are very young, parents often are reluctant to leave their children for any substantial amount of time. As children get older, their requirements change substantially. The degree of involvement of both partners in the parenting process and their competence in handling parenting have a significant impact on the relationship (Sanders, Nicholson, & Floyd, 1997).

RELOCATION

A generation ago many people were raised, educated, worked, and died in the same general area; now we have increased social mobility (McDonald, 1995). The effect of relocation on couples is substantial. Relocation to another city usually reduces the contact the couple have with their extended family. The informal advice and support of their parents is often less accessible for a couple raising children. The sense of connection with extended family is lowered. All this throws extra demands on the partners to support each other and to meet each other's needs.

Relocation also changes people's social networks. As people move from city to city, often in pursuit of jobs and career advancement, friendships that are formed outside work are often broken off. People become increasingly involved with those people they meet through their work for their social network. If people remain in the same industry, this can often result in primarily knowing other individuals who work in the same profession or industry. If the person then leaves that industry, it can often be devastating as it disrupts the social network as well as the professional network.

Common Variations in Couple Relationships

There are some common variations in couple relationships which involve specific challenges. All relationships are unique, but particular types of couple relationships may have variations in context and life events that are somewhat different from those in other relationships. I want to consider three general categories: stepfamilies, living together, and gay relationships.

Stepfamilies

An individual whose first marriage ended unsuccessfully probably has an overrepresentation of individual vulnerabilities and difficulties with adaptive couple processes, as these factors are likely to have contributed to the breakdown of the first relationship. These factors probably put second marriages at higher risk for problems than first marriages. A challenge for partners entering a second relationship is to avoid the errors that may have contributed to the breakup of the first relationship. Children from the first marriage add some further, specific challenges in negotiating stepparenting arrangements. In stepfamilies, parenting often necessitates ongoing contact with the ex-partner, and the relationship with the ex-partner can be a source of difficulty to the new relationship in some instances.

It is important to recognize that the new partner may have difficulties in interacting with the child, or children. New partners may not have any direct experience in parenting. Consequently, they will not have had the opportunity to develop the skills and knowledge of normal developmental processes that often accompany having one's own children. Knowledge deficits may include not knowing what language to use to a child of a given age or what sorts of things interest children of particular ages. Combining this lack of child-care knowledge with a lack of any relationship history with the child often makes those early interactions difficult. Moreover, if the stepparents are committed to the relationship with their new partners, the stepparents often desperately want to form a bond with the child and may feel distraught if the children are unresponsive or even negative toward them.

The role of the new partner in parenting is an important issue that needs to be negotiated within a relationship. Research has shown that disagreements between partners about the role of stepparents in caring for children are a core source of conflict in reconstituted families (Lawton & Sanders, 1994). Furthermore, conflict around this issue often is associated with relationship dissolution, even if other things within the relationship are working well (Nicholson, Halford, & Sanders, 1996). Table 8.2 identifies some key issues that are often problematic for couples to negotiate about the role of stepparent. If stepparenting looks as if it is a core issue in the couple's relationship, it can be useful to review this handout with couples and have them discuss their assumptions and expectations about these issues. For example, within relationship psychoeducation it is useful to explore the impact on the stepparent of suddenly acquiring additional responsibilities for a child or children whom they do not know very well.

A common complication in reconstituted families is that ongoing contact

---

TABLE 8.2. Special Issues for Stepfamilies

Developing the role of the new partner in:
1. Disciplining of children
   - Determining behavior limits
   - Giving instructions
   - Enacting penalties

2. Major decisions about children
   - Schooling
   - Medical care
   - Child rules (e.g., who can visit, where, how late away from home)
   - Negotiations with ex-partner about parenting

3. Activities of child
   - School events
   - Birthdays
   - Friends
   - Special outings with biological parent

---

with an ex-partner is required about issues of sharing parenting. Issues such as the responsibilities of each of the biological parents for child care, access visits, and financial support of children can be sources of major disagreement between the ex-partners. Bearing in mind that the original marriage may have broken up because of difficulties in managing conflict, it is easy to imagine why there is often heated disagreement around these issues of sharing parenting. These conflicts present a stress to the current relationship in numerous forms such as the effect on the mood of the spouse, impact on children, and the financial implications of changes in child support payments. Table 8.3 provides a list of common issues confronting people who are attempting to negotiate coparenting arrangements after the end of a couple relationship. In circumstances in which the relationship with the ex-partner is having a major stressful impact on the current relationship, it can often be useful to focus the couple on each of these issues and see whether further negotiation can occur between the current parent and the ex-partner.

There is a consistent finding that conflict between parents which is directly observed by the children is distressing to children (Grych & Fincham, 1993). To minimize the deleterious effects of a relationship breakup on children, I emphasize the importance to partners of managing conflict effectively and minimizing the amount of conflict that spills over to children. This may involve the current partner being supportive of his or her spouse during interactions with the ex-partner, at least while the children are present. Major disagreements about child care and management should be discussed, if the children are young, privately between the parents to reach an agreement. Once they have a common understanding of what they are trying to achieve, it is appropriate to try to discuss these issues with the children.

Living Together

In the last generation in many Western countries, it has become much more common for couples to live together without going through the legal steps of marriage. In some countries living together is now more popular among young people than getting married. For example, in Australia, over 60% of young people live with a partner in a committed relationship (Edgar, 1997). Some people prefer to stay living together rather than ever marry, and other people use living together as a transitional point to decide whether they wish to make the transition to marriage (McDonald, 1995).

There is considerably less research on relationships in which couples cohabit than on couples that are formally married. In part, this may be because it is harder to identify couples living together than it is to identify people who are married. What research has been done suggests that there are more commonalities between cohabiting and married couples than differences. Couples that choose to cohabit generally endorse assumptions that they should be mo-

TABLE 8.3. Parenting after Divorce: A Checklist of Issues

Visitation
- Schedule of regular arrangements for child
- Transport between parents' homes
- Consequences for late dropoff or pickup
- Who has responsibility for sick children? (i.e., Who would stay home from work, etc.?)

Changes to regular visitation procedure
- How are changes for visitation to be negotiated?
- How do vacations, and other special occasions, impact on regular visitation?

Telephone calls
- When is acceptable for parent to initiate call?
- When is acceptable for child to initiate call?

Special occasions
- Who has child during holiday periods?
- Who has child on birthdays? (Two celebrations are possible.)

Health care
- Who schedules regular dentist, doctor appointments?
- Advising each other of medications or other health care required

School
- Who decides choice of school?
- Who has contact with the school, attends meetings with teachers?
- Who attends school events?
- Who gets report cards?

Vacations
- Are there limits on travel on vacations (out of state, out of country)?
- Contact telephone numbers for holiday absences.

Note. Adapted from Baris and Garrity (1997). Copyright 1997 by John Wiley & Sons, Inc. Adapted by permission.

nogamous, and that love, intimacy, good communication, and support for each other are all important characteristics of the relationship that they want (McDonald, 1995).

Given all the commonalities between cohabitation and marriage, I believe that almost all the procedures that have been described for couple therapy are equally applicable to couples that are married or living together. However, it is important to note that couples that choose to live together often do attach some significance to the fact that they are not married. I find that it is often useful to ask couples whether they see any important differences between themselves as a couple now versus how they would be if they were married. Some couples see no significant differences between marriage and cohabiting and attach little importance to the legal act of marriage. However, other couples refer to advantages they see in not getting married. In particular, some couples refer to the advantage of living together as preventing social pressure to conform to other people's ideas about marriage. For example, a number of couples report that if they married, they believe relatives would pressure them to have children, or to buy a house, or in some other way to alter their lives together. The expectations of others are less crucial for other couples, but they associate marriage with particular values to which they do not adhere. For example, couples may aspire to a more open relationship than that which they associate with marriage. Other people have had negative views of marriage and have simply resolved that they do not want to enter that institution.

Gay and Lesbian Relationships

Like living together, gay and lesbian relationships have much in common with married relationships. For example, the available research on gay and lesbian relationships suggests that most partners endorse a desire for intimacy, support, and closeness in their relationships (Julien et al., 1997). Although the amount of research on gay and lesbian relationships is somewhat limited, the research available suggests that those relationships suffer from many of the same challenges that relationships between heterosexual couples suffer (Julien et al., 1997). I have seen numerous gay and lesbian couples for whom issues of difficulties in communication, managing conflict, resolving household routines, developing a greater sense of shared intimacy, and problems with relationships with ex-partners and stepparenting issues have all been difficulties. In my experience, the procedures described in this book generally work equally as well for gay relationships and lesbian relationships as they do for heterosexual relationships. However, I would caution that there is a need for more systematic research to evaluate the effectiveness of these approaches with homosexual relationships.

One obvious difference between gay and lesbian relationships, on one hand, and heterosexual relationships, on the other hand, is that in the former you have same-sex pairs. Given that much of the research about difficulties in conflict management has identified important gender differences, it is interesting to examine how conflict is managed in same-sex relationships. Julien et al. (1997) did a thorough review of the available research. It was noted earlier in this book that the approach–withdraw pattern is quite common in conflict in distressed couples, and often it is the woman who demands and the male who withdraws. In studies of both gay and lesbian relationships it has been found that the approach–withdraw pattern also is evident (Julien et al., 1997). There does not seem to be any clear difference between the way that distressed gay and lesbian couples mismanage conflict and the way that heterosexual couples mismanage conflict.

One difference colleagues and I found between lesbian and heterosexual relationships was in terms of the standards held about boundaries. We found that lesbian couples desired significantly greater intimacy and closeness, or significantly fewer boundaries between the partners, than did heterosexual couples (Hannah et al., 2000). The standards that gay male couples hold for their relationships have not been systematically investigated, and this warrants further research.

Another difference between homosexual and heterosexual relationships is the degree of prejudice to which couples may be exposed. Almost all homosexuals report experiencing some degree of prejudice about their sexual orientation during their upbringing. How these individuals respond to homophobic responses by people around them varies considerably. When the partners differ in the way that they manage their homosexual identity it can be a source of distress. For example, if one partner is openly gay and the other person has tended to be much more discreet, it can lead to clashes in the way that they present themselves in public. As with other issues about which couples disagree, it can often be useful to trace the developmental course of how they as individuals arrived at their coping strategies. A greater appreciation of each person's perspective can often lead to greater respect for the differences that may exist between the partners.

Linking Relationship Psychoeducation to the Next Steps in Therapy

Relationship psychoeducation is intended to provide knowledge to assist partners to specify self-change goals and to overcome the effects of negative thoughts and feelings. Relationship psychoeducation is complete when these goals are achieved. Couple therapy can then proceed in one of two directions. The couple can move to self-change or to therapist-guided change. The therapist should follow the procedures listed in Chapters 6 and 7 to determine whether self-change is a viable option. If self-change is not viable and skills training is required, the procedures described in the next chapter are used.

9

Therapist-Guided Change

Therapist-guided change occurs when a couple have defined shared relationship goals and know the self-change they wish to implement but are unable to achieve self-change because they lack certain relationship skills. For example, suppose a couple want to increase their sense of intimacy through better communication. If one or both partners find it hard to express feelings, this can inhibit the achievement of their relationship goal. The therapist guides the partners to develop greater expressiveness of emotion.

This chapter describes therapist-guided change in four key areas of couple adaptive processes: positive day-to-day behavior, communication, conflict management, and helping partners to change negative thoughts and feelings. As noted in Chapter 1, problems in these areas are the most common complaints of distressed couples seeking therapy. The therapy procedures described are largely adaptations of procedures from behavioral couple therapy (BCT). However, in self-regulatory couple therapy (SRCT) therapist-guided change is a skill-building process used to empower the partners to engage in self-change. In SRCT each partner is assisted not only to acquire particular relationship skills but also to self-regulate use of that skill. In other words, partners are assisted to self-appraise their skills, to set goals for behavioral change, and to implement and evaluate self-change. The ultimate goal is for couples to move to self-change. Once the procedures described in this chapter are completed, the partners move to the procedures for self-change described in Chapter 7.

If couples need assistance in two or more of the areas described in this chapter, then the sequence in which areas are addressed needs to be negotiated with the couple. The sequence is determined predominantly by the expressed priorities of the partners. In addition, the therapist may recommend addressing areas that he or she believes are central to the relationship difficulties.

Increasing Positivity in Day-to-Day Interactions

An important element of my approach to behavioral change in couple therapy is to encourage positive behaviors that promote intimacy within the relationship. The small day-to-day behaviors that occur between partners are a crucial element of intimacy. The gentle hug, the kiss to farewell and greet, the shared smile expressing pleasure to see each other, and holding hands on a walk together are all examples of expressions of intimacy and closeness. Table 9.1 lists some of the key classes of daily behavior related to relationship satisfaction.

The early theoretical formulations of BCT were based on social exchange theory (Thibaut & Kelley, 1959), which hypothesizes that social relationships are formed and maintained as the result of the availability *and reciprocation* of reinforcement. Couple relationship satisfaction and a sense of intimacy resulted from each partner's immediately reinforcing positivity by his or her partner by reciprocating positivity. The reciprocity hypothesis proved to be wrong. Happy relationships are not reciprocal, or at least not in the short term (Jacobson et al., 1982). Rather, happy partners tend not to respond to their spouse's negativity, and they maintain positivity even when it is not reciprocated (Jacobson et al., 1982). Negative reciprocity is a key characteristic of relationship distress. The temporal form of the behavior of satisfied couples is analogous to a bank account. Positive behavior results in relationship credit, which can be drawn on in the form of negative behavior. Negative behaviors will not be reciprocated until relationship credit is low. Eventually persistent negative behavior will exceed relationship credit in most, if not all, relationships, but a long history of positive behavior will lead to much greater tolerance for negativity.

The problem for distressed couples is that they lack a "credit balance." Therapeutically, the task is to help the partners develop a credit balance by being positive toward their partner. Furthermore, this positivity needs to be done unilaterally. In other words, each partner needs to be positive in the absence of immediate reciprocation. The long-term goal is to develop a positive relationship, one in which there is substantial relationship credit. Some people find a contract such as that in Figure 9.1 useful for structuring their attempts to be more positive. Note that the wording at the top of the contract emphasizes the relationship goal. Such wording promotes attributions about each partner's efforts along the line of the following: "These positive acts are being done to express caring and to improve the relationship."

TABLE 9.1. Classes of Behavior Most Strongly Related to Relationship Satisfaction

Class of behavior	Examples
Affection	Saying "I love you" Giving a hug or kiss Enjoying a shared laugh or joke Saying he or she enjoys partner's company
Respect	Listening to the partner's opinion Telling partner of admiration/respect Saying/showing confidence in partner's abilities Introducing partner to others with pride
Support and assistance	Doing errands for partner Making self available to do work for partner Asking partner about their day Doing something to save partner time/energy
Shared quality time	Spending an hour or more just talking Work together on a project Take a drive or walk Go out together, just the two of you Discuss personal feelings

Attempts to build positive, intimate relationship behaviors revolve around the appraisal of current behavior, goal setting of appropriate positive behaviors to increase, and implementing and evaluating changes. In conducting this process it is important to challenge partners to be more creative in their relationship and to put effort into making the relationship more fun, more supportive, and more interesting for their partner. In enhancing partners' creativity in setting goals, it is useful to review how the partners generate self-change goals. One option is to sit and think alone. Another is to ask one's partner. A third is to reflect on couples perceived as being happy in their relationship and to attempt to identify behaviors that are intimacy enhancing. Another option is to ask friends or relatives what they do which is romantic or intimacy enhancing in their relationship. Reading books, watching other people, and getting tips from the therapist all are possibilities. Different clients will respond to different suggestions.

One homework task that often is useful for enhancing partners' creativity in relationship positivity is to ask them to generate new ideas for positivity. The handout presented in Figure 9.2 offers suggestions of possible caring behaviors. This can be a useful start in developing self-change goals for enhancing positivity, but it is also important to have people use resources available outside therapy to enhance relationship creativity, such as asking friends or reading. These resources will be available to the partner

Support for the partner's leisure pursuits also can be important. I routinely ask each partner to identify activities which the other partner enjoys (but may not currently engage in), and how he or she could support the partner in this interest. Often it is useful for the individual to learn a little about the interest, so he or she can discuss this with the partner. This does not mean that football-phobic women must learn the details of all games played this century by their husband's favorite team, or that men who have never heard of the gentle arts should suddenly be engrossed in their wife's passion for needlework. In fact, some level of independent interests probably is desirable in any relationship. However, the couple can provide support for those separate interests.

Promoting Better Communication

Good communication builds a deep sense of intimacy, whereas bad communication erodes commitment and positivity in relationships. When there is poor communication partners begin to escape or avoid painful communication. Escape and avoidance can take various guises, including physical withdrawal from interaction, extreme verbal aggression or physical aggression that terminates the interaction, avoiding each other, using distractions such as television, or avoiding discussion of certain topics.

Self-Regulation of Good Communication

Effective communication differs as a function of numerous variables, including culture, setting, and the individual characteristics of the partners and the couple. Yet many approaches to couple therapy seem based on the assumption that there are specific communication skills that are generally adaptive in promoting better couple communication. For example, traditional BCT taught couples a series of specific communication skills that were assumed to reflect effective communication, and the use of these responses was assumed to improve the relationship. Bornstein and Bornstein (1986), Jacobson and Margolin (1979), and Baucom and Epstein (1990) describe various sets of communication skills, and recommend that couples be taught the skills described.

In research on couple communication, most studies *do* find consistent differences between distressed and happy couples at the level of broad classes of communication behavior. Specifically, almost all studies find that distressed couples use more negative speaking and listening and less positive speaking and listening than do happy couples (Weiss & Heyman, 1997). However, the findings about the differences between distressed and happy couples at the level of specific communication behaviors are highly inconsistent (Weiss & Heyman, 1997). There is little evidence that the use of any specific communication behavior (e.g., self-disclosure, paraphrasing, or behavioral pinpointing) consistently is associated with relationship satisfaction or global quality of the relationship (Weiss & Halford, 1996; Weiss & Heyman, 1997).

In other words, what works as effective communication for one couple does not necessarily work for another. For example, like many other therapists, I have taught partners to paraphrase their partner's thoughts and feelings. This seems very helpful for some couples. But for other couples it never feels like a comfortable or genuine response no matter how much they try paraphrasing. In one case both partners were social workers and the woman became incensed with the man if paraphrasing occurred. She saw this as "becoming like a therapist to me," which she interpreted as the man detaching emotionally from her.

In essence, the behaviors that constitute good communication need to be defined within a specific relationship and context. A self-regulation approach is helpful as it focuses on helping partners to appraise how they currently are communicating, to identify specific changes each wishes to make in their communication, to implement those changes, and to evaluate the effects on communication. There is no simple formula, such as learning to paraphrase, that will universally improve relationship communication.

The need to define good communication for a given relationship does not mean that there are no general guidelines to help couples appraise their communication. Good couple communication combines effective speaking, listening, and taking turns to speak or listen. The therapist helps the partners to use these general classes of communication to select specific communication behaviors they wish to change. The specific behaviors they wish to change also vary according to the function of their communication.

Functions of Communication

Table 9.2 sets out some of the most common functions that communication serves for couples. I have ordered the communication functions from those tasks most couples find less difficult at the top of the table to those often found most difficult toward the bottom of the table. At the top is discussion, in which couples talk about how they spend their time apart, or other everyday topics of mutual interest. The exchange of everyday experiences and ideas gradually builds an understanding of each other's lives and world views. A related function of communication is expressing interest in the other person's interests. Most couples have individual as well as couple interests. Asking partners about their individual interests can enhance a sense of mutual closeness and respect. This does not mean that partners must suddenly be transformed to share the same passions. However, the man who truly understands his wife's love of sewing will be less likely to suggest throwing away old sewing patterns, and the woman who truly understands a

Name: _____   Date: _____

The aim of this form is for you to identify your strengths and weaknesses in communication and to specify goals for improvement. Rate each of the skills below using this code:

0—Very poor use of skill
1—Unsatisfactory use of skill
2—Satisfactory use of skill, but room for improvement
3—Good use of skill
N/A—Not applicable

Skill	0	1	2	3	N/A
Speaking					
Specific description of events					
Self-disclosure of feelings					
Clear expression of positives					
Assertive expression of negatives					
Suggestions					
Other (specify):					
Listening					
Attending to partner					
Accepting					
Asking open questions					
Summarizing					
Reserving judgment					
Other (specify):					

Strengths in communication: _____
_____

Weaknesses in communication:_____
_____

Self-change goal(s):_____
_____

Appraisal of self-change effort

Behavior changes I succeeded in doing:_____
_____

Behavior changes I did not do:_____
_____

Effect(s) of behavior change on interaction:_____
_____

FIGURE 9.4. Self-evaluation of communication skills checklist.

your communication. I am going to ask each of you to focus on what you did, not what your partner did, but what *you* did. I will ask you to identify at least one thing that you felt you did well, and to identify one thing that you could improve in terms of the communication. One thing is difficult with this exercise. If you get into the topic it can be hard to stop talking about that topic and to focus on *how* you are talking. So, when I ask you to stop talking about the topic, please do stop talking about it.

SANDRA: So we just talk about what we might like to do together?

THERAPIST: That's right, and at the end of 3 or 4 minutes I'll ask you to comment on how you spoke to Guy. Why don't you take it away? (*Pushes chair back and signals to the two partners to look at and talk to each other.*)

SANDRA: What would you like to do?

GUY: I don't mind. Go out to dinner, I guess. We haven't done that for a while.

SANDRA: Yeah, dinner would be OK. But I am trying to lose weight, and we always go to restaurants where there is such tempting stuff. Couldn't we do something that's not to do with eating?

GUY: OK. Well I thought of the first thing, what do you suggest?

SANDRA: Well, we have been talking about getting some new furniture for the kitchen. Maybe we could go looking for a kitchen table and chairs together, maybe Saturday morning.

GUY: It's supposed to be fun Sandra, you know that I hate those sorts of places.

SANDRA: I know, I know, but you seem not to be very keen on anything that I like doing. Shopping is fun for me.

GUY: Look, I suggest going eating, and you reckon it's too much, and then you want me to go shopping instead. (*His voice is sounding increasingly irritated.*)

THERAPIST: OK, I want to stop you there. What I would like to do . . . is consider what has just happened between the two of you. It seemed to me that toward the end you two were getting a bit irritated with each other. But, early on, it started quite well. I'd like to turn to each of you and ask you to appraise how you thought you individually were doing. Guy, have a look at the checklist that I gave you for ideas, and can you tell me one thing that you thought you did that was helpful communication.

GUY: Well, I did make suggestions to Sandra about what we could do. I suggested dinner at the beginning. When she wasn't keen on that, then I put a question to her, which was what did she want to do.

THERAPIST: Excellent, so you asked her for her point of view and you also made specific suggestions yourself. I'd agree, those were two very helpful things that you did. Was there anything that you did that you thought was unhelpful?

GUY: Well, I was not very keen about going shopping for kitchen furniture.

THERAPIST: OK, so you responded negatively to a suggestion from Sandra. However, we were trying to find things that both of you would like to do. It sounds like that is something that you weren't really very keen on. Yet, when you said that to Sandra, it seemed like the conversation seemed to go downhill. I wonder if there was any other way that you might have expressed yourself, that might have made it easier for the conversation to stay on track.

GUY: Well, I guess I did get kind of irritated at that point. I'd suggested something, Sandra wasn't happy, and then I felt she suggested something that she should have known I wouldn't like. It would have been better if I had just said that there are probably other things I'd rather do.

In this transcript you can see that Guy is being prompted to attend to process, to reflect on the communication behaviors he used in the interaction. It is also important to notice that the therapist intervened quickly when the communication process started to go wrong. It is crucial that therapists are assertive so that there are not prolonged negative interchanges. We are attempting to help people to recognize when things first start to go wrong in their communication and then to correct it. This process would then be extended by asking Sandra also to self-appraise.

SELF-SELECTION OF GOALS

At the end of the foregoing interaction with Guy and Sandra, we would then move to goal setting. I omit the interaction I had with Sandra and just focus on the discussion with Guy.

THERAPIST: So, Guy, if you were to have this conversation again, what would you like to do differently?

GUY: Well, I would like to keep making suggestions, and I think it was a good idea to ask the question of Sandra. I want to avoid immediately disagreeing with Sandra or putting her ideas down. It might be better if I suggest that we generate a whole list of possibilities, and then we can try and pick something that both of us would like.

THERAPIST: Excellent. So you want to keep doing the positive things such as making suggestions and asking questions, but you also want to hold back from immediately disagreeing with suggestions from Sandra. That is a terrific idea.

Sometimes clients have more difficulty in self-identifying goals for change. For example, when I asked Sandra to appraise her behavior during the foregoing interaction, Sandra mentioned that she had made useful suggestions and asked questions. However, she was struggling to think of what she might do further to enhance communication. The therapist tried to help her out in the following manner.

THERAPIST: Sandra, you are saying that it got stuck, but you are not quite sure what you could do to make it any different. I noticed that when Guy said that he didn't particularly want to go shopping, you came back with a comment about him not wanting to do things that you like. I wonder if there is a different way that you could have responded there?

SANDRA: But it is true, he doesn't like going shopping with me, and I really want to do some of those things.

THERAPIST: I am not disagreeing with you. I hear that getting some new kitchen furniture is something that you would like to do, and you would like Guy to be involved. However, remember that the point of the exercise here was to try and find something that both of you would like to do in the next couple of weeks. It was meant to be something that both of you thought would be fun. So, how might you be able to identify something that both of you would enjoy?

SANDRA: Well, I guess I could ask him. I asked him once and he came up with something that I didn't particularly like, but maybe I need a longer list from him. Yeah, I could ask some more, couldn't I?

THERAPIST: Yeah you could. And if you have some fun together, and things start to work out better, then it may be that Guy gets more responsive to your needs . . .

IMPLEMENTATION AND EVALUATION

The couple continue with their conversation, trying to implement the changes. Once they had finished the next part of the interaction, the therapist asked them if they had successfully implemented their self-selected change goals. For example, Sandra was asked whether or not she had posed additional questions to Guy about what he might like to do. Then they were asked to appraise the impact of that behavioral change on their interactions. In other words,

"What happened when you asked Guy those questions?" Throughout this process, the therapist is prompting and shaping the couple's attention to self-directed change. Particular focus needs to be placed on reviewing successes, as it provides reinforcement for change efforts.

This self-regulation approach is compatible with traditional behavioral skills training. If someone is struggling to think of an appropriate change, a mixture of instruction, modeling, and feedback can be used to shape up appropriate skills. If someone says to me "I really am stuck, I don't know what to do," I would show them possible responses. For example, I might say: "Well, let me talk to your partner about this and I'll show you a couple of possible ways to respond. I want you to comment on which you prefer." Once I have modeled some alternative responses, I ask the client to select a response and to say that to his or her partner.

NONVERBAL EXPRESSION

Nonverbal encoding and decoding of feelings are some of the more difficult aspects of communication to change. In a number of controlled trials of couple communication training, nonverbal behavior did not change much whereas the verbal aspects of communication changed a lot (e.g., Halford, Sanders, & Behrens, 2001; Markman, Renick, Floyd, Stanley, & Clements, 1993). Nonverbal behavior seems to be under less immediate voluntary control than verbal behavior. When asked to deliberately portray their communication in a positive manner, distressed couples can "fake good" verbal behavior but not nonverbal behavior (Vincent, Friedman, Nugent, & Messerly, 1979).

Nonverbal behavior makes a huge difference in the impact of messages between partners (Noller, 1981). Thus shifting distressed couples' nonverbal communication potentially is important. However, I am not persuaded that skills training is necessarily the best means by which to change nonverbal behavior. I have found often that nonverbal behavior reflects the affect of the partners, and the affect itself usually needs to be changed. Suppose a partner uses few active listening nonverbal behaviors while their partner is talking (e.g., they look away, and show slight grimacing and other signs of impatience while the spouse talks). One approach to this problem would be to model and rehearse the desired nonverbal behaviors (lean forward, nod, smile, etc.). Another option is to attempt to induce an emotional and cognitive state in the person that is focused on listening.

Usually a listening cognitive set can be induced by posing questions to the listener, questions that prompt listening behavior. For example, Denise was expressing anger that her husband Angelo did not help out when friends or relatives came over for a meal. Angelo would roll his eyes, and look away as Denise spoke, which prompted her to get even angrier. I intervened with Angelo in the following manner.

THERAPIST: Angelo, I notice that you rolled your eyes and looked away as Denise started to talk about her anger toward you. What were you feeling as she spoke?

ANGELO: I was thinking, here we go again. Denise wishes she married a chef. She always carries on about me not cooking, I cannot cook. My mother was a good Italian woman, she didn't let her son into the kitchen.

THERAPIST: So you think Denise just wants you to cook. Is that your understanding?

ANGELO: Of course, that is what she is always on about. Angelo do something in the kitchen, Angelo you're a lazy so and so . . .

THERAPIST: Angelo, you may be right. Let's check this with Denise. Denise, is Angelo right? Is it just that you want him to cook? Is there nothing else about this situation that angers you?

Denise: No, it's not the cooking. I know he can't cook. But . . .

THERAPIST: (*Holds hand up toward Denise*) Denise, stop there for just a moment. Angelo, Denise is saying there is more to this than you think. Are you interested in her point of view? Do you really want to know what it is that upsets her?

ANGELO: Yeah. I guess.

THERAPIST: I think if you two are to sort out your problems each of you has to really want to understand the other. Angelo, do you really want to know what is bugging Denise here?'

ANGELO: Yeah, yeah I do.

THERAPIST: Will you really try to listen here? Focus on her, let her talk, really try to understand what she is saying. You don't have to agree with what she's saying, just understand it.

ANGELO: Sure, I'll give it another try.

It is important to note that Angelo begins the interaction by defending his position. He assumes he understands Denise and replays the same justifications he has used in the past. I drew to his attention that Denise has more to say, other things he may not understand. I then got him to talk to her. Another option would be for the therapist to draw Denise out, to get the rest of her message from her, then to ask Angelo to describe what the therapist did to get the extra information. In essence, I am advocating attempting to develop a mind-set of wanting to listen to the partner and assuming that the nonverbal expression of affect will reflect this set of listening. Simply teaching people to lean forward or to maintain eye contact is, in my experience, less effective than trying to get the partners to value listening to each other.

Some Useful Structured Exercises

Some couples require a large degree of structure in order to develop communication skills. For those couples I provide highly structured tasks in therapy sessions to facilitate learning. Next I describe some exercises that are useful with couples.

THE FLOOR EXERCISE

The floor exercise was originally described by Gottman, Notarius, Gonso, and Markman (1976). It is intended to facilitate effective turn taking in couples. For couples in which partners tend to interrupt and over talk each other, the floor exercise can be particularly useful. The basic idea of the floor exercise is that speaker and listener roles are clearly separated. One partner is defined as the listener and is asked to engage only in listener behaviors. The listener is not permitted to use any of the specific speaking behaviors, such as offering an opinion. To ensure that the listener is actively processing the information the speaker is conveying, I often suggest that the listener summarize what the speaker said.

When couples are finding it really difficult to take turns, I use a physical cue to turn taking. I have a small piece of carpet in my office, which I describe to them as the floor. I hand the floor to the speaker. While the speaker holds the piece of carpet, he or she literally has the floor. The individual continues in the speaker role until such a time as he or she feels understood and then hands the floor across to the listener. I do not expect couples regularly to pull out a piece of floor covering when they are talking to each other at home. However, the symbolic importance of the floor often cues people to better turn taking. It can be useful to get people to take the piece of floor home and to use it in a homework task to promote generalization. Ultimately, we fade out this contrived structure but prompt the couple to sustain balanced turn taking.

PINPOINTING

Some people have great difficulty in precision of explanation. They may describe their thoughts, feelings, and desires in wordy and abstract terms. For such people, learning to be more specific in their descriptions can be useful. For example, in the following transcript I am working with a man who found it difficult to give specific positive feedback. To enhance his ability to give positive feedback, we had been discussing what first attracted him to his wife. Given that his initial answer was vague, I helped him be more specific.

JOHN: Well, the first thing I remember noticing about Caroline was how bubbly she was. Very effervescent.

THERAPIST: Bubbly and effervescent. They sound very positive. What do you remember noticing that made you feel that she was bubbly?

JOHN: Oh I don't know, she was just sort of positive, you know, smiley.

THERAPIST: You noticed her smile. Any other things you noticed?

JOHN: Well, Caroline did smile a lot, and she laughed, and was often looking at people and touching them, and she had a lively way of telling stories that I really liked. She had a great sense of humor.

THERAPIST: OK, so she smiled a lot, she talked enthusiastically, she looked at people, she told stories, she had a great sense of humor. When you noticed all of those things about her, how did that make you feel?

JOHN: Attracted (*laughs*).

ENHANCING EMOTIONAL EXPRESSIVENESS

Some partners find it difficult to express their emotions clearly. Sometimes this unexpressiveness reflects an inability to monitor or label internal emotional states. For example, I regularly have clients who report they are not aware of any strong emotion even when the circumstances suggest strong emotional arousal. For example, recently a woman told her husband in the therapy session that she seriously doubted that their relationship could work, largely because he seemed so emotionally unresponsive to her. I asked the husband how he felt when she made that statement, and he said, "Not sure, a bit concerned, I guess." Despite several other attempts to solicit any other feelings (despair, hopelessness, relief, sadness), mild concern was all the man could report. Yet, this man seemed genuinely committed to making his relationship work.

Sometimes the presence of emotional arousal will seem evident to the therapist, but the person does not report experiencing any emotion. For example, I often have seen couple conflict in which one partner's nonverbal behavior becomes progressively more tense and voice volume increases, and yet if I ask "Are you angry?," the partner says "No." Often these partners report occasionally being overwhelmed by rage, which they assert occurs without warning. I believe such people find it hard to recognize or label their emotional states, and only when the emotion becomes extreme do they notice how they are responding.

Increasing attention to internal emotional states can be achieved in a variety of ways. I find that working with emotion which is aroused in the therapy session is the most helpful. If a partner is struggling to identify emotion, I often use experiential techniques to increase attention to internal cues. For example, I might ask the partners to pause during a discussion and ask each of them internally to scan how they are feeling. The therapist can ask the partners to "freeze" in their current positions and to report on how they are sitting and how various parts of their body feel. During interactions I monitor the behaviors of the partners. If someone is tensing his hand, or jiggling her leg, or raising his voice, I might draw his or her attention to the relevant behavior. Sometimes it is useful to ask the person to repeat and even exaggerate the verbal and nonverbal behaviors in which he or she is engaging and then report on what he or she feels. In all the various procedures to increase attention to internal states, the point is to increase the person's monitoring and awareness of his or her internal state. The intent is not to interpret, justify, or analyze the behavior. Consequently I do not ask why people are doing something. Rather, I focus on "Are you aware that you are doing X?"

A useful element of emotional expressiveness training is teaching people to label emotions with precision. Guerney (1977) provides couples with tables of feeling words. When asking people about feelings, he invites them to select words that best capture their feelings. In my experience some people seem to have limited emotional vocabularies; they describe emotions in terms of positive or negative. However, rather than provide a formal handout on feeling words, I ask the person to generate words that convey a similar emotional state but vary in intensity. For example, if someone is feeling positive about how his relationship with his partner felt in the last week, I might ask him if he feels ecstatic. If he says no, I ask for a range of less extreme words and ask him to identify which label best captures his emotional state.

As described in Chapters 1 and 2, a primary function of emotion is to direct behavior. When someone is fearful of his or her partner, the individual often selectively attends to threat cues and is primed to respond in self-defense by attack or escape. I conceptualize awareness of one's emotional state as a self-regulation skill. If one is fearful and aware of being afraid, then active coping attempts to manage the source of threat can be made. If the person is unaware of his or her emotional state, the person is unable to monitor or change ineffective adaptations.

EMOTIONAL EXPLORATION

Perhaps the most sophisticated skill, and a form of communication which in my experience produces huge increases in emotional intimacy, is the notion of emotional exploration. These are discussions between the partners where they try hard to understand issues which are really important to the other person. At the beginning of this book, I began with a quote from John Butler Yeates: "I think a man and a woman should choose each other for life, for the simple reason that a long life with all its accidents is barely enough for a man and a woman to understand each other, and in this case to understand is to love. "I can offer no empirical evidence to support what I see as the implicit truth in this quote. For me, committed relationships become increasingly intimate as the couples get to know more and more about each other.

Table 9.3 provides a list of potential topics about which couples might talk together. Some of these topics relate more to general beliefs and values outside the relationship, and others are focused more on the partners as individuals, or on their interaction within the relationship. All involve a degree of self-disclosure and emotional expression. I often invite couples to review this list and to talk to each other about one or more of the topics. I cannot provide any data that these processes improve communication or enhance intimacy, but it has been my repeated clinical experience that if couples engage effectively in talking with each other, and discover more about each other, their intimacy develops in a very important way.

LEVELING AND EDITING

My emphasis on self-disclosure and mutual emotional expression does not mean that I believe that unlimited openness is necessarily healthy in relationships. Some people work on the assumption that total openness is highly desirable in relationships. I value honesty, and I value self-disclosure. However, that does not mean that relationships are healthier if partners always say the

---

TABLE 9.3. Topics for Couple Emotional Exploration

What would you like to achieve in your job in the next 10 years?

What do you most wish for our children?

Are there things about yourself you want to change?

What is it about your body that you like?

Tell me about a dream or wish you have not yet fulfilled.

If you won the lottery, would you want to stop work? Why?

How would you most like to be remembered after you're gone?

Whom do you most admire, and why?

Is there a cause about which you feel passionate? What is it?

What experiences do you think had the most impact on you growing up?

What is your greatest asset?

What does "leading a good life" mean to you?

How could I support you better in what you want to do?

---

first thing that pops into their mind. Some partners are extremely rude in talking to their spouses and express themselves in ways that they would never do to a stranger. Notarius and Markman (1993) refer to the need to edit out aggressive, rude, and destructive communication to the spouse. If partners are being rude to their spouse, often I suggest that it is helpful to edit some of the things that they say.

Editing can mean reformulating an answer so that the emotional impact is supportive of the partner. For example, I was working with a couple in which the woman had undergone a bilateral mastectomy for breast cancer. She felt self-conscious about her physical appearance and asked her partner whether he still found her sexually attractive. The husband responded by saying that he had loved her for 25 years, he expected to love her for another 25 years, and that expressing his love sexually toward her was something that was really important to him. At that point they hugged each other.

Previously the man told me that initially he had been shocked and somewhat repulsed by the extent of his wife's scarring after the operation. Subsequently the couple talked further about the impact of the woman's operation on the two of them. The man told her that he had struggled to accept the scarring but that he was adjusting now. I am not convinced that a blunt statement initially saying "Well, to be honest, the scar has been fairly off-putting to me" would have been good communication. The husband responded to the more subtle nuance of his wife's question, reassuring her that she was still a loved and valued partner.

Some people are so avoidant of disclosing their feelings that they may need to engage in what Notarius and Markman (1993) call leveling. Leveling means increasing the level of self-disclosure so the spouse really does know what the other person feels. Some partners who are highly avoidant of self-disclosure are that way because self-disclosure makes people somewhat vulnerable. The fear of making oneself vulnerable and being rejected often dominates distressed relationships, and neither partner takes the risk of leveling. The therapist then needs to structure therapy to create a sufficient sense of safety that partners will begin to level with each other. This can be done by asking partners to self-disclose about less threatening topics initially (e.g., an opinion of a current affairs topic) and building up to more personally revealing topics (e.g., how one partner feels after rejection of his or her sexual advances to the spouse). The notions of leveling and editing and the need to get the balance between editing and leveling right make sense to most couples. This often assists couples to self-select communication goals in terms of increasing leveling or editing.

Conflict Management

Most distressed couples experience destructive conflict. To this point in the book I have described a number of levels of intervention to help couples manage conflict effectively. First, the processes of assessment, feedback, and negotiation are intended to help partners reformulate problem areas that are sources of conflict into shared relationship goals. For many couples this is sufficient to allow them to implement self-change to resolve conflict. Other couples will manage conflict better after relationship psychoeducation. The psychoeducation provides information that can allow better formulation of relationship goals, or cognitive-affect restructuring can help couples manage negative thoughts and feelings that are associated with destructive conflict. Enhancement of couple communication also assists many couples to manage conflict. This works in two ways. First, the better communication can allow couples to better understand each other's perspectives when talking about conflict issues, and this can help couples resolve conflict. Second, frequent good communication about other topics reduces the likelihood of destructive conflict about conflict topics (Gottman, 1994). However, some couples have difficulty with conflict management even if they communicate well. There are three other conflict management skills that are useful to consider teaching couples with ongoing destructive conflict: conflict management rules, problem solving, and managing negativity before and after conflict.

Developing Conflict Management Rules

As Notarius and Markman (1993) described, couples usually develop implicit rules about how to manage conflict within their relationship. Rules might include when or how difficult issues should be raised with the partner. For example, my partner and I do not raise things with each other on weekday mornings, particularly close to the time either of us is due to leave for work. The sense of pressure from needing to get to work seems to be incompatible with really listening to each other about anything important. Rules might include what is considered "fair fighting," what sort of form criticism can take, or how one can reasonably express oneself.

Couples rarely explicate the rules of conflict within their relationship, and often it can be useful to get the partners to discuss their relationship conflict rules. They can then appraise the helpfulness of existing rules and implement changes in the rules. For example, some couples implicitly adopt the rule that either partner should be able to raise any issue that concerns him or her at any time with the partner. While having such open access to raise issues might appeal in some ways, it does not always lead to productive discussion. It may be preferable for individuals to signal that they wish to talk about something important and to select a quiet time and place for such a discussion.

In Table 9.8 I describe some of the common rules couples apply to their conflicts. It is useful to have couples read through this set of potential conflict rules and discuss which rules they want to adopt. These self-selected rules can then be applied in order to establish if they are effective in managing conflict.

Managing Negativity Before and After Conflict

Many distressed couples think of conflict only in terms of a heated argument, when the strength of emotion is most obvious. However, as Christensen and Pasch (1993) highlighted, distressed couples often exhibit negativity in anticipation of, and after, conflict. Negativity at these times often can exacerbate destructive conflict. Many couple disagreements are at least somewhat predictable. For example, if finances have been a source of conflict and there are times when large bills are due, the couple may anticipate arguing about money. Particular times and places also can become associated with conflict. For example, in families with young children late afternoon and early evening often are associated with the need to do a variety of household and child-care tasks, and many couples find they have disagreements at those times (Halford et al., 1992). Many distressed couples anticipate destructive arguments and avoid the times, places, and topics they associate with conflict. For example, the couple may avoid discussing certain difficult topics, (e.g., money), or the partners avoid high-risk times and places for arguments (e.g., arriving home late from work). Some couples have such widespread avoidance of conflict that they rarely, if ever, argue. Apart from the sense of distance this often engenders in the relationship, conflict avoidance fails when the couple need to make a conjoint decision.

Some distressed couples anticipate negative conflict but still engage in discussion. However, if one or both partners anticipate that the ensuing interaction will be negative, it may arouse particular emotions within them that make that prediction self-fulfilling. Relative to satisfied couples, distressed couples showed much higher levels of physiological arousal while awaiting a discussion of a conflict topic (Gottman, 1994). This finding has been interpreted as the distressed partners anticipating negative conflict. To the extent that couples have negative emotional arousal and anticipate conflict as threatening, this will predispose them to see their partner in a negative light and to respond by either escalating or attempting to escape from the conflict.

Once a conflict is over it is likely that both partners will show some continuing affect arousal. This often prompts them to reflect on the interaction that has occurred. In my experience distressed couples often replay in their minds the injustices and hurts that they feel have been perpetuated on them. These cognitive rehearsals of negativity frequently serve to maintain the anger and distress associated with the conflict. I have clients report to me that they can walk around for days after an argument feeling upset, hurt, and angry.

Many distressed couples report that reengagement after severe conflict is difficult. For example, some couples report that the argument flares up again when the partners see each other. Often one partner will restate some aspect of the original argument, which then restarts the argument. Other couples report that they are distant and withdrawn from each other for days after an argument. In contrast, happy couples often make specific, positive efforts to over-

Managing Negativity Before and After Conflict

Many distressed couples think of conflict only in terms of a heated argument, when the strength of emotion is most obvious. However, as Christensen and Pasch (1993) highlighted, distressed couples often exhibit negativity in anticipation of, and after, conflict. Negativity at these times often can exacerbate destructive conflict. Many couple disagreements are at least somewhat predictable. For example, if finances have been a source of conflict and there are times when large bills are due, the couple may anticipate arguing about money. Particular times and places also can become associated with conflict. For example, in families with young children late afternoon and early evening often are associated with the need to do a variety of household and child-care tasks, and many couples find they have disagreements at those times (Halford et al., 1992). Many distressed couples anticipate destructive arguments and avoid the times, places, and topics they associate with conflict. For example, the couple may avoid discussing certain difficult topics, (e.g., money), or the partners avoid high-risk times and places for arguments (e.g., arriving home late from work). Some couples have such widespread avoidance of conflict that they rarely, if ever, argue. Apart from the sense of distance this often engenders in the relationship, conflict avoidance fails when the couple need to make a conjoint decision.

Some distressed couples anticipate negative conflict but still engage in discussion. However, if one or both partners anticipate that the ensuing interaction will be negative, it may arouse particular emotions within them that make that prediction self-fulfilling. Relative to satisfied couples, distressed couples showed much higher levels of physiological arousal while awaiting a discussion of a conflict topic (Gottman, 1994). This finding has been interpreted as the distressed partners anticipating negative conflict. To the extent that couples have negative emotional arousal and anticipate conflict as threatening, this will predispose them to see their partner in a negative light and to respond by either escalating or attempting to escape from the conflict.

Once a conflict is over it is likely that both partners will show some continuing affect arousal. This often prompts them to reflect on the interaction that has occurred. In my experience distressed couples often replay in their minds the injustices and hurts that they feel have been perpetuated on them. These cognitive rehearsals of negativity frequently serve to maintain the anger and distress associated with the conflict. I have clients report to me that they can walk around for days after an argument feeling upset, hurt, and angry.

Many distressed couples report that reengagement after severe conflict is difficult. For example, some couples report that the argument flares up again when the partners see each other. Often one partner will restate some aspect of the original argument, which then restarts the argument. Other couples report that they are distant and withdrawn from each other for days after an argument. In contrast, happy couples often make specific, positive efforts to over-

es of assessment, feedback,
formulate problem areas that
goals. For many couples this
lf-change to resolve conflict.
fter relationship psychoeduca-
on that can allow better formu-
ct restructuring can help cou-
ings that are associated with
le communication also assists
ks in two ways. First, the better
understand each other's perspec-
nd this can help couples resolve
cation about other topics reduces
t conflict topics (Gottman, 1994).
with conflict management even if
e other conflict management skills
ples with ongoing destructive con-
m solving, and managing negativity

t Rules

cribed, couples usually develop implicit
ithin their relationship. Rules might in-
ould be raised with the partner. For ex-
hings with each other on weekday morn-
ither of us is due to leave for work. The
et to work seems to be incompatible with
anything important. Rules might include
what sort of form criticism can take, or how
f.

rules of conflict within their relationship,
he partners to discuss their relationship con-
e the helpfulness of existing rules and imple-
ample, some couples implicitly adopt the rule
to raise any issue that concerns him or her at
having such open access to raise issues might
t always lead to productive discussion. It may
signal that they wish to talk about something
t time and place for such a discussion.
me of the common rules couples apply to their
couples read through this set of potential conflict
they want to adopt. These self-selected rules can
stablish if they are effective in managing conflict.

Our Physicians:

Regular Physicians:

- Bert Lopansri, M.D., Internal Medicine, Infectious Diseases
- Brad Lewis, M.D., General Surgery, Urgent Care
- Bryan Tuner, M.D., Holistic Medicine, Urgent Care
- Denise Provost, M.D., Family Medicine, Urgent Care
- Eileen Hyde, FNP, Urgent Care
- Elisabeth Kryway, PA, Urgent Care
- Elmer Sisneros, PA, Urgent Care
- Rachot Vacharothone, M.D., Internal Medicine, Urgent Care
- Renee Neff, FNP, Urgent Care
- Todd Wilcox, M.D., Orthopedic Surgery Training, Urgent Care

- Lacerations, sprains, and fractures
- X-ray & labs
- Any emergency or non-emergency situations

To get the most out of your visit, please let our physician know clearly the main concern as to why you are here today. Our goals are to stabilize the present situation, give appropriate treatment and/or referral, and deliver comfort measures.

first thing that pops into their mind. Some partners are extremely rude in talking to their spouses and express themselves in ways that they would never do to a stranger. Notarius and Markman (1993) refer to the need to edit out aggressive, rude, and destructive communication to the spouse. If partners are being rude to their spouse, often I suggest that it is helpful to edit some of the things that they say.

Editing can mean reformulating an answer so that the emotional impact is supportive of the partner. For example, I was working with a couple in which the woman had undergone a bilateral mastectomy for breast cancer. She felt self-conscious about her physical appearance and asked her partner whether he still found her sexually attractive. The husband responded by saying that he had loved her for 25 years, he expected to love her for another 25 years, and that expressing his love sexually toward her was something that was really important to him. At that point they hugged each other.

Previously the man told me that initially he had been shocked and somewhat repulsed by the extent of his wife's scarring after the operation. Subsequently the couple talked further about the impact of the woman's operation on the two of them. The man told her that he had struggled to accept the scarring but that he was adjusting now. I am not convinced that a blunt statement initially saying "Well, to be honest, the scar has been fairly off-putting to me" would have been good communication. The husband responded to the more subtle nuance of his wife's question, reassuring her that she was still a loved and valued partner.

Some people are so avoidant of disclosing their feelings that they may need to engage in what Notarius and Markman (1993) call leveling. Leveling means increasing the level of self-disclosure so the spouse really does know what the other person feels. Some partners who are highly avoidant of self-disclosure are that way because self-disclosure makes people somewhat vulnerable. The fear of making oneself vulnerable and being rejected often dominates distressed relationships, and neither partner takes the risk of leveling. The therapist then needs to structure therapy to create a sufficient sense of safety that partners will begin to level with each other. This can be done by asking partners to self-disclose about less threatening topics initially (e.g., an opinion of a current affairs topic) and building up to more personally revealing topics (e.g., how one partner feels after rejection of his or her sexual advances to the spouse). The notions of leveling and editing and the need to get the balance between editing and leveling right make sense to most couples. This often assists couples to self-select communication goals in terms of increasing leveling or editing.

Conflict Management

Most distressed couples experience destructive conflict. To this point in the book I have described a number of levels of intervention to help couples the beginning of this book, I began with a quote from John Butler Yeates: "I think a man and a woman should choose each other for life, for the simple reason that a long life with all its accidents is barely enough for a man and a woman to understand each other, and in this case to understand is to love. "I can offer no empirical evidence to support what I see as the implicit truth in this quote. For me, committed relationships become increasingly intimate as the couples get to know more and more about each other.

Table 9.3 provides a list of potential topics about which couples might talk together. Some of these topics relate more to general beliefs and values outside the relationship, and others are focused more on the partners as individuals, or on their interaction within the relationship. All involve a degree of self-disclosure and emotional expression. I often invite couples to review this list and to talk to each other about one or more of the topics. I cannot provide any data that these processes improve communication or enhance intimacy, but it has been my repeated clinical experience that if couples engage effectively in talking with each other, and discover more about each other, their intimacy develops in a very important way.

LEVELING AND EDITING

My emphasis on self-disclosure and mutual emotional expression does not mean that I believe that unlimited openness is necessarily healthy in relationships. Some people work on the assumption that total openness is highly desirable in relationships. I value honesty, and I value self-disclosure. However, that does not mean that relationships are healthier if partners always say the

TABLE 9.3. Topics for Couple Emotional Exploration

What would you like to achieve in your job in the next 10 years?

What do you most wish for our children?

Are there things about yourself you want to change?

What is it about your body that you like?

Tell me about a dream or wish you have not yet fulfilled.

If you won the lottery, would you want to stop work? Why?

How would you most like to be remembered after you're gone?

Whom do you most admire, and why?

Is there a cause about which you feel passionate? What is it?

What experiences do you think had the most impact on you growing up?

What is your greatest asset?

What does "leading a good life" mean to you?

How could I support you better in what you want to do?

Our Physicians:

- Lacerations, sprains, and fractures
- X-ray & labs
- Any emergency or non-emergency situations

Regular Physicians:

- Bert Lopansri, M.D., Internal Medicine, Infectious Diseases
- Brad Lewis, M.D., General Surgery, Urgent Care
- Bryan Tuner, M.D., Holistic Medicine, Urgent Care
- Denise Provost, M.D., Family Medicine, Urgent Care
- Eileen Hyde, FNP, Urgent Care
- Elisabeth Kryway, PA, Urgent Care
- Elmer Sisneros, PA, Urgent Care
- Rachot Vacharothone, M.D., Internal Medicine, Urgent Care
- Renee Neff, FNP, Urgent Care
- Todd Wilcox, M.D., Orthopedic Surgery Training, Urgent Care

To get the most out of your visit, please let our physician know clearly the main concern as to why you are here today. Our goals are to stabilize the present situation, give appropriate treatment and/or referral, and deliver comfort measures.

Welcome to
After Hours Medical, Urgent Care

Our Billing Process:

After Hours Medical is a walk-in emergency clinic where you have the luxury of being seen instantly without going through the usual process of waiting for an appointment or paying the fees from the higher Emergency Room co-pay. The clinic's fees are based upon the fees from the Physician Fee Schedule by the American Medical Association. **After submitting the charges to your insurance, we accept only what your insurance determines to be the appropriate amount, the allowed amount. The rest is a write-off by After Hours Medical and you should not be billed for it.** The charge for the "Emergency Visit" is always attached because the clinic is considered an emergency clinic. It is up to your insurance to accept it or deny it. You are not responsible for this charge if your insurance denies it. The billing and collection process is out-sourced to an independent billing company, All Medical Billing. For any billing issues, problems or questions, please let us know or call the billing department directly at 801-294-5921.

Our objectives:

- Little waiting
- Friendly and relaxing atmosphere
- Quality medical services

Our Services:

manage conflict effectively. First, the processes of assessment, feedback, and negotiation are intended to help partners reformulate problem areas that are sources of conflict into shared relationship goals. For many couples this is sufficient to allow them to implement self-change to resolve conflict. Other couples will manage conflict better after relationship psychoeducation. The psychoeducation provides information that can allow better formulation of relationship goals, or cognitive-affect restructuring can help couples manage negative thoughts and feelings that are associated with destructive conflict. Enhancement of couple communication also assists many couples to manage conflict. This works in two ways. First, the better communication can allow couples to better understand each other's perspectives when talking about conflict issues, and this can help couples resolve conflict. Second, frequent good communication about other topics reduces the likelihood of destructive conflict about conflict topics (Gottman, 1994). However, some couples have difficulty with conflict management even if they communicate well. There are three other conflict management skills that are useful to consider teaching couples with ongoing destructive conflict: conflict management rules, problem solving, and managing negativity before and after conflict.

Developing Conflict Management Rules

As Notarius and Markman (1993) described, couples usually develop implicit rules about how to manage conflict within their relationship. Rules might include when or how difficult issues should be raised with the partner. For example, my partner and I do not raise things with each other on weekday mornings, particularly close to the time either of us is due to leave for work. The sense of pressure from needing to get to work seems to be incompatible with really listening to each other about anything important. Rules might include what is considered "fair fighting," what sort of form criticism can take, or how one can reasonably express oneself.

Couples rarely explicate the rules of conflict within their relationship, and often it can be useful to get the partners to discuss their relationship conflict rules. They can then appraise the helpfulness of existing rules and implement changes in the rules. For example, some couples implicitly adopt the rule that either partner should be able to raise any issue that concerns him or her at any time with the partner. While having such open access to raise issues might appeal in some ways, it does not always lead to productive discussion. It may be preferable for individuals to signal that they wish to talk about something important and to select a quiet time and place for such a discussion.

In Table 9.8 I describe some of the common rules couples apply to their conflicts. It is useful to have couples read through this set of potential conflict rules and discuss which rules they want to adopt. These self-selected rules can then be applied in order to establish if they are effective in managing conflict.

The rules in Figure 9.5 generally are self-explanatory, except perhaps the last rule. Immediate relationship crises describes problems that need to be solved now; relationship rules or standards describe general principles of how the partners believe they should usually relate and share responsibilities. For example, if a child is sick and cannot go to school, one parent needs to be around to look after that child. The immediate issue is who will look after the child today. A related but broader topic is the relationship standard of how the partners generally should share parenting responsibilities. Unfortunately, some couples rarely discuss standards, and standards get raised when there is an immediate issue to resolve. For example, the couple with the sick child may argue just as each is due to leave for work about who should do what share of household and parenting responsibilities. The immediate issue becomes confused with the standard, and conflict results.

The purpose of this guide is to decide which rules may help you manage conflict. Place a tick beside those rules you wish to implement.

1. Either person can raise a topic for discussion at any time.
2. If the other person does not want to talk, he or she can say "no" but must suggest another time within the next day.
3. If either person feels the conversation is not working he or she can suggest either (a) a brief time out to calm down and collect thoughts or (b) to reschedule the discussion.
4. Regularly (at least once per month) we will do some relationship planning.
5. A partner who wishes to raise a topic that has been a source of conflict should pick a good time and place to raise the issue. Good times for discussion include
   Alone together
   No distractions
   With time
6. If we have a difficult topic to discuss we will try to eliminate distractions: for example, turn off the TV, radio, music; switch on the telephone answering machine or take the telephone off the hook; no reading or other activities while talking.
7. Do not offer solutions when we have disagreed, first talk till we understand each other.
8. If an argument occurs, use the speaker–listener strategy.
9. Do not raise conflict topics in front of other people.
10. No criticisms of each other in public.
11. Set aside time to discuss relationship rules; do not just respond to relationship crises.

FIGURE 9.5. Rules for managing relationship conflict.

Distressed couples often avoid discussing relationship standards as they have been a source of destructive conflict, and repeated destructive conflict prompts avoidance of discussion. When a pressing relationship issue is raised, the standard gets mixed up with the immediate issue. It is important to encourage couples to distinguish between immediate issues and negotiating relationship standards. If couples set aside time to discuss relationship standards, then trying to negotiate standards within the context of a relationship crisis becomes less likely.

Problem Solving

Problem-solving training has been a cornerstone of the management of conflict within BCT from the late 1970s (e.g., Jacobson & Margolin, 1979; Baucom & Epstein, 1990). Problem-solving training involves teaching couples a set of rational decision-making steps, which are intended to help the couple negotiate decisions. The major advantage of problem-solving training is that it provides a high degree of structure for couples, which helps couples to make complex or important decisions. The major disadvantages of problem solving are twofold. First, it attempts to impose a rational decision-making process on issues which often are highly emotionally charged. Second, implicitly it is presumed that reaching a decision about actions to be taken will resolve the relationship problem. However, as noted in Chapter 1, negative thoughts and feelings may be the essence of some relationship conflict, and negotiated behavioral change does not resolve all conflict.

Problem solving can be useful when two preconditions are met. First, the couple emotionally are ready to collaborate. If that precondition does not exist, further assessment and negotiation of goals or relationship psychoeducation is needed. Second, the conflict is about a complex decision that is likely to be resolved by negotiated behavioral change.

STRUCTURE OF PROBLEM SOLVING

Figure 9.6 sets out the basic steps of problem solving. Usually I give this handout to couples and have them work through an issue they are trying to resolve following these steps. The first step is to define the problem. The problem needs to be defined as specifically as possible. Once the couple has the problem defined in a mutually acceptable, constructive manner, the next challenge is to generate options available to the couple. Creativity is central to this phase of problem solving. Sometimes couples get stuck because they cannot generate any options that are acceptable to both partners. I encourage partners to brainstorm at this point. The basic rules of brainstorming are as follows: (1) Generate as many options as you can in a limited time; (2) do not censor your-

1. Define problem: _____

2. Generate options	3. Evaluate options	
	Advantages	Disadvantages
(a)		
(b)		
(c)		
(d)		
(e)		
(f)		
(g)		
(h)		
(i)		
(j)		
(k)		

4. Define solution: _____

FIGURE 9.6. Problem solving worksheet.

self or hold back, as ideas that initially seem crazy may lead to a good solution; (3) all options are recorded; and (4) there is no criticizing of suggestions at this point. This phase can often be fun, and it is interesting how saying ideas out loud often inspires extra ideas from the partner.

The generated options are each considered in terms of their advantages and disadvantages. There are several useful guidelines for this phase. First, both advantages and disadvantages of each option must be identified. Exploring options not only identifies the value of this option but also often generates ideas for evaluating other options. Also, each partner must have the chance to identify both advantages and disadvantages of each option. It is important that each partner's evaluation of each option be explicated. Second, options must be asked about in such a manner that existing assumptions are tested. If one partner strongly believes that action X should be taken, that partner should be asked first to identify the disadvantages of option X. If one partner strongly believes that X is a terrible solution, that partner must be asked to identify the advantages of X. In my experience, distressed couples often become polarized in their view of conflict issues; they adopt extreme views and refuse to accede any validity to the other person's perspective. Gently challenging partners' viewpoints can increase flexibility.

Once all the options are examined the action to be taken needs to be negotiated. There is more to this final phase than just selecting one of the options generated in the second phase. The therapist helps the couple to pull together the issues the couple has explored and to creatively try to maximize the benefits to all concerned with an action plan. The therapist needs to be active in prompting and shaping the active listening of each partner to the other. Integrating summaries are often useful to draw together the issues and come up with a short list of possible solutions. Sometimes the best solution is a combination of options that have been considered.

IMPLEMENTING SELF-REGULATION OF PROBLEM SOLVING

Once a couple are familiar with the general steps of problem solving, I have them adapt the model to their needs. One issue to discuss is when problem solving is likely to be useful. Couples generally do not report implementing formal problem solving after couple therapy (Jacobson, 1989). It is unrealistic to imagine couples routinely using this very structured process, but the structure of problem solving can be useful for complex decisions. Many couples benefit from problem solving when deciding about buying a house or car or whether to accept an interstate job.

If a couple have a history of difficulty making key decisions, then focusing on their problem-solving skills is particularly valuable. In such cases I ask the couple to do a series of problem-solving tasks. Consistent with the self-regulation approach, I ask each partner to self-evaluate his or her skills during problem solving and to self-select goals for change. In this process the partners evolve means of problem solving that work for them.

Given that problem solving is rational, it requires the partners to define the problem conjointly. If couples are arguing heatedly about an issue, problem solving probably is not appropriate. Rather, the couple should seek to understand each other's perspective before trying to identify solutions. I prompt couples to apply communication skills as described earlier in the chapter. If they are having difficulty listening effectively, I propose the speaker–listener structure. If the couple try this and still are not able to resolve the issue, cognitive-affect reconstruction may help them move beyond destructive conflict.

Managing Negativity Before and After Conflict

Many distressed couples think of conflict only in terms of a heated argument, when the strength of emotion is most obvious. However, as Christensen and Pasch (1993) highlighted, distressed couples often exhibit negativity in anticipation of, and after, conflict. Negativity at these times often can exacerbate destructive conflict. Many couple disagreements are at least somewhat predictable. For example, if finances have been a source of conflict and there are times when large bills are due, the couple may anticipate arguing about money. Particular times and places also can become associated with conflict. For example, in families with young children late afternoon and early evening often are associated with the need to do a variety of household and child-care tasks, and many couples find they have disagreements at those times (Halford et al., 1992). Many distressed couples anticipate destructive arguments and avoid the times, places, and topics they associate with conflict. For example, the couple may avoid discussing certain difficult topics, (e.g., money), or the partners avoid high-risk times and places for arguments (e.g., arriving home late from work). Some couples have such widespread avoidance of conflict that they rarely, if ever, argue. Apart from the sense of distance this often engenders in the relationship, conflict avoidance fails when the couple need to make a conjoint decision.

Some distressed couples anticipate negative conflict but still engage in discussion. However, if one or both partners anticipate that the ensuing interaction will be negative, it may arouse particular emotions within them that make that prediction self-fulfilling. Relative to satisfied couples, distressed couples showed much higher levels of physiological arousal while awaiting a discussion of a conflict topic (Gottman, 1994). This finding has been interpreted as the distressed partners anticipating negative conflict. To the extent that couples have negative emotional arousal and anticipate conflict as threatening, this will predispose them to see their partner in a negative light and to respond by either escalating or attempting to escape from the conflict.

Once a conflict is over it is likely that both partners will show some continuing affect arousal. This often prompts them to reflect on the interaction that has occurred. In my experience distressed couples often replay in their minds the injustices and hurts that they feel have been perpetuated on them. These cognitive rehearsals of negativity frequently serve to maintain the anger and distress associated with the conflict. I have clients report to me that they can walk around for days after an argument feeling upset, hurt, and angry. Many distressed couples report that reengagement after severe conflict is difficult. For example, some couples report that the argument flares up again when the partners see each other. Often one partner will restate some aspect of the original argument, which then restarts the argument. Other couples report that they are distant and withdrawn from each other for days after an argument. In contrast, happy couples often make specific, positive efforts to overcome the negativity associated with a destructive conflict. For example, one partner may apologize for the interaction or frame what has happened as a mutual problem to be overcome.

In summary, distressed couples seem to have difficulties with conflict management not only during interaction with their partner but also in anticipation of conflict and after conflict has occurred. The whole process of conflict management employed by the couple may need to be explored with the therapist. Sometimes identifying negativity before or after the conflict is sufficient to allow the person to engage in self-change of this unhelpful negativity. Other times the person may need additional assistance to overcome persistent negative thoughts and feelings. The next section addresses overcoming negative thoughts and feelings, and these strategies can be applied to the anticipation and recovery phases of conflict management.

Changing Negative Thoughts and Feelings

Couple therapy is, in large part, helping partners to feel differently about their relationships. In traditional BCT, changes in affect were believed to result from behavioral change. If the distressing behaviors of your partner decreased and the pleasing behaviors increased, then positive feelings and relationship satisfaction would result. In the cognitive-behavioral approach to couple therapy it was assumed that thoughts interacted with behavior to determine feelings. For example, changing attributions, standards, and expectations were all seen as means for enhancing positive emotions about the relationship.

I do not believe that affect is the final product of behavioral and cognitive processes but, rather, that emotion interacts with cognition and behavior. Research on couple interaction consistently points to affect as a powerful predictor of future thoughts and behaviors within the relationship (Gottman, 1994; Johnson & Greenberg, 1994). This is inconsistent with the view that affect is the end product of thoughts and feelings. The implication is that sometimes affect needs to be targeted as the primary focus of therapy.

In one sense all methods reviewed thus far are methods of affect change in that some affect change is expected as part of the interventions. For example, cognitive-affect reconstruction explicitly is targeted on drawing out the experience of "cooler" emotional vulnerabilities. Affect change also is an important part of many other procedures with less explicit focus on affect. For example, I emphasized in the chapters on assessment and goal setting that developing a shared model of the relationship with the couple is a crucial initial task in therapy. This shared model is intended to increase feelings of cooperation and to decrease anger and hostility. In this section I describe some key procedures to change negative thoughts and feelings: contingency management of affect, affect exposure, and rational self-analysis.

Contingency Management of Affect

Sometimes it is possible to rearrange the relationship environment to reduce inadvertent reinforcement that maintains negative affect. If partners are to apply contingency change procedures I believe two conditions must be met. First, the partners must agree that the negative emotion is the problem. Understandably, partners are unlikely to agree to reduce a negative emotion that they feel reflects a real problem in their relationship. However, some partners do report extreme negative emotions that seem disproportionate to the actual event but find it hard to regulate their affect. Second, the therapist must be able to identify a coherent model of how contingencies may maintain the negative feelings. Contingencies that maintain negative feelings tend to be either inadvertent reinforcement provided by the spouse or escape or avoidance by the person with the negative feelings.

To illustrate how partners inadvertently may reinforce negative affect, consider the following case example. Gayle and John had been married for 4 years and living together for 3 years prior to that. Each described the relationship as being very happy until approximately 6 months before presenting for couple therapy. At that time Gayle had met some old friends of John, who had described John's lifestyle as being sexually active prior to meeting Gayle. This came as a shock to Gayle. Gayle felt John had tricked her by presenting himself as a gentle, caring, and monogamous man. She said she was horrified to find her husband was a "womanizer." Gayle reported recurrent, intrusive feelings of jealousy and hurt; Gayle was jealous about the women John had had sex with before he met her and hurt in that she felt he had misled her.

Gayle believed that there were no behavioral changes she or he could make which would alter her new perception of her partner. It was possible to see the problem as exclusively cognitive, because there was no reported behavioral change by either partner to explain the development of the problem. The therapist did discuss with Gayle the evidence for the belief that John was a "womanizer and therefore always would be." Although Gayle acknowledged that people could change their behavior, she believed that these cognitive changes did not produce affect change. The strength of affect experienced by Gayle when reflecting on the possibility of John's having an affair was striking. I hypothesized that the affect was primary in the problem and that directly changing the affect might be crucial. I asked each partner to self-monitor interactions between them in which John's past sexual behavior was mentioned. At the next session both partners reported several interactions during the week. In each case Gayle had raised the topic and subsequently become upset. John then attempted to comfort and reassure Gayle that he loved her. The therapist developed the hypothesis that the recurrent feelings inadvertently were reinforced and maintained by the contingent attention of the husband. Gayle had mentioned that she felt a minor problem had developed in the relationship with John. She felt John was not being intimate enough with her; that he was being emotionally a little distant with her. Perhaps John's reassurance had particular value given that context.

In the session I posed the following question: "Given how often you have talked about this issue, do you think talking about it one more time will solve your problem?" Both partners reported that that would not help, and they reported that discussing things often made them feel worse. I suggested to John that he not discuss the issue and if Gayle raised the issue to say "We have agreed talking about this does not help" and to leave the room for 2 minutes. Moreover, I suggested that in order to reassure Gayle that this action did not reflect a lack of caring by John, John should try to be especially expressive of his feelings toward Gayle at other times. In a single case it can be difficult to determine what causes change. However, in the next session both partners reported that the first time Gayle raised the issue of jealousy it had been difficult not to talk about it, but after that John had declined to discuss it further. Gayle reported that by the end of the week she felt much less concern about the issue and had had a major reduction in the frequency of intrusive images and jealous feelings.

Extreme emotional responses also may be reduced by extinction by the partners themselves. For example, Kim and Eric had multiple problems including a long history of drug abuse by Kim, severe sexual abuse of Kim as a child, depression in Eric, and relationship problems. One major problem for Eric was that he was hypersensitive to criticism by Kim of his role as husband and father. In the course of relationship psychoeducation Eric described how his father had left the family when Eric was 7 years old. Eric related how his mother repeatedly told him as a young man that he must be a good husband and father and that he must never be like his dreadful father. Kim sometimes used a phrase, "You're just like all men," when she was angry. This phrase reflected her feeling that men had abused her much of her life. Eric felt he had stood by Kim through her drug problems and tried hard to be a good husband. Her criticisms often led him to feel very depressed.

Despite Kim's learning through communication enhancement to tone down her negativity when expressing dissatisfactions, and despite Eric's developing an understanding of where his sensitivity might have came from, he still became distressed when Kim criticized him. A number of sessions of rational challenging of his dire fear of failure as a partner did not shift his feelings substantially. We decided that learning to feel differently in response to criticism was important but cognitive procedures did not seem to be working. I videotaped Kim making criticisms of Eric and copied them so that a tape contained dozens of similar criticisms. Eric watched the tape multiple times, initially in the session and then at home between sessions. The structure in these viewing sessions was negotiated as follows: Eric would watch the tape alone. He had to watch the tape until his level of upset reduced. I also had him write a letter to his mother, who was now dead, describing his shortcomings as a husband but also describing his good qualities. He was asked to read and reread this letter, sometimes to me and sometimes privately to himself. His level of extreme response to criticism abated over the course of three sessions.

I conceptualized watching the videotape and reading the letter as an extinction process. The affect was expressed in a controlled manner so that no reinforcement for negative affect was available, either through inadvertent positive reinforcement from a partner or therapist or negative reinforcement through escape from the feelings. Often the extreme negative emotions in the relationship would lead Eric to escape, for example, to exit an argument with Kim. It was hard to rearrange the contingencies to alter that. It was impossible for Eric truly to communicate with his dead mother, but it seemed that the strong affect he felt in response to the belief that she would disapprove of him as a husband was difficult for him to change. Thus we used extinction.

Rational Self-Analysis

Some individuals need to increase their proficiency in identifying, challenging, and replacing the negative thoughts that affect their relationship. The form presented in Figure 9.7 is a useful structure for clients to conduct rational self-analysis. The example presented can be used to illustrate the process partners are asked to follow. The process of rational self-analysis is used when the client experiences a high level of upset about a relationship event. First, as soon as practicable after the upset, the person records his or her feelings at the top of the page. The second step is to write a brief description of the sequence of events leading up to that set of feelings. Most of the rest of the form is divided into two halves labeled "existing thoughts" and "new and challenging thoughts," respectively. In the "existing thoughts" column clients record all the thoughts they had during the event. In the "challenges" column the client does three steps. The thoughts already recorded are reviewed. Any thoughts that the client perceives as being accurate, rational, and appropriate about the situation are simply ticked. Thoughts seen as unhelpful are then identified and challenged. For example, unsupported or unrealistic assumptions about the meaning or likely consequences of the event, or catastrophizing about negative outcomes, are labeled as such. Then the client writes in a set of more rational and adaptive ways of thinking about the event. Finally, the client records the effects of the rational challenging on his or her feelings.

Reviewing clients' completed rational self-analysis forms can be used to provide feedback on their rational challenging skills. For example, a woman client returned a rational self-analysis form that focused on her upset and anger with her husband when he did not come to her house on the day she expected him. She and her partner had separated prior to the start of therapy and now were spending weekends together to attempt to improve their relationship

Name: _____ Date: _____

1. Describe your feelings that are a problem: I was angry, and hurt, crying

2. Describe the events that led up to you feeling this way: Jeff was late home for dinner on his birthday, I had prepared a special dinner and it was ruined.

3. My existing thoughts	4. New and challenging thoughts
Where the hell is he? The dinner will be ruined.	The dinner will be ruined, that is true.
He might have had an accident, he may be dead or injured somewhere.	It is possible, but not very likely. Getting worried about something unlikely is not helpful.
This special event is ruined, we never can seem to do anything right together.	The dinner has not worked out as I planned, but perhaps we can still rescue something. It is not true that we never do anything right together.
He was boozing with his work mates! He cares more about them than me. How can he be so selfish?	He was drinking with friends, but it is his birthday. It does not prove he cares more for them. It would have been better if he let me know if he was going to be late.
Why does everything I try to do to improve things with Jeff fail? There is no hope for us.	It is untrue that everything fails. It is true that tonight did not work as planned. The idea that our marriage is hopeless is just me overreacting to the disappointment. It probably is true that we will need to work harder to make the marriage right, and things still might not work out. All I can do is give this my best shot.

5. The effect on you of these new and challenging thoughts: I was still disappointed, but not as angry. It probably would have been better to tell Jeff about the dinner. I still want him to call me if he's late in the future, so I'll talk to him about that.

FIGURE 9.7. The rational self-analysis form: An example.

before taking the step of living together again. The rational self-analysis form was the basis of the discussion reported next.

JULIE: As I wrote on the form, it is clear that Tony does not care about me, or the children . . .

TONY: Julie, you know I care about us, I want it to work.

JULIE: If you cared you would have been there, obviously you don't care . . . What other conclusion can I draw?

TONY: I didn't even know you expected me on Friday night. I was bushed after work, and didn't fancy the drive on the bike.

THERAPIST: OK, so Tony you are saying it was not clear to you that you were expected on Friday night?

TONY: Well no, not really . . .

JULIE: You could have rung me, if you were really tired, let me know, at least thought of how I might be feeling . . .

THERAPIST: Julie, it seems clear that what upsets you was the thought that Tony did not see being with you as important. But he is saying it was a misunderstanding.

JULIE: I still think the weekend begins on Friday night, he should have let me know if he wasn't coming.

The foregoing interaction continued for some time. The final result was that Julie came to conclude that her thoughts had made the problem worse. She agreed that there was little evidence from this occasion that things would not work out. Another of Julie's beliefs also discussed, was the idea that if the marriage were not reconstituted it would be a disaster and a failure on her part. She came to believe that she would simply give the marriage a reasonable try and if things did not work out she would accept it and get on with her life. In the end she wrote on her form: "I will give this relationship my best shot. It is important to me, and I will do what I can. If it works, that is great, that is what I want. If it does not work out, then at least I know I tried. If we end, that does not mean either of us failed, just that maybe the relationship is not meant to be. That would be hard to get used to as an idea, but we have separated before and I survived. I will get by."

After Therapist-Guided Change

Therapist-guided change is intended to provide the partners with relationship skills that allow them to then engage in self-change. Once the couple has worked with the therapist to achieve the required skills, therapy moves to the self-change procedures described in Chapter 7. At this point couples are assisted to identify further changes they wish to make in their relationship and to use self-change procedures to achieve those changes. The couple also are assisted to generalize and maintain their gains using the procedures described in Chapter 7.

The couple depart from what we believe is their final session. Ideally at this point each partner has a broad understanding of the diverse influences on their relationship. This knowledge, combined with the capacity to self-regulate thoughts, feelings, and behaviors acquired across the process of therapy, empowers the partners to self-direct change in their relationship. When a couple leave therapy I do not know the long-term fate of their relationship. I know that therapy can only contribute a part of the variance that determines their relationship future. The couple may face severe future stresses that undermine their relationship or they may be blessed with better luck. The effort each extends to succor their relationship, and their collective ability to support each other also determine their individual and collective fates.

I have savored and been enriched by a loving partnership with my wife, Barbara, for more than 20 years. I have seen and felt the suffering of clients and friends when relationships come to painful ends. As I watch the figures of a couple receding from my office, I always hope that this couple will transcend the pain of relationship distress and experience the joy of truly loving, and being loved by, their spouse. If this book helps couple therapists to help more couples achieve loving relationships, then I have done what I set out to do.

References

Achenbach, T. M., & Edelbrock, C. S. (1983). *Manual for the Child Behavior Checklist and Revised Child Behavior Profile.* Burlington: Department of Psychiatry, University of Vermont.

Acitelli, L. K., & Antonucci, T. C. (1994). Gender differences in the link between marital support and satisfaction in older couples. *Journal of Personality and Social Psychology, 67,* 688–698.

American Psychological Association. (1993, October). *Final report of the task force on promotion and dissemination of psychological procedures.* New York: American Psychological Association, Division of Clinical Psychologists (Division 12).

Annon, J. S. (1975). *The behavioral treatment of sexual problems. Volume 1: Brief therapy.* Honolulu: Kapiolani Health Services.

Arnold, D. S., Wolff, L. S., O'Leary, S. G., & Acker, M. M. (1993). The Parenting Scale: A measure of dysfunctional parenting in discipline situations. *Psychological Assessment, 5,* 137–144.

Australian Institute of Family Studies. (1997, April 3). What we want in marriage. *The Courier Mail,* p. 4.

Bandura, A. (1977). *Social learning theory.* Englewood Cliffs, NJ: Prentice-Hall.

Bandura, A. (1986). *Social foundations of thought and action: A social cognitive theory.* Englewood Cliffs, NJ: Prentice-Hall.

Baris, M. A., & Garrity, C. B. (1997). Co-parenting post-divorce: Helping parents negotiate and maintain low-conflict separations. In W. K. Halford & H. J. Markman (Eds.), *Clinical handbook of marriage and couples intervention* (pp. 619–649). Chichester, UK: Wiley.

Barrowclough, C., & Tarrier, N. (1992). *Families of schizophrenic patients: Cognitive-behavioural interventions.* London: Chapman & Hall.

Baucom, D. H., & Aiken, P. A. (1984). Sex role identity, marital satisfaction and response to behavioral marital therapy. *Journal of Consulting and Clinical Psychology, 52,* 438–444.

Baucom, D. H., & Epstein, N. (1990). *Cognitive-behavioral marital therapy.* New York: Brunner/Mazel.

Baucom, D. H., Epstein, N., Daiuto, A. D., Carels, R. A., Rankin, L. A., & Burnett, C. K. (1996). Cognitions in marriage: The relationship between standards and attributions. *Journal of Family Psychology, 10,* 209–222.

Baucom, D. H., Epstein, N., Rankin, L. A., & Burnett, C. K. (1996). Assessing relationship standards: The Inventory of Specific Relationship Standards. *Journal of Family Psychology, 10,* 72–88.

Baucom, D. H., & Hoffman, J. A. (1986). The effectiveness of marital therapy: Current status and application to the clinical setting. In N. S. Jacobson & A. S. Gurman (Eds.), *Clinical handbook of marital therapy* (pp. 597–620). New York: Guilford Press.

Baucom, D. H., & Lester, G. W. (1986). The usefulness of cognitive restructuring as an adjunct to behavioral marital therapy. *Behavior Therapy, 17,* 385–403.

Baucom, D. H., Sayers, S. L., & Sher, T. G. (1990). Supplementing behavioral marital therapy with cognitive restructuring and emotional expressiveness training: An outcome investigation. *Journal of Consulting and Clinical Psychology, 58,* 636–645.

Baucom, D. H., Shoham, V., Mueser, K., Daiuto, A. D., & Stickle, T. R. (1998). Empirically supported couple and family interventions for marital distress and adult mental health problems. *Journal of Consulting and Clinical Psychology, 66,* 53–88.

Baumeister, R. F., & Bratlavsky, E. (1999). Passion, intimacy, and time: Passionate love as a function of change in intimacy. *Personality and Social Psychology Bulletin, 3,* 49–67.

Baumeister, R. F., & Leary, M. R. (1995). The need to belong: Desire for interpersonal attachments as a fundamental human motivation. *Psychological Bulletin, 117,* 497–529.

Baxter, L. A. (1986). Accomplishing relationship disengagement. In S. Duck & D. Perlman (Eds.), *Understanding personal relationships: An interdisciplinary approach* (pp. 243–265). London: Sage.

Beach, S. R. H., Arias, I., & O'Leary, K. D. (1986). The relationship of marital satisfaction and social support to depressive symptomatology. *Journal of Psychopathology and Behavioural Assessment, 8,* 305–316.

Beach, S. R. H., Sandeen, E. E., & O'Leary, K. D. (1990). *Depression in marriage.* New York: Guilford Press.

Bebbington, P. E. (1987a). Marital status and depression: A study of English national admission statistics. *Acta Psychiatrica Scandinavica, 76,* 640–650.

Bebbington, P. E. (1987b). The social epidemiology of clinical depression. In A. S. Henderson & G. Burrows (Eds.), *Handbook of studies on social psychiatry* (pp. 51–78). Melbourne, Australia: Blackwell.

Beck, A. T. (1976). *Cognitive therapy and the emotional disorders.* New York: International Universities Press.

Beck, J. S. (1995). *Cognitive therapy: Basics and beyond.* New York: Guilford Press.

Behrens, B. C., Sanders, M. R., & Halford, W. K. (1990). Generalization of communication skills training during behavioural marital therapy. *Behavior Therapy, 21,* 423–433.

Belsky, J., & Kelly, J. (1994). *Transition to parenthood.* New York: Delacorte Press.

Belsky, J., & Rovine, M., (1990). Patterns of marital change across the transition to parenthood. *Marital and Family Review, 52,* 5–19.

Birchler, G. B., & Weiss, R. L. (1977). *Inventory of Rewarding Activities.* Eugene: Oregon Marital Studies Program, University of Oregon.

Birchler, G. B., Weiss, R. L., & Vincent, J. P. (1975). Multimethod analysis of social reinforcement exchange between maritally distressed and non-distressed spouse and stranger dyads. *Journal of Personality and Social Psychology, 31,* 349–360.

Birchnall, J., & Kennard, J. (1983). Does marital maladjustment lead to mental illness? *Social Psychiatry, 18,* 79–88.

Black, L. E., & Sprenkle, D. H. (1991). Gender differences in college students' attitudes toward divorce and their willingness to marry. *Journal of Divorce and Remarriage, 14,* 47–60.

Block, J., Block, J. H., & Keyes, S. (1988). Longitudinally foretelling drug usage in adolescence: Early childhood personality and environmental precursors. *Child Development, 59,* 336–355.

Bloom, B. L. (1985). A factor analysis of self-report measures of family functioning. *Family Process, 24,* 225–239.

Bloom, B., Asher, S. J., & White, S. W. (1978). Marital disruption as a stressor: A review and analysis. *Psychological Bulletin, 85,* 867–894.

Booth, A., & Edwards, J. N. (1992). Starting over: Why remarriages are more unstable. *Journal of Family Issues, 13,* 179–194.

Bornstein, P. H., & Bornstein, M. T. (1986). *Marital therapy: A behavioral-communications approach.* New York: Pergamon.

Boughner, S. R., Hayes, S. F., Bubenzer, D. L., & West, J. D. (1994). Use of standardized assessment instruments by marital and family therapists: A survey. *Journal of Marital and Family Therapy, 20,* 69–75.

Bowlby, J. (1969). *Attachment and loss: Vol. 1. Attachment.* New York: Basic Books.

Bradbury, T. N. (1995). Assessing the four fundamental domains of marriage. *Family Relations, 44,* 459–468.

Bradbury, T. N. (Ed.). (1998). *The developmental course of marital dysfunction.* New York: Cambridge University Press.

Bradbury, T. N., & Fincham, F. D. (1987). Affect and cognition in close relationships: Towards an integrative model. *Cognition and Emotion, 1,* 59–87.

Bradbury, T. N., & Fincham, F. D. (1990). Attributions in marriage: Review and critique. *Psychological Bulletin, 107,* 3–33.

Bradbury, T. N., & Fincham, F. D. (1992). Attributions and behavior in marital interaction. *Journal of Personality and Social Psychology, 63,* 613–628.

Browne, A., & Williams, K. R. (1993). Gender, intimacy and lethal violence: Trends from 1976 through 1987. *Gender and Society, 7,* 78–98.

Burman, B., & Margolin, G. (1992). Analysis of the association between marital relationships and health problems: An interactional perspective. *Psychological Bulletin, 112,* 39–63.

Buss, D. M. (1994). *The evolution of desire: Strategies of human mating.* New York: Basic Books.

Cascardi, M., Langhinrichsen, J., & Vivian, D. (1992). Marital aggression, impact, injury and health correlates for husbands and wives. *Archives of Internal Medicine, 152,* 1178–1184.

Catania, A. C. (1975). The myth of self-reinforcement. *Behaviorism, 3,* 192–199.

Chambless, D. L., & Hollon, S. D. (1998). Defining empirically supported therapies. *Journal of Consulting and Clinical Psychology, 66,* 7–18.

Christensen, A. (1988). Dysfunctional interaction patterns in couples. In P. Noller & M. A. Fitzpatrick (Eds.), *Perspectives on marital interaction* (pp. 31–52). Clevedon, UK: Multilingual Matters.

Christensen, A., & Pasch, L. A. (1993). The sequence of marital conflict: An analysis of seven phases of marital conflict in distressed and nondistressed couples. *Clinical Psychology Review, 13,* 3–13.

Christensen, A., & Shenk, J. L. (1991). Communication, conflict and psychological distance in non-distressed, clinic and divorcing couples. *Journal of Consulting and Clinical Psychology, 59,* 458–463.

Clements, M., & Markman, H. J. (1996). The transition to parenthood: Is having children hazardous to marriage? In S. Duck (Ed.), *A lifetime of relationships* (pp. 290–310). Pacific Grove, CA: Brooks/Cole.

Cowen, C. P., & Cowen, P. A. (1992). *When partners become parents.* New York: Basic Books.

Coyne, J. C., Kahn, J., & Gotlib, I. H. (1987). Depression. In T. Jacob (Ed.), *Family interaction and psychopathology* (pp. 509–534). New York: Plenum Press.

Cutrona, C. E., & Suhr, J. A. (1992). Controllability of stressful events and satisfaction with spouse supportive behaviors. *Communication Research, 19,* 154–176.

Dadds, M. R., & Powell, M. B. (1991). The relationship of inter-parental conflict and global marital adjustment to aggression, anxiety and immaturity in aggressive and non-clinic children. *Journal of Abnormal Child Psychology, 19,* 553–567.

Davis, D. I., Berenson, D., Steinglass, P., & Davis, S. (1974). The adaptive consequences of drinking. *Psychiatry, 37,* 209–215.

De Guibert-Lantoine, C., & Monnier A. (1992, July–August). La conjoncture demographie: L'Europe et les pays développés d'Outre-Mer. *Population,* 27–38.

Derogatis, L. R. (1975). *Derogatis Sexual Functioning Inventory.* Baltimore: Clinical Psychometrics Research.

Derogatis, L. R., & Melisaratos, N. (1979). The DSFI: A multidimensional measure of sexual functioning. *Journal of Sex and Marital Therapy, 5,* 244–281.

Dickson, F. C. (1997). Aging and marriage: Understanding the long-term, later-life marriage. In W. K. Halford & H. J. Markman (Eds.), *Clinical handbook of marriage and couples intervention* (pp. 255–269). Chichester, UK: Wiley.

Dobson, K. S. (1987). Marital and social adjustment in depressed and remarried women. *Journal of Consulting and Clinical Psychology, 43,* 261–265.

Eddy, J. M., Heyman, R. E., & Weiss, R. L. (1991). An empirical evaluation of the Dyadic Adjustment Scale: Exploring the differences between marital "satisfaction" and "adjustment." *Behavioral Assessment, 13,* 199–220.

Edelstein, B. A. (1989). Generalization: Terminological, methodological and conceptual issues. *Behavior Therapy, 20,* 311–324.

Edgar, D. (1997). *Men, mateship and marriage.* Sydney, Australia: Harper Collins.

Eidelson, R. J., & Epstein, N. (1982). Cognition and relationship maladjustment: Development of a measure of dysfunctional relationship beliefs. *Journal of Consulting and Clinical Psychology, 50,* 715–720.

Emery, R. E. (1982). Interparental conflict and the children of discord and divorce. *Psychological Bulletin, 9,* 310–330.

Emery, R. E., Joyce, S. A., & Fincham, F. D. (1987). The assessment of child and marital problems. In K. D. O'Leary (Ed.), *Assessment of marital discord* (pp. 223–262). Hillsdale, NJ: Erlbaum.

Emmelkamp, P. M. G., De Haan, E., & Hoogduin, C. A. I. (1990). Marital adjustment and obsessive–compulsive disorder. *British Journal of Psychiatry, 156,* 55–60.

Emmelkamp, P. M. G., van Linden van den Heuvell, C., Ruphan, M., Sanderman, R., Scholing, A., & Stroink, F. (1988). Cognitive and behavioral interventions: A comparative evaluation with clinically distressed couples. *Journal of Family Psychology, 1,* 365–377.

Emmelkamp, P. M. G., van Linden van den Heuvell, C., Sanderman, R., & Scholing, A. (1988). Cognitive marital therapy: The process of change. *Journal of Family Psychology, 1,* 385–389.

Ewart, C. K., Taylor, C. B., Kraemer, H. C., & Agras, W. S. (1991). High blood pressure and marital discord: Not being nasty matters more than being nice. *Health Psychology, 10,* 155–163.

Eyberg, S. M., & Robinson, E. A. (1983). Conduct problem behavior: Standardization of a behavior rating scale with adolescents. *Journal of Clinical Child Psychology, 12,* 347–354.

Feeney, J., & Noller, P. (1996). *Adult attachment.* Thousand Oaks, CA: Sage.

Fincham, F. D., Beach, S. R. H., & Kemp-Fincham, S. I. (1997). Marital quality: A new theoretical perspective. In R. J. Sternberg & M. Hojjat (Eds.), *Satisfaction in close relationships* (pp. 275–304). New York: Guilford Press.

Fincham, F. D., & Bradbury, T. N. (Eds.). (1990). *The psychology of marriage: Basic issues and applications.* New York: Guilford Press.

Fincham, F. D., & Bradbury, T. N. (1992). Assessing attributions in marriage: The relationship attribution measure. *Journal of Personality and Social Psychology, 62,* 457–468.

Fincham, F. D., Garner, P. C., Gano-Phillips, S., & Osborne, L. N. (1995). Preinteraction expectations, marital satisfaction and accessibility: A new look at sentiment override. *Journal of Family Psychology, 9,* 3–14.

Floyd, F. J., & Markman, H. J. (1983). Observational biases in spouse observation: Toward a cognitive/behavioral model of marriage. *Journal of Consulting and Clinical Psychology, 51,* 450–457.

Fowers, B. J., Applegate, B., Olson, D. H., & Pomerantz, B. (1994). Marital conventionalization as a measure of marital satisfaction: A confirmatory factor analysis. *Journal of Family Psychology, 8,* 98–103.

Fowers, B. J., Lyons, E. M., & Montel, K. H. (1996). Positive marital illusions: Self-enhancement or relationship enhancement? *Journal of Family Psychology, 10,* 192–208.

Fowers, B. J., & Olson, D. H. (1989). ENRICH marital inventory: A discriminant validity and cross-validation assessment. *Journal of Marital and Family Therapy, 15,* 65–69.

Furman, W., & Flanagan, A. S. (1997). The influence of earlier relationships on marriage: An attachment perspective. In W. K. Halford & H. J. Markman (Eds.), *Clinical handbook of marriage and couples intervention* (pp. 179–202). Chichester, UK: Wiley.

Gabardi, L., & Rosen, L. A. (1991). Differences between college students from divorced and intact families. *Journal of Divorce and Remarriage, 15,* 175–191.

Gallup, O. (1989, October 3). Marriage satisfaction in America. *Los Angeles Times,* p. 4.

Gallup, G. Jr. (1990). *The Gallup poll: Public opinion 1990.* Wilmington, DE: Scholarly Resources.

Gallup, G. Jr. (1996). *The Gallup poll: Public opinion 1996.* Wilmington, DE: Scholarly Resources.

Glass, S. P., & Wright, T. L. (1997). Reconstructing marriages after the trauma of infidelity. In W. K. Halford & H. J. Markman (Eds.), *Clinical handbook of marriage and couples intervention* (pp. 471–507). Chichester, UK: Wiley.

Glenn, N. D., & Kramer, K. B. (1987). The marriages and divorces of the children of divorce. *Journal of Marriage and the Family, 49,* 811–825.

Glick, P. C. (1989). Remarried families, stepfamilies and stepchildren: Brief demographic profile. *Family Relations, 38,* 24–27.

Goodnow, J. J., & Bowes, J. M. (1994). *Men, women and household work.* New York: Oxford University Press.

Gottman, J. M. (1990). How marriages change. In G. R. Patterson (Ed.), *Depression and aggression in family interaction* (pp. 75–102). Hillsdale, NJ: Erlbaum.

Gottman, J. M. (1993a) A theory of marital dissolution and stability. *Journal of Family Psychology, 7,* 57–75.

Gottman, J. M. (1993b). The roles of conflict engagement, escalation, and avoidance in marital interaction: A longitudinal view of five types of couples. *Journal of Consulting and Clinical Psychology, 61,* 6–15.

Gottman, J. M. (1994). *What predicts divorce.* Hillsdale, NJ: Erlbaum.

Gottman, J. M., & Krokoff, L. J. (1989). Marital interaction and marital satisfaction: A longitudinal view. *Journal of Consulting and Clinical Psychology, 57,* 47–52.

Gottman, J. M., & Levenson, R. W. (1988). The social psychophysiology of marriage. In P. Noller & M. A. Fitzpatrick (Eds.), *Perspectives on marital interaction* (pp. 182–200). Clevedon, UK: Multilingual Matters.

Gottman, J. M., Markman, H. J., & Notarius, C. I. (1977). The topography of marital conflict: A sequential analysis of verbal and non-verbal behavior. *Journal of Marriage and the Family, 39,* 461–477.

Gottman, J. M., Notarius, C. I., Gonso, J., & Markman, H. J. (1976). *A couple's guide to communication.* Champaign, IL: Research Press.

Greenberg, J. M., & Johnson, S. M. (1988). *Emotionally focused therapy for couples.* New York: Guilford Press.

Grych, J. H., & Fincham, F. D. (1990). Marital conflict and children's adjustment: A cognitive-contextual framework. *Psychological Bulletin, 108,* 267–290.

Grych, J. H., & Fincham, F. D. (1993). Children's appraisals of marital conflict: Initial investigations of the cognitive-contextual framework. *Child Development, 64,* 215–230.

Guerney, B. G. (1977). *Relationship enhancement*. San Francisco: Jossey-Bass.

Hafner, R. J. (1986). *Marriage and mental illness: A sex-roles perspective*. New York: Guilford Press.

Hahlweg, K., & Klan, N. (1997). The effectiveness of marital counseling in Germany: A contribution to health services research. *Journal of Family Psychology, 11,* 410–421.

Hahlweg, K., & Markman, H. J. (1988). Effectiveness of behavioral marital therapy: Empirical status of behavioral techniques in preventing and alleviating marital distress. *Journal of Consulting and Clinical Psychology, 56,* 440–447.

Hahlweg, K., Schindler, L., Revenstorf, D., & Brengelmann, J. C. (1984). The Munich marital therapy study. In K. Hahlweg & N. S. Jacobson (Eds.), *Marital interaction: Analysis and modification* (pp. 3–19). New York: Guilford Press.

Halford, W. K. (1995). Marriage and the prevention of psychiatric disorder. In B. Raphael & G. D. Burrows (Eds.), *Handbook of studies preventive psychiatry* (pp. 121–138). Amsterdam: Elsevier.

Halford, W. K. (1997). Empirically validated psychological treatment: What does it mean in the domain of relationship problems? *Behaviour Change, 14,* 9–14.

Halford, W. K. (1998). The ongoing evolution of behavioral couples therapy: Retrospect and prospect. *Clinical Psychology Review, 18,* 613–633.

Halford, W.K. (1999). *Australian couples in Millennium Three: A research development agenda for marriage and relationship education*. Canberra, Australia: Department of Family and Community Services.

Halford, W. K., Bouma, R., Kelly, A. B., & Young, R. (1999). The interaction of individual psychopathology and marital problems: Current findings and clinical implications. *Behavior Modification, 23,* 179–216

Halford, W. K., Gravestock, F. M., Lowe, R., & Scheldt, S. (1992). Towards a behavioural ecology of stressful marital interactions. *Behavioral Assessment, 14,* 199–217.

Halford, W. K., Hahlweg, K., & Dunne, M. (1990). The cross-cultural consistency of marital communication associated with marital distress. *Journal of Marriage and the Family, 52,* 109–122.

Halford, W. K., & Hayes, R. L. (1991). Psychological rehabilitation of chronic schizophrenic patients: Recent findings on social skills training and family psychoeducation. *Clinical Psychology Review, 11,* 23–44.

Halford, W. K., Kelly, A., & Markman, H. J. (1997). The concept of a healthy marriage. In W. K. Halford & H. J. Markman (Eds.), *Clinical handbook of marriage and couples intervention* (pp. 3–12). Chichester, UK: Wiley.

Halford, W. K., & Markman, H. J. (Eds.). (1997). *Clinical handbook of marriage and couples intervention*. Chichester, UK: Wiley.

Halford, W. K., & Osgarby, S. M. (1993). Alcohol abuse in individuals presenting for marital therapy. *Journal of Family Psychology, 11,* 1–13.

Halford, W. K., Osgarby, S. M., & Kelly, A. (1996). Brief behavioural couples therapy: A preliminary evaluation. *Behavioural and Cognitive Psychotherapy, 24,* 263–273.

Halford, W. K., & Sanders, M. R. (1988a). Dyadic behavior and requests for change in Australian maritally distressed and non-distressed couples. *Australian Journal of Psychology, 40,* 45–52.

Halford, W. K., & Sanders, M. R. (1988b). Assessment of cognitive self-statements during marital problem solving: A comparison of two methods. *Cognitive Therapy and Research, 12,* 515–530.

Halford, W. K., & Sanders, M. R. (1990). The relationship of cognition and behavior during marital interaction. *Journal of Social and Clinical Psychology, 9,* 489–510.

Halford, W. K., Sanders, M. R., & Behrens, B. C. (1993). A comparison of the generalization of behavioral marital therapy and enhanced behavioral marital therapy. *Journal of Consulting and Clinical Psychology, 61,* 51–60.

Halford, W. K., Sanders, M. R., & Behrens, B. C. (1994). Self-regulation in behavioral couples therapy. *Behavior Therapy, 25,* 431–452.

Halford, W. K., Sanders, M. R., & Behrens, B. C. (2000). *Can skills training prevent relationship problems in at-risk couples? 4-year effects of relationship education on high- and low-risk couples.* Manuscript under review.

Halford, W. K., Sanders, M. R., & Behrens, B. C. (2000). Repeating the errors of our parents? Family of origin spouse violence and observed conflict management in engaged couples. *Family Process, 39,* 219–236.

Halford, W.K, Scott, J., & Smythe, J. (in press). Couples and cancer. In K. Schmaling & T. Sher (Eds.), *Couples and illness.* Washington, DC: American Psychological Association.

Halford, W. K., Moore, E., Wilson, K., & Farrugia, C. (2000). *Flexi-PREP Telephone Facilitator's Manual.* Brisbane, Australia: School of Applied Psychology, Griffith University.

Hannah, J., Halford, W. K., & Dadds, M. R. (2000). *Relationship standards, communication patterns and relationship satisfaction in lesbian couples.* Manuscript submitted for publication.

Haynes, S. N., Jensen, B. J., Wise, E., & Sherman, D. (1981). The marital intake interview: A multi-method criterion validity assessment. *Journal of Consulting and Clinical Psychology, 49,* 379–387.

Heavey, C. L., Christensen, A., & Malmuth, N. M. (1995). The longitudinal impact of demand and withdrawal during marital conflict. *Journal of Consulting and Clinical Psychology, 63,* 797–801.

Heavey, C. L., Layne, C., & Christensen, A. (1993). Gender and conflict structure in marital interaction: A replication and extension. *Journal of Consulting and Clinical Psychology, 61,* 16–27.

Heyman, R. E., Sayers, S. L., & Bellack, A. S. (1994). Global marital satisfaction vs. marital adjustment: An empirical comparison of three measures. *Journal of Family Psychology, 8,* 432–446.

Hill, M. S., (1988). Marital stability and spouse's shared time: A multidisciplinary hypothesis. *Journal of Family Issues, 9,* 427–451.

Holtzworth-Munroe, A., Jacobson, N. S., DeKlyn, M., & Whisman, M. A. (1989). Relationship between behavioral marital therapy outcome and process variables. *Journal of Consulting and Clinical Psychology, 57,* 658–662.

Holtzworth-Munroe, A., Smutzler, N., Bates, L., & Sandin, E. (1997). Husband violence: Basic facts and clinical implications. In W. K. Halford & H. J. Markman (Eds.), *Clinical handbook of marriage and couples intervention* (pp. 129–156). Chichester, UK: Wiley.

Hooley, J. M., Orleay, J., & Teasdale, J. D. (1986). Levels of expressed emotion and relapse in depressed patients. *British Journal of Psychiatry, 148,* 642–647.

Houseknecht, S. K. (1987). Voluntary childlessness. In M. B. Sussman & S. K. Steinmetz (Eds.), *Handbook of marriage and the family* (pp. 369–395). New York: Plenum Press.

Howes, P., & Markman, H. J. (1989). Marital quality and child functioning: A longitudinal investigation. *Child Development, 60,* 1044–1051.

Iverson, A., & Baucom, D. H. (1990). Behavioral marital therapy outcomes: Alternative interpretations of the data. *Behavior Therapy, 21,* 129–138.

Jacobson, N. S. (1989). The maintenance of treatment gains following social learning-based marital therapy. *Behavior Therapy, 20,* 325–336.

Jacobson, N. S. (1991). Toward enhancing the efficacy of marital therapy and marital therapy research. *Journal of Family Psychology, 4,* 373–393.

Jacobson, N. S., & Addis, M. E. (1993). Research on couples and couple therapy: What do we know? Where are we going? *Journal of Consulting and Clinical Psychology, 61,* 85–93.

Jacobson, N. S., & Christensen, A. (1996). *Integrative behavioral couple therapy.* New York: Norton.

Jacobson, N. S., Follette, W. C., & McDonald, D. W. (1982). Reactivity to positive and negative behavior in distressed and non-distressed couples. *Journal of Consulting and Clinical Psychology, 49,* 269–277.

Jacobson, N. S., Follette, W. C., & Pagel, M. (1986). Predicting who will benefit from behavioral marital therapy. *Journal of Consulting and Clinical Psychology, 54,* 518–522.

Jacobson, N. S., Follette, W. C., Revenstorf, D., Baucom, D. H., Hahlweg, K., & Margolin, G. (1984). Variability in outcome and clinical significance of behavioral marital therapy: A reanalysis of outcome data. *Journal of Consulting and Clinical Psychology, 52,* 497–567.

Jacobson, N., & Margolin, G. (1979). *Marital therapy: Strategies based on social learning and behavior exchange principles.* New York: Brunner/Mazel.

Jacobson, N. S., McDonald, D. W., Follette, W. C., & Berley, R. A. (1985). Attributional processes in distressed and nondistressed married couples. *Cognitive Therapy and Research, 9,* 35–50.

Jacobson, N. S., & Moore, D. (1981). Spouses as observers of the events in the relationships. *Journal of Consulting and Clinical Psychology, 49,* 269–277.

Jacobson, N. S., Schmaling, K. B., & Holtzworth-Munroe, A. (1987). Component analysis of behavioral marital therapy: Two-year follow-up and prediction of relapse. *Journal of Marital and Family Therapy, 13,* 187–195.

Jaffe, P., Wolfe, D. A., Wilson, S. K., & Zak, L. (1986). Emotional and physical health problems of battered women. *Canadian Journal of Psychiatry, 31,* 625–629.

Johnson, P. I., & O'Leary, D. K. (1996). The behavioral components of marital satisfaction: An individualized assessment approach. *Journal of Consulting and Clinical Psychology, 64,* 417–423.

Johnson, S. M., & Greenberg, L. S. (1985). Differential effects of experiential and problem-solving interventions in resolving marital conflict. *Journal of Consulting and Clinical Psychology, 53,* 175–184.

Johnson, S. M., & Greenberg, L. S. (1988). Relating process to outcome in marital therapy. *Journal of Marital and Family Therapy, 14,* 175–183.

Johnson, S. M., & Greenberg, L. S. (1994). Emotion in intimate interactions: a synthesis. In S. M. Johnson & L. S. Greenberg (Eds.), *The heart of the matter: Perspectives on emotion in marital therapy* (pp. 297–324). New York: Brunner/Mazel.

Johnson, S. M., & Greenberg, L. S. (1995). The emotionally focused approach to problems in adult attachment. In N. S. Jacobson & A. S. Gurman (Eds.), *Clinical handbook of couple therapy* (pp. 121–141). New York: Guilford Press.

Johnson, S. M., & Talitman, E. (1997). Predictors of success in emotionally focused couples therapy. *Journal of Marital and Family Therapy, 23,* 135–152.

Jones, A. C., & Chao, C. M. (1997). Racial, ethnic and cultural issues in couples therapy. In W. K. Halford, & H. J. Markman (Eds.), *Clinical handbook of marriage and couples intervention* (pp. 157–178). Chichester, UK: Wiley.

Julien, D., Arellano, C., & Turgeon, L. (1997). Gender issues in heterosexual, gay and lesbian couples. In W. K. Halford & H. J. Markman (Eds.), *Clinical handbook of marriage and couples intervention* (pp. 107–127). Chichester, UK: Wiley.

Julien, D., Markman, H. J., Léveillé, S., Chartrand, E., & Bégin, J. (1994). Networks' support and interference with regard to marriage: Disclosures of marital problems to confidants. *Journal of Family Psychology, 8,* 16–31.

Kanfer, F. H. (1970). Self-monitoring: Methodological limitations and clinical applications. *Journal of Consulting and Clinical Psychology, 35,* 148–152.

Kanfer, F. H., & Karoly, P. (1972). Self-control: A behavioristic excursion into the lion's den. *Behavior Therapy, 3,* 389–416.

Kanfer, F. H., & Schefft, B. K. (1988). *Guiding the process of therapeutic change.* Champaign, IL: Research Press.

Karney, B. R., & Bradbury, T. N. (1995). The longitudinal course of marital quality and stability: A review of theory, method and research. *Psychological Bulletin, 118,* 3–34.

Karoly, P. (1993). Mechanisms of self-regulation: A systems view. *Annual Review of Psychology, 44,* 23–52.

Kazdin, A. E., & Bass, D. (1989). Power to detect differences between alternative treatments in comparative psychotherapy outcome research. *Journal of Consulting and Clinical Psychology, 57,* 138–147.

Kelly, A. B., & Halford, W. K. (1995). The generalisation of cognitive-behavioural marital therapy in behavioural, cognitive and physiological domains. *Behavioural and Cognitive Psychotherapy, 23,* 381–398.

Khavari, K. A., & Farber, P. D. (1978). A profile instrument for the quantification and assessment of alcohol consumption. *Journal of Studies on Alcohol, 39,* 1525–1539.

Kiecolt-Glaser, J. K., Kennedy, S., Malkoff, S., Fisher, L., Speicher, C. E., & Glaser, R. (1988). Marital discord and immunity in males. *Psychosomatic Medicine, 50,* 213–229.

Klerman, G. L., & Weissman, M. M. (1982). Interpersonal psychotherapy: Theory and research. In A. J. Rush (Ed.), *Short-term psychotherapy for depression: Behavioural, interpersonal, cognitive and psychodynamic approaches* (pp. 121–146). New York: Guilford Press.

Lange, A., Schaap, G., & van Widenfelt, B. (1993). Family therapy and psychopathology: Developments in research and approaches to treatment. *Journal of Family Therapy, 15,* 113–146.

Lawton, J. M., & Sanders, M. R. (1994). Designing effective behavioural family interventions for stepfamilies. *Clinical Psychology Review, 5,* 463–496.

LeBow, J. L., & Gurman, A. S. (1995). Research assessing couple and family therapy research. *Annual Review of Psychology, 46,* 27–57.

Levinger, G., & Huston, T. L. (1990). The social psychology of marriage. In F. D. Fincham & T. N. Bradbury (Eds.), *The psychology of marriage* (pp. 19–58). New York: Guilford Press.

Locke, H. J., & Wallace, K. M. (1959). Short marital adjustment and prediction tests: Their reliability and validity. *Marriage and Family Living, 21,* 251–255.

Lovibond, S. H., & Lovibond, P. F. (1995). *Manual for the Depression Anxiety Stress Scale.* Sydney: Psychology Foundation of Australia.

Mahoney, M. J., & Thoreson, C. E. (1974). *Power to the person.* Pacific Grove, CA: Brooks/Cole.

Maisto, S. A., O'Farrell, T. J., Connors, G. J., McKay, J. R., & Pelcovits, M. (1988). Alcoholics' attributions of factors affecting their relapse to drinking and reasons for terminating relapse episodes. *Addictive Behavior, 13,* 79–82.

Margolin, G., Fernandez, V., Talovic, S., & Onorato, R. (1983). Sex role considerations and behavioral marital therapy: Equal does not mean identical. *Journal of Marital and Family Therapy, 9,* 131–145.

Markman, H. J., Floyd, F. J., Stanley, S. M., & Storaasli, R. D. (1988). Prevention of marital distress: A longitudinal investigation. *Journal of Consulting and Clinical Psychology, 56,* 210–217.

Markman, H. J., & Hahlweg, K. (1993). The prediction and prevention of marital distress: An international perspective. *Clinical Psychology Review, 13,* 29–43.

Markman, H. J., Halford, W. K., & Cordova, A. D. (1997). A grand tour of future directions in the study and promotion of healthy relationships. In W. K. Halford & H. J. Markman (Eds.), *Clinical handbook of marriage and couples intervention* (pp. 695–716). Chichester, UK: Wiley.

Markman, H. J., & Kraft, S. A. (1989). Men and women in marriage: Dealing with gender differences in marital therapy. *Behavior Therapist, 12,* 51–56.

Markman, H. J., Renick, M. J., Floyd, F. J., Stanley, S. M., & Clements, M. (1993). Preventing marital distress through communication and conflict management training: A 4- and 5-year follow-up. *Journal of Consulting and Clinical Psychology, 61,* 70–77.

Markman, H. J., Stanley, S. M., & Blumberg, S. L. (1991). *Fighting for your marriage, Tape 1: Ground rules for fighting and loving* [Videotape]. Denver: PREP Educational Videos.

Martin, T. C., & Bumpass, L. L. (1989). Recent trends in marital disruption. *Demography, 26,* 37–51.

McCabe, M. P. (1994). The influence of the quality of relationship on sexual dysfunction. *Australian Journal of Marriage and the Family, 15,* 2–8.

McDonald, P. (1995). *Families in Australia.* Melbourne: Australian Institute of Family Studies.

Medalie, J. H., & Goldbourt, U. (1976). Angina pectoris among 10,000: II. Psycho-social and other risk factors as evidenced by a multivariate analysis of a five-year incidence study. *American Journal of Medicine, 60,* 910–921.

Millward, C. (1990). Expectations of marriage of young people. *Family Matters, 28,* 1–12.

Montgomery, R. B., & Evans, L. (1989). *Living and loving together.* Melbourne, Australia: Penguin.

Murphy, C. M., & O'Leary, K. D. (1989). Psychological aggression predicts physical aggression in early marriage. *Journal of Consulting and Clinical Psychology, 57,* 579–582.

National Committee on Violence. (1990). *Violence: Directions for Australia.* Canberra: Australian Institute of Criminology.

Nesdale, D., Rooney, R., & Smith, L. (1997). Migrant ethnic identification and psycho-logical distress. *Journal of Cross Cultural Psychology, 28,* 569–588.

Nicholson, J. M., Halford, W. K., & Sanders, M. R. (1996). Prevention of marital health problems in step-families. In *Proceedings of the First Australian Conference on Prevention and Health Promotion in Mental Health.* Sydney, Australia: Sydney University.

Noller, P. (1981). Nonverbal communication in marriage. In R. S. Feldman (Ed.), *Applications of nonverbal behavioral theories and research* (pp. 31–59). Hillsdale, NJ: Erlbaum.

Notarius, C. I., Benson, P. R., Sloane, D., Vanzetti, N. A., & Hornyak, L. M. (1989). Exploring the interface between perception and behavior: An analysis of marital interaction in distressed and nondistressed couples. *Behavioral Assessment, 11,* 39–64.

Notarius, C. I., & Markman, H. J. (1993). *We can work it out: Making sense of marital conflict.* New York: Putnam.

O'Farrell, T. J. (1989). Marital and family therapy in alcoholism treatment. *Journal of Substance Abuse Treatment, 6,* 23–29.

O'Farrell, T. J., & Birchler, G. R. (1987). Marital relationships of alcoholic, conflicted and non-conflicted couples. *Journal of Marital and Family Therapy, 13,* 259–274.

O'Farrell, T. J., & Rotunda, R. J. (1997). Couples interventions and alcohol abuse. In W. K. Halford & H. J. Markman (Eds.), *Clinical handbook of marriage and couples interventions* (pp. 555–588). Chichester, UK: Wiley.

O'Leary, K. D. (1987). *Assessment of marital discord: An integration for clinical research and practice.* Hillsdale, NJ: Erlbaum.

O'Leary, K. D. (1988). Physical aggression between spouses: A social learning theory perspective. In V. B. Van Hasselt & R. L. Morrison (Eds.), *Handbook of family violence* (pp. 31–55). New York: Plenum Press.

O'Leary, K., Barling, J., Arias, I., Rosenbaum, A., Malone, J., & Tyree, A. (1989). Prevalence and stability of physical aggression between spouses: A longitudinal analysis. *Journal of Consulting and Clinical Psychology, 57,* 263–268.

O'Leary, K. D., & Beach, S. R. H. (1990). Marital therapy: A viable treatment for de-pression and marital discord. *American Journal of Psychiatry, 147,* 183–186.

O'Leary, K. D., & Vivian, D. A. (1990). Physical aggression in marriage. In F. D.

Fincham & T. N. Bradbury (Eds.), *The psychology of marriage: Basic issues and applications* (pp. 323–348). New York: Guilford Press.

O'Leary, K. D., Vivian, D., & Malone, J. (1992). Assessment of physical aggression against women in marriage: The need for multi-modal assessment. *Behavioral Assessment, 14,* 5–14.

Olson, D. H., & Fowers, B. J. (1986). Predicting marital success with PREPARE: A predictive validity study. *Journal of Marital and Family Therapy, 12,* 403–413.

Olson, D. H., & Larsen, A. S. (1989). Predicting marital satisfaction using PREPARE: A replication study. *Journal of Marital and Family Therapy, 15,* 311–322.

Osgarby, S. M., & Halford, W. K. (2000a). *Positive intimacy skills and couple relationship satisfaction.* Manuscript submitted for publication.

Osgarby, S. M., & Halford, W. K. (2000b). *Memory bias and couple relationship distress.* Manuscript submitted for publication.

Overall, J. E., Henry, B. W., & Woodward, A. (1974). Dependence of marital problems on parental family history. *Journal of Abnormal Psychology, 83,* 446–450.

Pasch, L. A., & Bradbury, T. N. (1998). Social support, conflict, and the development of marital dysfunction. *Journal of Consulting and Clinical Psychology, 66,* 219–230.

Pasch, L. A., Bradbury, T. N., & Davila, J. (1997). Gender, negative affectivity, and observed social support behavior in marital interaction. *Personal Relationships, 4,* 361–378.

Prado, L., & Markman, H. J. (1998). For better or worse the second time around: Analyzing the communication patterns of remarried couples. In M. Cox & J. Brooks-Gunn (Eds.), *Conflict and cohesion* (pp. 117–141). Hillsdale, NJ: Erlbaum.

Raush, H. L., Barry, W. A., Hertel, R. K., & Swain, M. A. (1974). *Communication, conflict and marriage.* San Francisco: Jossey-Bass.

Reich, J., & Thompson, W. D. (1985). Marital status of schizophrenic and alcoholic patients. *Journal of Nervous and Mental Disease, 173,* 499–502.

Reissman, C., Aron, C., & Bergen, M. R. (1993). Shared activities and marital satisfaction: causal direction and self-expansion versus boredom. *Journal of Social and Personal Relationships, 10,* 243–254.

Rogge, R. D., & Bradbury, T. N. (1999). Till violence does us part: The differing roles of communication and aggression in predicting adverse marital outcomes. *Journal of Consulting and Clinical Psychology, 67,* 340–351.

Rounsaville, B. J., Weissman, M. M., Prusoff, B. A., & Herceg-Baron, R. L. (1979). Marital disputes and treatment outcome in depressed women. *Comprehensive Psychiatry, 20,* 483–490.

Ruscher, S. M., & Gotlib, I. H. (1988). Marital interaction patterns of couples with and without a depressed partner. *Behavior Therapy, 19,* 455–470.

Sanders, M. R., & Dadds, M. R. (1993). *Behavioral family intervention.* Boston: Allyn & Bacon.

Sanders, M. R., Halford, W. K., & Behrens, B. C. (1999). Parental divorce and premarital couple communication. *Journal of Family Psychology, 13,* 60–74.

Sanders, M. R., Markie-Dadds, C., & Nicholson, J. M. (1997). Concurrent interventions for marital and children's problems. In W. K. Halford & H. J. Markman

(Eds.), *Clinical handbook of marriage and couples intervention* (pp. 509–536). Chichester, UK: Wiley.

Sanders, M. R., Nicholson, J. M., & Floyd, F. J. (1997). Couples' relationships and children. In W. K. Halford & H. J. Markman (Eds.), *Clinical handbook of marriage and couples intervention* (pp. 225–253). Chichester, UK: Wiley.

Saunders, J. B., Aasland, O. G., Babor, T. F., de La Fuente, J. R., & Grant, M. (1993). Development of the Alcohol Use Disorders Identification Test (AUDIT): WHO collaborative project on early detection of persons with harmful alcohol consumption: II. *Addiction, 88,* 791–804.

Sayers, S. L., Baucom, D. H., Sher, T. G., Weiss, R. L., & Heyman, R. E. (1991). Constructive engagement, behavioral marital therapy, and changes in marital satisfaction. *Behavioral Assessment, 13,* 25–49.

Schenk, J., Pfrang, H., & Raushe, A. (1983). Personality traits versus the quality of the marital relationship as the determinant of marital sexuality. *Archives of Sexual Behavior, 12,* 31–42.

Schmaling, K. B., & Sher, T. G. (1997). Physical health and relationships. In W. K. Halford & H. J. Markman (Eds.), *Clinical handbook of marriage and couples intervention* (pp. 323–345). Chichester, UK: Wiley.

Seligman, M. E. P. (1995). The effectiveness of psychotherapy: The *Consumer Reports* study. *American Psychologist, 50,* 965–974.

Shadish, W. R., Montgomery, L. M., Wilson, P., Wilson, M. R., Bright, I., & Okwumabua, T. (1993). Effects of family and marital psychotherapies: A meta-analysis. *Journal of Consulting and Clinical Psychology, 61,* 992–1002.

Sharpley, C. F., & Cross, D. G. (1982). A psychometric evaluation of the Spanier Dyadic Adjustment Scale. *Journal of Marriage and the Family, 44,* 739–747.

Shelton, J. L., & Levy, R. L. (1981). *Behavioral assignments and treatment compliance: A handbook of clinical strategies.* Champaign, IL: Research Press.

Skinner, B. F. (1953). *Science and human behavior.* New York: Macmillan.

Skuja, K., & Halford, W. K. (2000). *Repeating the errors of our parents? II: Parental spouse abuse in men's family of origin and conflict management in dating couples.* Manuscript submitted for publication.

Snyder, D. K. (1998, July). Beyond behavioral couples therapy: Affective reconstruction of relationship dispositions. In W. K. Halford (Chair), *Beyond traditional behavioral couples therapy: New directions in the treatment of relationship problems.* Symposium conducted at the World Congress of Behavioral and Cognitive Therapies, Acapulco, Mexico.

Snyder, D. K., Mangrum, L. F., & Wills, R. M. (1993). Predicting couples' response to marital therapy: A comparison of short- and long-term predictors. *Journal of Consulting and Clinical Psychology, 61,* 61–69.

Snyder, D. K., & Wills, R. M. (1989). Behavioral versus insight-oriented marital therapy: Effects on individual and interspousal functioning. *Journal of Consulting and Clinical Psychology, 57,* 39–46.

Snyder, D. K., Wills, R. M., & Grady-Fletcher, A. (1991a). Long term effectiveness of behavioral versus insight-oriented marital therapy: A 4-year follow-up study. *Journal of Consulting and Clinical Psychology, 59,* 138–141.

Snyder, D. K., Wills, R. M., & Grady-Fletcher, A. (1991b). Risks and challenges of long-term psychotherapy outcome research: Reply to Jacobson. *Journal of Consulting and Clinical Psychology, 59,* 146–149.

Spanier, G. B. (1976). Measuring dyadic adjustment: New scales for assessing the quality of marriage and similar dyads. *Journal of Marriage and the Family, 37,* 63–275.

Spence, S. H. (1997). Sex and relationships. In W. K. Halford & H. J. Markman (Eds.), *Clinical handbook of marriage and couples intervention* (pp. 73–105). Chichester, UK: Wiley.

Stanley, S., Lobitz, C., & Markman, H. J. (1989, May). Marital therapy in Colorado. *Colorado Psychological Association Bulletin,* 12–18.

Stanley, S., & Markman, H. J. (1996). [National survey of U. S. married couples]. Unpublished raw data, University of Denver, Denver, CO.

Stanway, A. (1991). *The lovers' guide: How to enhance your loving and sexual relationship.* London: Lifetime Vision.

Stanway, A. (1992). *The lovers' guide 2.* London: Lifetime Vision.

Stanway, A. (1993). *The lovers' guide 3.* London: Lifetime Vision.

Stark, E., & Flitcraft, A. (1988). Violence among intimates. In V. B. Van Hasselt, R. L. Morrison, A. S. Bellack, & M. Hersen (Eds.), *Handbook of family violence* (pp. 293–317). New York: Plenum Press.

Stets, J. E., & Straus, M. A. (1990). Gender differences in reporting marital violence and its medical-psychological consequences. In M. A. Straus & R. J. Gelles (Eds.), *Physical violence in American families: Risk factors and adaptation to violence in 8145 families* (pp. 151–166). New Brunswick, NJ: Transaction.

Stokes, T. F., & Baer, D. M. (1977). An implicit technology of generalization. *Journal of Applied Behavior Analysis, 10,* 349–367.

Stokes, T. F., & Osnes, P. G. (1988). The developing applied technology of generalization and maintenance. In R. H. Horner & G. Dunlop (Eds.), *Generalization and maintenance: Life-style changes in applied settings* (pp. 5–19). Baltimore: Brookes.

Straus, M. A., & Gelles, R. J. (1986). Societal change and change in family violence from 1975 to 1985 as revealed by two national surveys. *Journal of Marriage and the Family, 48,* 465–479.

Straus, M. A., Gelles, R. J., & Steinmetz, S. K. (1980). *Behind closed doors: Violence in the American family.* Garden City, NJ: Doubleday.

Straus, M. A., Hamby, S. L., Boney-McCoy, S., & Sugarman, D. B. (1996). The revised Conflict Tactics Scales (CTS2): Development and preliminary psychometric data. *Journal of Family Issues, 17,* 283–316.

Stuart, R. B. (1980). *Helping couples change.* New York: Guilford Press.

Terman, L. M. (1939). *Psychological factors in marital happiness.* New York: McGraw-Hill.

Thibaut, J. W., & Kelley, H. H. (1959). *The social psychology of groups.* New York, UK: Wiley.

Thomas, L. T., & Ganster, D. C. (1995). Impact of family supportive work variables on work-family conflict and strain: A control perspective. *Journal of Applied Psychology, 80,* 6–15.

Thompson, B. M. (1997). Couples and the work-family interface. In W. K. Halford &

H. J. Markman (Eds.), *Clinical handbook of marriage and couples intervention* (pp. 273–290). Chichester, UK: Wiley.

Vannicelli, M., Gingerich, S., & Ryback, R. (1983). Family problems related to the treatment and outcome of alcoholic patients. *British Journal of Addiction, 78,* 193–204.

Vanzetti, N. A., Notarius, C. I., & NeeSmith, D. (1992). Specific and generalized expectancies in marital interaction. *Journal of Family Psychology, 6,* 171–183.

Vincent, J. P., Friedman, L. C., Nugent, J., & Messerly, L. (1979). Demand characteristics in observations of marital interactions. *Journal of Consulting and Clinical Psychology, 47,* 557–566.

Volker, T., & Olson, D. H. (1993). Problem families and the circumplex model: Observational assessment using the Clinical Rating Scale (CRS). *Journal of Marital and Family Therapy, 19,* 159–175.

Walsh, F., Jacob, L., & Simons, V. (1995). Facilitating healthy divorce processes: therapy and mediation issues. In N. S. Jacobson & A. S. Gurman (Eds.), *Clinical handbook of couple therapy* (pp. 340–368). New York: Guilford Press.

Weiss, R. L. (1984). Cognitive and strategic interventions in behavioral marital therapy. In K. Hahlweg & N. S. Jacobson (Eds.), *Marital interaction: Analysis and modification* (pp. 337–355). New York: Guilford Press.

Weiss, R. L. (1989). Marital violence: Issues in conception, assessment and intervention. Special Issue: Behavioural marital therapy. *Behaviour Change, 6,* 153–164.

Weiss, R. L., & Aved, B. M. (1978). Marital satisfaction and depression as predictors of physical health status. *Journal of Consulting and Clinical Psychology, 46,* 1379–1384.

Weiss, R. L., & Birchler, G. R. (1975). *Areas of change.* Unpublished manuscript, University of Oregon at Eugene, OR.

Weiss, R. L., & Cerreto, M. C. (1980). The Marital Status Inventory: Development of a measure of dissolution potential. *American Journal of Family Therapy, 8,* 80–86.

Weiss, R. L., & Halford, W. K. (1996). Managing couples therapy. In V. Van Hasselt & M. Hersen (Eds.), *Sourcebook of psychological treatment manuals for adult disorders* (pp. 489–537). New York: Plenum Press.

Weiss, R. L., & Heyman, R. E. (1990). Marital distress. In A. S. Bellack, M. Hersen, & A. E. Kazdin (Eds.), *International handbook of behavior modification* (pp. 475–502). New York: Plenum Press.

Weiss, R. L., & Heyman, R. E. (1997). A clinical-research overview of couples interactions. In W. K. Halford & H. J. Markman (Eds.), *Clinical handbook of marriage and couples intervention* (pp. 13–41). Chichester, UK: Wiley.

Weiss, R. L., Hops, H., & Patterson, G. R. (1973). A framework for conceptualizing marital conflict: A technology for offering it; some data for evaluating it. In L. A. Hamerlynck, L. C. Handy & E. J. Mash (Eds.), *Behavior change: Methodology, concepts and practice* (pp. 309–342). Champaign, IL: Research Press.

Weiss, R. L., & Perry, B. A. (1983a). *Assessment and treatment of marital dysfunction.* Unpublished manuscript, University of Oregon, Eugene, OR.

Weiss, R. L., & Perry, B. A. (1983b). The Spouse Observation Checklist. In E. E. Filsinger (Ed.), *A sourcebook of marriage and family assessment* (pp. 65–84). Beverly Hills, CA: Sage.

Weissman, M. M. (1987). Advances in psychiatric epidemiology: Rates and risk for major depression. *American Journal of Public Health, 77,* 445–451.

Whisman, M. A. (1990). The efficacy of booster maintenance sessions in behavior therapy: Review and methodological critique. *Clinical Psychology Review, 10,* 155–170.

Whisman, M. A., & Jacobson, N. S. (1990). Power, marital satisfaction, and response to marital therapy. *Journal of Family Psychology, 4,* 202–212.

Whisman, M. A., & Snyder, D. K. (1997). Evaluating and improving the efficacy of conjoint couple therapy. In W. K. Halford & H. J. Markman (Eds.), *Clinical handbook of marriage and couples intervention* (pp. 679–693). Chichester, UK: Wiley.

Widom, C. S. (1989). Does violence beget violence? A critical examination of the literature. *Psychological Bulletin, 106,* 3–28.

Wiersma, U. J. (1994). A taxonomy of behavioural strategies for coping with work–home role conflict. *Human Relations, 47,* 211–276.

Wills, R. M., Faitler, S. L., & Snyder, D. K. (1987). Distinctiveness of behavioral versus insight-oriented marital therapy: An empirical analysis. *Journal of Consulting and Clinical Psychology, 55,* 685–690.

Winkler, I., & Doherty, W. J. (1983). Communication style and marital satisfaction in Israeli and American couples. *Family Process, 22,* 229–237.

Wolcott, I., & Glazer, H. (1989). *Marriage counselling in Australia: An evaluation.* Melbourne: Australian Institute of Family Studies.

Worthington, E. L., McCullough, M. E., Shortz, J. L., Mindes, E. J., Sandage, S. J., & Chartrand, J. M. (1995). Can couples assessment and feedback improve relationships?: Assessment as a brief relationship enrichment procedure. *Journal of Counseling Psychology, 42,* 466–475.

Zimmer, D. (1983). Interaction patterns and communication skills in sexually distressed, maritally distressed, and normal couples: Two experimental studies. *Journal of Sex and Marital Therapy, 9,* 251–265.

Index